also by Barbara Seaman and Laura Eldridge

The Greatest Experiment Ever Performed on Women
The Body Politic

also by Barbara Seaman

Lovely Me
For Women Only!
The Doctors' Case Against the Pill
Free and Female
Women and the Crisis in Sex Hormones

the no-nonsense guide to menopause

Barbara Seaman and
Laura Eldridge

Simon & Schuster Paperbacks
New York   London   Toronto   Sydney

Simon & Schuster Paperbacks
A Division of Simon & Schuster, Inc.
1230 Avenue of the Americas
New York, NY 10020

First Simon & Schuster trade paperback edition July 2009

SIMON & SCHUSTER PAPERBACKS and colophon are registered trademarks of Simon & Schuster, Inc.

For information about special discounts for bulk purchases, please contact Simon & Schuster Special Sales at 1-866-506-1949 or business@simonandschuster.com.

The Simon & Schuster Speakers Bureau can bring authors to your live event. For more information or to book an event, contact the Simon & Schuster Speakers Bureau at 866-248-3049 or visit our website at www.simonspeakers.com.

Designed by Nancy Singer

Manufactured in the United States of America

10   9   8   7   6   5   4   3   2   1

The Library of Congress has cataloged the hardcover as follows:

Seaman, Barbara.
   The no-nonsense guide to menopause / Barbara Seaman and Laura Eldridge.
      p.   cm.
   1. Menopause—Popular works.   I. Eldridge, Laura.   II. Title.
RG186.S426   2008
618.1'75—dc22   2007042420

ISBN: 978-0-7432-7678-8
ISBN: 978-0-7432-7679-5 (pbk)
ISBN: 978-1-4165-6483-6 (e-book)

Barbara: To my daughter Shira Jean Seaman

Laura: To Paul and Susan Eldridge

acknowledgments

First and foremost, thanks to our agent, Valerie Borchardt, whose patience and calm set the right tone for the writing of the book, and also to Ann and Georges Borchardt.

Big thanks to our editor, Sydny Miner, for her invaluable advice and encouragement. Without her clarity of vision and rigorous and careful editing this book would most certainly never have been finished. Her assistant, Michelle Rorke, was helpful, reassuring, and generous with her time. Thanks also to copyeditor Gill Kent and Mara Lurie at Simon and Schuster.

Many thanks for their expertise and advice to:

- Gordon Guyatt, MD, for evidence-based medicine.
- The late, great Romano Deghgenghi, PhD, for his wide range of knowledge and contribution to the study of hormones. He will be missed. Also to Susan Love, MD, for her study of breast cancer and hormones.
- Vivian Pinn, MD, Jacques Rossouw, MD, Sylvia Smoller, PhD, Marcia Stefanik, PhD, and Ross Prentice, PhD, for their clear explanations of the science behind menopause.
- Gill Sanson, Sherry Sherman, PhD, and Bruce Stadel, MD, for their information on osteoporosis.
- Artemis Simopoulos, MD, for defying the diet fads of her time.
- Fredi Kronenberg, PhD, and Adriane Fugh-Berman, for their dedication to alternative medicine.
- William Parker, MD, for defining the rights and wrongs of hysterectomies and oophorectomies.

Barbara thanks her co-founders of the National Women's Health Network: Alice Wolfson, Belita Cowan, Phyllis Chessler, PhD, and Mary Howell, MD. She also thanks Cindy Pearson, Olivia Cousins, PhD, and Amy Allina, who carried on our goals. Also, we are grateful to Phil Corfman, MD, and Richard Crout, MD (who stood up for informed consent in women's health care), Judy Norsigian

(OBOS), Pat Cody and Sybill Shainwald (on behalf of DES families), Maryann Napoli (Center for Medical Consumers), Susan Wood, PhD (formerly of the FDA), and Nancy Krieger, PhD.

We are grateful also to Andrea Tone, Leonore Tiefer, Shere Hite, Gloria Steinem, Congresswoman Carolyn Maloney, Minna Elias, Sheryl Burt Ruzek, Barbara Brenner, Barbara Ehrenreich, Alice Yaker, Suzanne Parisian, MD, Byllye Avery, David Michaels, PhD, Devra Lee Davis, PhD, Carolyn Westhoff, MD, Elizabeth Siegel Watkins, PhD, Pat Cody, Gordon Guyatt, MD, Bruce Stadel, Diane Meier, MD, Ben Loehnen, Jennifer Baumgardner, Nikki Scheuer, Sheila and Donald Bandman, Judge Emily Jane Goodman, Daniel Simon, Thomas Hartman, E. Neil Schachter, Debra Chase, Tara Parker-Pope, Senator Ron Wyden, Nora Coffey, Warren Bell, MD, Alan Cassels, Wendy Armstrong, Colleen Fuller, Anne Rochon-Ford, Leora Tanenbaum, Abby Lippman, PhD, Harriet Rosenberg, PhD, Amy Richards, Pam Martens, Ariel Olive, Ann Fuller, Barbara Mintzes, Aubrey Blumsohn, MD, Frances C. Whittelsey, K-K Seaman, Ronnie Eldridge, Mavra Stark, Joan Michel, Linda K. Nathan, and Dominic Carter.

For their excellent, unique scholarship that inspired us at different points in the writing process, we thank Madeline Gray, Andrea Tone, Elizabeth Siegel Watkins, Jerrilyn Prior, Lynnette Leidy Sievert, Dan Hurley, Michael Pollan, John Abramson, Cathryn Jakobson Ramin, and Margaret Morganroth Gullette.

Thanks to our top-notch assistants: Sara Germain (who helped extensively with the hysterectomy chapter), Megan Buckley, Helen Lowery, and Reed Eldridge—your dedication to the project, patience with a hectic environment, and writing and editing skills beyond your years helped at every stage of the process. Also, to David Eldridge, who provided an excellent edit of the appendix at a crucial time, and Michael Patrick Hearn and Noah Seaman, who gave vital help with the notes. To Kim Chung, who against all odds kept our computers running, and Maria Tylutki, who made sure everything else around the office was organized and efficient as possible. And as always, we are grateful to Agata Rumprecht-Behrens, who knows where things are better than either of us and who helps with whatever project we are working on, despite her own busy schedule.

• • •

Additionally Barbara would like to thank:

My exercise teachers: Tom Compo (yoga), Tai Chi master Arthur Lin, and Blanca Cubillos-Roman (salsa).

My deepest graditude to Dr. Susan Love, Dr. Neil Schachter, Deborah Chase, Dr. Diane Meier.

Ruth Gruber, my stepmother; my sisters Elaine Rosner Jerria and Jerri Drucker and her husband, Ernest Drucker, PhD; my children, Noah, Shira, and Elana; my sons-in-law Urs Bammert and Timothy Walsh; my cousins Emilia Rosner and Richard Hyfler, Jesse Drucker, Nell Casey, and Henry Jerria.

My grandchildren, who were always willing to help with secretarial duties: Sophia Bammert, Idalia Bammert, Liam Walsh, and Ezekiel Walsh.

Additionally Laura would like to thank:

Irene Xanthoudakis, Rebecca Kraut, Lauren Porsch, Molly Barry, Rachel Fisher, Rumela Mitra, Zachary Johnson, April Timko, Nicole Richman, Stephanie Kirk, Rabbi Leora Kaye, Tom Mizer, Travis McGhie, Chi-Hyun Kim, and Rabbi Sari Laufer. I am grateful to my aunts, Nancy Dilworth and Laurie Reed, who shared their stories, and also to Lois Cromwell. Special thanks goes to Rob Tennant, whose invaluable friendship and support I always feel with me in whatever project I undertake.

I want to express my thanks to my brothers: David, my alter ego, without whom I wouldn't get through a week, let alone the writing of a book; Reed, whose creativity and wit challenge and inspire me; and Peter, whom I couldn't be more proud of. Thanks also to my grandfather Paul Eldridge Sr.

My gratitude to the Seaman family—Shira for her good advice and sense of humor, Elana for her generosity and hospitality, and Noah whose friendship throughout this project got me through some dark moments in the writing process, and who on a day-to-day basis has cheered me up, gotten me thinking, and basically been an important part of my life.

A special thanks to the Weinberg/Josell family, and especially

Beth Weinberg for her wonderful stories, willingness to give personal insights on the book and constant helpful conversations on various chapter topics. I haven't words enough to thank my darling, Jeremy Weinberg, for his seemingly endless support, patience, and love. I could not ask for more in a friend, partner, and husband. I wouldn't have finished this project without you, and indeed wouldn't want to dream up future ones.

Finally, I cannot overstate my gratitude to Paul and Susan Eldridge, my parents, who imagined this book as a finished project before I could, who helped me when it took longer than I expected, and who have always been willing to make sacrifices so that I could take chances. They are also my best friends.

disclaimer

This publication contains the opinions and ideas of its authors. It is intended to provide helpful and informative material on the subjects addressed in the publication. It is sold with the understanding that the authors and publisher are not engaged in rendering medical, health, or any other kind of personal professional services in the book. The reader should consult her medical, health, or other competent professional before adopting any of the suggestions in this book or drawing inferences from it.

The authors and publisher specifically disclaim all responsibility for any liability, loss, or risk, personal or otherwise, that is incurred as a consequence, directly or indirectly, of the use and application of any of the contents of this book.

contents

introduction

Arm in arm, the women walked toward the doors of the Natcher Auditorium at the National Institutes of Health. It was the end of February 2006. Dressed in brightly colored coats to keep out the late-winter chill, they entered the conference center and were handed rose boutonnieres to distinguish them from the fleets of doctors, scientists, and journalists who were also slowly making their way to their seats.

The occasion was a two-day summit to discuss the results of the Women's Health Initiative (WHI), a massive clinical trial that had studied possible preventative approaches to problems that plague aging women—primarily heart disease, osteoporotic fracture, and breast and colorectal cancer. When we call the trial massive, we mean in scope, duration, and expense. Started in 1991 and involving 161,808 participants, the WHI cost millions of government dollars and spanned fifteen years.[1]

The clusters of middle-aged women proudly sporting the flowers on their lapels were members of that 161,808-strong sisterhood. Although they looked like any other people their age, these women had accomplished an incredible feat. Though they might not have understood it at the time they signed up to take hormone replacement therapy, make changes in their diet, and commit to decades of calcium and vitamin D capsules, these women had transformed the way that women in North America, Europe, and indeed much of the world experience menopause. For at least a century, the transition from fertility to menopause had been medicalized and treated as a disease. For over five decades, hormone treatment (HT) drugs were assumed to be the first line of defense for all women against this presumed illness. The WHI confirmed what some daring scientists and women's health advocates had been saying for years: hormones weren't the answer, and beyond that, menopause itself was a natural process that wasn't necessarily in need of any medical intervention.

None of this would have been possible without the trial participants and the generations of women who have experienced and talked about menopause in spite of prevailing medical opinions, drug fads, and dangerous social taboos. This conference, as organizer Marcia Stefanik made explicit in her opening remarks, was to honor their contribution.

Although it was a scientific meeting, the atmosphere at the NIH was closer to a school reunion. Images of the quilts created by WHI participants flashed on the main screen between presentations heavy with charts, figures, and seemingly endless statistical analyses. On panels, WHI subjects sat side by side with experts, doctors, and scientists. The message could not have been more clear: after decades of women being told what to do about their menopause by doctors, scientists, and drugmakers, at last the voices of women themselves were being heard.

As we—Barbara and Laura, the authors of this book—watched the results of the WHI unfold between 2001 and 2003, we couldn't help but wonder how we had arrived at a cultural point where we needed to be reminded that menopause was part of a woman's natural life cycle. We were amazed by the shock women experienced as the WHI was publicized and were impressed by their desire to understand the seismic shifts in menopause medicine. There were so many questions that needed answers, and we wanted to give menopausal women an easy-to-read but thorough, honest but optimistic way to understand how "the change" has, well, changed.

Things That Were, Things That Might Have Been

As long as women have been around, they have been going through menopause. It is a bodily process that is as old as human birth, death, and, of course, menstruation. There is a cultural myth that before the twentieth century, women didn't live long enough to experience menopause in significant numbers. Such a claim is simply not born out by the facts; a visit to any cemetery thick with graves from centuries past reveals the fallacy of a history without old women. Anthropologist Margaret Lock debunks the widely held idea that "the existence of women over fifty years of age is a recent phenomenon,"[2] explaining that statistics that put mean life expectancy before the twentieth century at forty-nine years of age is a mean; that is, all the people who died in infancy and as young adults are averaged in with those who lived to ripe old ages. For example: there are three people, one who dies at the age of one, one who dies at seventy-five, and one who dies at one hundred. The mean age, or average age, is fifty-eight years old. Even though two of the three people in this group live to be senior citizens, the average age is still one that falls in midlife.

It is exceedingly difficult to recover a history of menopause before the twentieth century. While it is likely that women were talking privately with each other about their experiences, written records are few and far between. This, in combination with the fact that humans are one of the few species to experience a long postreproductive life, has contributed to the idea that menopause is "strange" or even "unnatural."

In pre-nineteenth-century thinking, this included the idea that when a woman ceased to menstruate, the blood that would formerly have left her body in a monthly bleed had nowhere to go and would fester and eventually poison her. Like many normal biological processes, such as birth, menopause was gradually medicalized in the nineteenth and twentieth centuries when mostly male doctors, uncomfortable with the differences of female bodies and their processes, were quick to pathologize every gynecological event. Charles Reed, the president of the American Medical Association in 1901 and 1902, wrote that menopause was a "mental condition."[3] In the twentieth century, with the rise of pharmaceutical medicine, smart women and smart doctors were convinced that the Change was an "estrogen deficiency disease" that could be treated by supplementing the body's declining estrogen with hormones from chemical and other biological sources. Generations of women matured assuming that "a choice about estrogen" was an inevitable part of getting older.

Of course menopause was already being treated with drugs long before the synthesis of oral estrogens. A European medical book dating from the Renaissance advised women having problems with menopause to combine "a decoction of myrrh and apples" with taking a walk. A more modern approach to "treatment" was pioneered by Merck, a drug company that still exists today but was founded in 1668 as an apothecary in Darmstadt, Germany. By the late nineteenth century, Merck suggested medicating women with, among other things, wine, cannabis, opium, and a product made out of the powdered ovaries of cows called Ovariin. It's hard to say what biological effect Ovariin would have had, but the effect of the opium and cannabis can be more easily imagined.

When Premarin, a pill made from the urine of pregnant horses, was accepted by the Food and Drug Administration (FDA) for the treatment of menopause in May 1942, it was approved primarily to treat hot flashes and vaginal dryness and atrophy. From the beginning, HT was prescribed for a host of other things. (When a drug is prescribed to deal with an ailment that the FDA hasn't approved it to treat, this prescribing is called "off label" use.) For example, for years women were told to take HT to protect their hearts, despite the fact that the drug was never conclusively shown to do that.

By 1990, HT had been on the market for forty-eight years but there had still never been serious clinical trials to demonstrate its effect on the heart, as well as other symptoms it was being used to treat. Despite this, Wyeth-Ayerst Laboratories (now Wyeth Pharmaceuticals), the makers of Premarin, attempted to get the drug officially approved for the prevention of heart disease, hoping to expand its already lucrative market. The FDA refused. Taking the advice of the National Women's Health Network, a grassroots group that eschews pharmaceutical funding and functions as an advocate for women's health rights, the FDA called for the creation of the WHI, a massive randomized double-blind clinical trial set to last for more than a decade and a half. Almost everyone was convinced that trial would affirm what everyone already knew: HT was a wonder drug for "women of a certain age" that should perhaps, as one doctor suggested, be put in the drinking water alongside fluoride.

When the Prempro (premarin and progestin) arm of the trial came to a screeching halt in 2002, doctors and patients alike were shocked by the reasons. Women taking hormones had *more* heart attacks, more breast cancer, more strokes, more pulmonary embolisms, and more blood clots than women taking sugar pills. The reigning paradigm of menopause management for over fifty years had fallen like a collapsing bridge, and legions of women and their doctors were left to scramble for solid ground and make sense of this brave new world.

A Word about Words

Recently, those in the know have started to use different names for hormone drugs known for decades as "HRT" and "ERT." Now experts will refer to "HT" and "ET," but they are talking about the same medications. "ERT," the grandmother of them all, stood for "estrogen replacement therapy." When progestin and testosterone were added for safety, the term *HRT* or *hormone replacement therapy* was added. These terms reflected the attitudes of the time. Doctors believed that women *needed* estrogen and were therefore "replacing" something the body had lost. Since the WHI, doctors have reminded themselves and their patients that it's normal for estrogen and progesterone levels to fall. Because of this, folks have started calling these drugs "ET," or estrogen treatment, and "HT," or hormone treatment. These terms convey the current beliefs that estrogen is an outside chemical being used in the body to help treat a certain problem, such as hot flashing, not to to "replace" something natural.

Menopause: What's in a Name?

The "menopause," the "climacteric," the "change," the "pause," entering middle age, becoming "a certain age," becoming a "crone," going through "that time," suffering "ovarian failure," becoming "estrogen deficient": over the years we have come up with countless ways to talk about, euphemize, characterize, and medicalize this part of women's lives. While each "way of seeing" menopause tells us something about the point in time or attitudes of the people who came up with it, the multiplicity of terms makes it very difficult to pin down exactly what we are talking about.

Technically, *menopause* is the "permanent cessation of menstruation resulting from the loss of ovarian follicular activity."[4]

As women age, periods gradually cease due to the end of ovulation. This means that the cells that make eggs run out, and reproduction by natural, nonmedical means becomes impossible. Menopause is determined only in retrospect. A woman has officially gone through the process when a full year has passed since her last period. Dr. Sherry Sherman points out that the word *menopause* "corresponds to a single point in time,"[5] that is, the date immediately following the last period. Yet when we use the word *menopause* in conversation, we are most likely talking about a long process, not a discrete moment.

Premenopause is technically the entire time between menarche (which is your first menstrual bleed and is pronounced, appropriately enough, like "anarchy") to the final menstrual period. *Perimenopause* is the time before the final bleed when the reproductive cycles are winding up and slowing down. During perimenopause, bleeding begins to become irregular, and other possible symptoms that can accompany menopause, like hot flashes, start to show up. Dr. Sherman and others admit that "an adequate independent biological marker for the event doesn't exist."

When we talk about menopause in this book, unless we specify that we are using the clinical definition, that "single point in time," we are talking about the whole transition. We want to encourage women to think about the entire process as a unified experience. We want to broaden the discussion and ask how this particular transition relates to the ones that came before it. In many ways, puberty and menopause are part of the same larger process. Most books assume that women won't think about menopause until they are about to go through it. We believe that as with puberty, understanding menopause is something that should begin long before the physical experience. The decisions that a young woman makes about her health can have huge repercussions later on. For example, taking calcium and getting proper exercise throughout youth can have a huge impact on bone quality in later years; and women who smoke seem to go through menopause earlier than nonsmokers and are more likely to have a host of complications.

What's the Big Idea?

The ancient Greeks, who wisely observed a similarity between the cycles of the moon and a woman's monthly menstruation, incorrectly believed that all women would bleed at the same time each month. While this seems silly to us, in many ways women are still dealing with the notion that we all experience reproductive changes in the same way at the same time. While it might be nice if this were true, nothing in life is this straightforward, particularly changes in the body. Women can begin the menopause transition as early as their mid to late thirties or as late as their upper fifties. It can happen quickly, in the course of a year or two, or take a decade to complete itself. This variability makes it hard to paint a picture of an "average" transition or to reassure women when so many different events and experiences can rightly be called "normal."

For these reasons, when it comes to asking questions like "Am I going through menopause?" there are no straightforward answers. And a question like "What do I do about menopause?" is even more complicated.

A lot of menopause books tell women that they should be excited about this time in their lives while happily reinforcing women's worst fears about the transition. Most menopause books start by assuming that women are going to have a hard time changing. We want to start by assuming that like the majority of women, you won't have anything more than the small discomforts that accompany any major biological endocrinological shift.

If you are a woman who *is* having a tough menopause—and around 15 percent of us will—we want to provide a comprehensive, easy-to-use resource that gives you the information you need to make smart health decisions. We want to help you become a no-nonsense patient. Self-education can be a challenge. In certain ways, the Internet and other modern information sources have made it much easier to learn about, well, anything. You can get access to journals, Web sites, and online communities of women discussing the very challenges you might be facing. On the other hand, it is harder than ever to judge the quality of the information you are receiving. It seems as though every day there is a new medical breakthrough blasting its way across the evening news and the banners of Web sites.

We want to help you feel confident in evaluating different information sources (including this book!). We'll show you how to read and understand different scientific studies and assess the information you see in the media and hear from friends. We'll look at Web sites and menopause groups and show you how to tell if a group is funded by a drug company or other source that might compromise or bias the information it is presenting. Most basically, we'll talk about doctors and how to have a confident, mutually beneficial conversation with your health care professional. In the old days, doctors would tell their female patients exactly what to do, and if the patient expressed concern or objection, she was told not to worry her pretty head about it. More and more, physicians and internists are looking to their patients to be informed and ask smart questions about their health.

Finally, we want to take a hard, honest look at what we know and what we don't know about menopause. We will look at the different "symptoms" women experience that, rightly or wrongly, have become associated with it. There is no reason for anyone to suffer discomfort unnecessarily, and we'll look at all the possible treatment options available and ask some tough questions about what we really know about each problem. For many years, doctors thought the answer was simple: hormones. Since the findings of the WHI, this is clearly no longer a responsible or comprehensive response to the menopause experience. We'll look thoroughly at HT and ask what we know of its benefits and risks. As estrogen falls under greater scrutiny, alternatives such as natural medicines gain in popularity. The same kinds of questions need to be asked about their safety. Other pharmaceuticals such as bisphosphonates, statins, and antidepressants have been all too ready to fill the void left by HT. What lessons have we learned from HT that can be applied to other potentially helpful, potentially harmful pills?

Women have emerged from the collapse of HT with a new skepticism about menopause advice and treatments. This new menopausal woman—the no-nonsense woman—is who Germaine Greer has triumphantly termed "noncompliant." She realizes the importance of self-education and the value of consistently challenging received medical wisdom, refusing to take a drug until sufficient studies on it are available. She gets mad when important news about a drug's medical risks are shuffled to the back pages of the newspaper while claims of its benefits are ballyhooed on the front page.

It is for this new reader that we are writing this book.

The Women's Health Initiative: A Brief Timeline

http://www.nhlbi.nih.gov/whi/ctos.htm

- 1991: The Women's Health Initiative is mandated by Congress.
- October 1992: The Trial begins operations; it is really several small trials under the umbrella of a larger one. The WHI seeks to look at the roles of various lifestyle factors in the health of aging women. It will last fifteen years and involve 161,808 postmenopausal women. Here is a brief summary of the design.
  - It had two main components—the clinical trial and the observational trial. The clinical trial was a randomized, controlled study that included 68,132 women between the ages of fifty and seventy-nine. The observational study included 93,676 women in the same age range, many of whom either didn't want to participate in the clinical trial or were ineligible to do so. (For more information on the differences between clinical and observation studies, see the Afterword.)
  - There are three major wings of the study: the Hormone Trial, the Dietary Modification Trial, and the Calcium/Vitamin D Supplementation Trial. All three wings have both clinical and observational parts.
  - The Hormone Trial has two arms: the Estrogen Only section that studied women taking Premarin alone, and the Estrogen Plus Progestin section that studied women taking Premarin plus progestin (Prempro). For the most part, the women in the Estrogen Only section had hysterectomies and the women in the Estrogen Plus Progestin section had intact uteri. Originally, there was a small group of women with intact uteri taking Premarin alone, but this ended in 1995 because of concerns about endometrial cancer. Both arms of this trial examined the effects of hormones on heart disease and osteoporosis. The clinical hormone trials contained 27,347 women, and although it received the most media attention, it had the fewest participants.
  - The Dietary Modification Trial: the largest of the clinical trials with 48,835 women participating, this section of the WHI

sought to evaluate the role of a low-fat diet in preventing chronic illnesses like heart disease and breast and colon cancer.

- The Calcium/Vitamin D Trial included 36,282 women and looked at the effect of calcium and vitamin D supplementation on fracture risk and colon cancer. It actually began two years after participants had joined one or both of the other trials.

⚙ December 1993: First Clinical Trial participants are randomized (from the Hormone and Dietary Modification trials).

⚙ September 1994: Observational Study begins.

⚙ 1995: First Calcium/Vitamin D participants randomized.

⚙ 1995: After the results of the Postmenopausal Estrogen/Progestin Interventions Trial (PEPI) emphasize the dangers of taking estrogen alone with an intact uterus—particularly of endometrial growths and even endometrial cancer—the unhysterectomized women in the Estrogen Only Trial are reassigned to the Estrogen Plus Progestin Trial.

⚙ April 2000 and May 2001: Participants in the Estrogen and Estrogen Plus Progestin trials receive letters informing them of unexpected findings, particularly more heart attacks, strokes, and blood clots in the legs and lungs. The findings receive media attention.

⚙ July 2002: Because of increased heart attacks, strokes, and blood clots, as well as higher breast cancer rates, the Estrogen Plus Progestin Trial is halted early. A media firestorm erupts and women everywhere are left wondering how to move forward.

⚙ March 2004: The Estrogen Only study is stopped, again because it is decided that the risks of ET outweigh the benefits for participants.

⚙ March 31, 2005: All components of the WHI end. This coincides with a National Institutes State-of-the-Science conference on the Management of Menopause Symptoms that concludes that menopause is a natural part of life and "not a disease state."

⚙ April 2005: The Extension Study, which will follow willing participants for an additional five years, begins.

⚙ February 2006: The WHI Legacy conference officially summarizes and synthesizes the various findings of the entire study.

are you going through menopause?

1

flashing back
a brief history of menopause

*A Story has no beginning or end:
arbitrarily one chooses that moment of
experience from which to look back or
from which to look ahead.*

— GRAHAM GREENE

What are the stories we tell ourselves and each other about menopause? Are they our own biographies, tales of individual women and their lives? Perhaps these narratives are cautionary: an early menopause endured as the result of an ill-advised tubal ligation, or a decade of blistering hot flashes and night sweats suffered without medical relief. Maybe they are practical: advice on herbs that can cure vaginal dryness or exercises to help prevent potentially dangerous falls. Often they are inspirational: relief from years of fear about unwanted pregnancy or crippling menstrual cramps. Tales of women finally realizing, in this next great phase of their lives, who they want to be or what significant work they want to do in the world.

For many years, women didn't feel they could tell their menopause stories out loud. The subject was considered at best inappropriate and at worst vulgar. Author Amber Coverdale Sumrall describes her own mother's tough transition: "I remembered my mother's rage and ensuing depression, the emotional unavailability of my father, her many prayers. Menopause was unmentionable, a taboo subject. There were no outlets. The feelings were all internalized." She contrasts this with her own experience: "Now we have books, resources, women doctors, women's voices, friends and lovers to guide us through this transition. We have choices."[1]

Indeed, today, most menopausal women are eager to share their experiences. When Laura attended a bridal shower in the summer of 2006, someone mentioned that she was writing a book about menopause. Suddenly, Laura was as popular as the bride, and more than a dozen guests took turns sharing their stories. The change has become the topic of talk shows and news reports. There is even a popular musical attracting women in several major cities to come and laugh about our common experiences. So long forced to stay silent, menopause has found its cultural voice, and it is a booming one.

How did this attitude adjustment take place? Well, for one thing, women started talking. The women's movement of the 1970s and 1980s totally changed the way that we as a culture think about women's bodies. In particular the women's health movement got lots of different women talking about their sex lives, their hysterectomies, their medical problems, and, of course, their menopause.

At some point, each woman goes in search of her own menopause story. Whether it will be an epic with a cast of thousands or a small drama involving just you and a few good friends, we'll give you a few background stories to spark your imagination and help you better decide where your own tale will start.

A Tale of One Monkey, or a (Pre)History of Menopause

We probably don't need to tell you that human beings are special and different from other animals. For women, there is one particular aspect of our biology that sets us apart from even our closest relatives in the animal kingdom. Although there is debate in the scientific community, it is generally agreed that humans are among a very small set of creatures that live long after our sexual reproductive capabilities end. There are a handful of other animals that may share this strange trait with us—among them certain whales and African elephants.[2]

Although some apes—chimpanzees, for example—have a maximum reproductive capacity of around twenty-five years, it is rare for those species to live more than a couple years beyond losing the ability to have babies. Lest you think that is simply a product of their harsh lives, scientists have found that upon death their organs are worn by age in a way that human bodies wouldn't be until old age. These primates aren't meant to outlive childbearing. Human females are.

So when did we become different from the other apes? It is possible that when humans first evolved, women were able to keep having babies until they died. It's hard to say exactly when this changed, but fossils suggest it was[3] perhaps 1.6 million years ago,[4] before *Homo sapiens* replaced their prehuman ancestors.

Why we became so different is another, even more confusing, matter. The idea of long life after reproduction flies in the face of a lot of evolutionary tenets. One popular idea about why this happened is called the "grandmother hypothesis," which says that women enjoy long postreproductive lives to give their offspring an advantage by providing additional caretaking for grandchildren. This allows a woman's daughter to reproduce at a younger age and have more children with the confidence that they would receive proper care. Also, in a time before written records, grandparents became repositories for important knowledge,[5] sort of human libraries handing out survival tips.

This idea has had its critics; anthropologist Jocelyn Scott Peccei is prominent among them. First and foremost, Peccei points out, the theory ignores the role of men in both helping to get food and aiding in child care. She cautions that "one cannot overlook male investment in an explanation of menopause,"[6] and adds that older men, who remain fertile to varying degrees until extreme old age or death, would have been just as capable as their aging female counterparts of providing extra family support.

Instead, Peccei advocates a competing idea called the "mother hypothesis." In this version of the story, as humans evolved, it took more and more energy to raise babies and keep them healthy and safe. Women who stopped reproducing at a young age were at an evolutionary advantage because they would have more energy to put in to their existing children.[7] It also increased the likelihood that they would live long enough to provide proper support to their young.

Regardless of which of these ideas is true, it seems that middle-aged women had great value in their families and societies. Menopause in ancient times, as today, became a vehicle through which women could transform themselves and do important work to improve both their own lives and those around them.

In Search of Menopause

The author Grace Paley writes that "menopause has had a poor press. The bad parts have been touted and the good parts have been kept a secret."[8] It would be fair to say that this is an understatement.

Although historical evidence about menopause is scarce before the fifteenth or sixteenth century, references can be found. An ancient Egyptian medical papyrus tells of a woman who hasn't menstruated in many years and is suffering from a battery of physical problems including nausea, vomiting, and burning in the stomach. Deborah Sweeney writes, "The diagnosis is not that the woman is growing older but that she has been bewitched."[9] In 1250 BCE, a Hittite king named Hattusilis wrote to Rameses II for help with his aging sister. Didn't the Egyptian ruler have some sort of medicine that could help his sixty-year-old sibling bear children? Rameses replied matter-of-factly that at that age there was probably nothing even his best doctors could do to help.[10] The first story shows that even millennia before the common era, menopause was already in the process of being medicalized and explained with ill-supported rationales. In the second story, it is clear from Rameses' response that it was common knowledge that aging women became infertile.

By the late Middle Ages, it was widely believed that menstruation was necessary for cleaning out the body. In twelfth-century Italy, a female doctor named Trotula of Salerno wrote about menopause, menstruation, and the differences between male and female health. Trotula believed that men and women were composed of converse but complementary biologies, with men bearing too much heat and women too much moisture. Her view—and it was popular for centuries afterward—was that this excess moisture (later specifically blood) collected in the body at unhealthy levels when not alleviated through monthly bleeds.

She noted that menstruation lasts "up to about the 50th year if (the patient) is lean; sometimes up to the 60th or 65th is she is moist; in the moderately fat up to about 45."[11] Here the good doctor observed something crucial: lifestyle factors play a role in when and how periods stop. She also writes that most women "dare not reveal the difficulties of their sickness to a male doctor."

Some female patients, however, had no trouble talking at length about their menopause problems with male doctors. Another Italian, the sixteenth-century doctor Giovanni Marinello, gave a laundry list of the potential problems awaiting a woman, including "pains ... apostemata, eye disorders, weak sight, vomiting, fever."[12] Perhaps most shockingly, he added, women desire sex more than ever. By this point, doctors believed that menstrual blood served an essential purgative function. When a woman failed to menstruate, toxins built up in the body and at best would make a woman sick. One theory held that the blood converted to fat, and that was why menopausal women gained weight. At worst, experts feared, the extra blood might actually kill the female patient.

There were dissenters to this alarmist view: in 1582, a Frenchman named Jean Liébault observed that the change "does no harm to woman's body."[13] Liébault wrote of more benign symptoms, including what he called "*petites rougeurs*"—"little reds"—most certainly what we now call hot flashes.

By the eighteenth century, the first menopause manuals were printed. They were exceedingly popular: it's very clear that when information is made available, women are hungry to receive it. This century also saw a boom in potentially dangerous pharmaceuticals. These preparations, including "pills of Rufus," "pills of Franck," "the sacred tincture," and "*elixir de propriété*" were wildly popular, despite the fact that doctors scorned them as the province of female health experts who were, in the opinion of most male physicians, little better than witches. The doctor's solution, it should be mentioned, was far worse than the mostly herbal and even narcotic ingredients in early pills: bleeding was recommended in the hope that letting blood from other parts of the body would relieve pressure on the reproductive organs.

It was in the second half of the ninetienth century that the term *menopause* became common parlance. It was originally coined by a French doctor named C. P. L. de Gardanne in his book treatise *On the Menopause, or the Critical Time for Women*. At the time, menopause was known in English as "the dodging time."[14]

The concept of "climacteric," popular in the nineteenth century, was an idea applied equally to men and women. This notion more closely resembled our "midlife crisis" and had been in circulation in educated circles[15] since the Middle Ages. Some nineteenth-century doctors observed that while women experienced climacteric, it was much worse and much more pronounced in male patients.

After centuries of purgation and bleeding as the main treatments for a bad menopause, late-nineteenth-century doctors, full of their growing power and new knowledge, came up with what they thought represented a true advance in medicine for midlife women: the prophylactic hysterectomy. For a doctor like the American gynecologist Edward Curry, the growing popularity of "female castration" represented a leap into modernity, the opening of centuries of shuttered dustiness in women's medicine.[16] Curry became a great advocate for the procedure, explaining that if you were going to remove the uterus and fallopian tubes, you might as well take the ovaries too. This idea has had a particularly persistent popularity with modern doctors.

Around the same time Curry was taking out his patients' organs, other doctors were jumping on the pill bandwagon, employing more traditional herbs and opiates as well as newer drugs based on animal reproductive organs. In the early twentieth century, drug companies would take on this effort to find new and better ways to medicate menopause.

The growing field of psychoanalysis offered its own answers about midlife women. Janice Delaney, Mary Jane Lupton, and Emily Toth explain, "Victorian medicine men knew in their hearts that during the menopause, a woman could expect to have mental problems."[17] No less an authority than Sigmund Freud wrote that women "become quarrelsome and obstinate, petty and stingy, show typical sadistic . . . features which they did not show before."[18]

These three growing forces in the medical world—surgery, pharmaceuticals, and psychotherapy—combined to create the menopausal perfect storm in the twentieth century, and one hundred years later we are beginning undo some of the damage done by thousands of years of misunderstanding, misdiagnosis, and mistreatment.

So What *Is* Going On in There?

When periods stop coming, it is really just the outward sign of changes that have been taking place in the body's reproductive system over the course of decades. Reproductive aging in women happens in part because the number of oocytes (pre-egg cells) gradually lessens over time. Human females make *all* of the cells needed for reproduction during gestation; female fetuses produce millions of oocytes, only a small fraction of which will become mature eggs. To put this in perspective, compare these millions with the five hundred or so eggs a woman will produce during her reproductive years. The initial millions are cut in half by the time a baby is born and continues to decline over the woman's lifetime.

Like getting taller or putting on weight, the loss of eggs happens constantly but unevenly. The time in the womb is one time of substantial loss. Another moment happens sometime between the early forties and the early to mid-fifties, when the number of oocytes drops from somewhere in the thousands to nearly zero.

When a woman has her period, her brain sends out hormones to stimulate the development of ovarian follicles (which contain the oocytes). Like a message over a loudspeaker, a brain chemical called gonadotropin-releasing hormone (GnRH) glides down to the pituitary gland. Reacting to this call to arms, the pituitary makes another chemical, follicles-stimulating hormone (FSH). FSH in turn causes several egg follicles to develop. Of these follicles, one or two eventually spit out an egg.

If the egg goes unfertilized, hormone levels fall and the woman has her period. The next month, this cycle repeats itself.

In the time right before menopause—what many people call "perimenopause"—the brain continues sending out signals to the body to cause a period. Like an increasingly hard-of-hearing person in a crowded restaurant, the ovaries begin to respond erratically, sometimes answering the brain's call as always and at other times acting as though no message was sent. This is because the oocytes, the pre-egg cells, have dwindled to low levels. When this happens, the brain responds as you would to someone who wasn't hearing you: it raises its voice, as it were, and makes more of the chemical FSH, desperately trying to kick-start the stalling ovaries.

Periods don't stop all at once, of course. They taper off and sputter and start and stop. They get lighter and lighter and then come flooding through like Niagara Falls—until one day the eggs are all spent and the bleeding stops once and for all.

Far from now being a useless organ, however, the ovary continues to make hormones, including estrogen and testosterone.

We do want to make a distinction between natural and induced menopause. There are two things that cause women to go through the transition: biology (both early and normal menopause) and medical intervention. Induced menopause is most commonly caused by surgical removal of the ovaries and/or uterus but can also result from radiation therapy and chemotherapy. Other gynecological procedures, such as tubal ligation and uterine embolization, can unintentionally bring on menopause by blocking blood flow to the ovaries. As many as one in four women experience this kind of menopause. And it is a very different experience from a natural transition.

In Our Own Words

Why some women have such terrible problems associated with menopause and others barely notice theirs remains a matter of speculation and the source of some very interesting questions.

Dena Taylor and Amber Coverdale Sumrall describe the multiplicity of voices they encountered when they set out to collect women's stories about menopause:

> We expected to find common experiences of hot flashes, a sense of loss and a general feeling of the blahs. Instead we found tremendous diversity and individuality in the women's accounts. Some had terrible hot flashes. Some had incredible dreams. Some went through a period of important self-discovery, often realizing a profound sense of spirituality.

Some left long-standing relationships, and some found new ones. Some laughed about what was happening. For some, menopause lasted one year; for others, ten years. Some had very heavy bleeding. Some couldn't get by without taking estrogen and others wouldn't hear of it. Many came through it much stronger. And some told us they had nothing to write because they hardly noticed their menopause.[19]

Maybe this diversity is one reason a medical model of the change will always fail. When you try to set strict parameters on any human experience, physical or otherwise, you are doomed to failure. To think of menopause as a strictly biological, medical occurrence underestimates the role of culture in generating physical experiences and our attitudes about them. To understand menopause as something made only culturally denies the unavoidable truths that our body tells us. Grace Paley says, "Our insides do know something about what is happening to our outsides. Our bodies live in this world and are picked up, shaken, and what is natural becomes difficult."[20]

Think back to adolescence: there were bodily changes—the periods, the skin trouble, the variable moods—but there were other issues. For example, how a culture feels about sex can make it harder or easier to deal with burgeoning sexuality. If your parents greet your first period with excitement and congratulations, you will feel very differently about your monthly cycles from someone whose first menstruation was met with fear and anxiety.

Asking the Right Questions

So if menopause is natural and not a disease, why do we call the physical experiences that accompany it "symptoms"?

Nancy Fugate Woods and Ellen Mitchell define *symptom* as a sensation that a person perceives as being out of the ordinary.[21] Because these physical experiences are out of the ordinary doesn't mean they are unnatural. And the fact that they're natural doesn't mean that they aren't disruptive and confusing or even potentially frightening. The reality is that many women do experience something they aren't used to during the menopausal transition: 85 percent of women report one or more symptoms, with 30 to 50 percent of women reporting hot flashes. In talking about "symptoms," we are acknowledging these experiences, not suggesting they are a mark of illness or abnormality.

The truth is that doctors and scientists aren't sure that many symptoms frequently attributed to the menopause transition have any actual connection to the process. It is very difficult to show what is caused by hormone fluctuation, what is caused by changing lifestyle factors, and what is just the result of normal aging. Serious health problems like heart disease and osteoporosis, which are often associated with menopause, increase in men, too, as the body ages. Until we better understand what questions we are asking, it is very hard to be certain about our answers. Treating the symptoms of menopause is like trying to prune a plant leaf by leaf when the problem lies in the root system.

This question is even more interesting when we consider that women in different societies, even in diverse ethnic groups in the same society, experience menopause in drastically different ways. Anthropologist Yewoubdar Beyene observed women in rural Guatemala and found that not only did they view menopause as an overwhelmingly positive thing, but not one of the women she worked with experienced a hot flash.[22] Anthropologist Marcia Flint studied five hundred women in India and reported a complete lack of any menopause symptoms.[23]

We will look together at many of these medical and cultural questions.

In the meantime, we want to encourage you to start writing your own story. Keep a journal. It may include a record of hot flashes or other physical events, or you may never have any physical issues in menopause other than the eventual end to your periods but you may be going through big changes in your life—a new job, relationship issues, basic transformations in the way you see and understand yourself. These, too, are worthy of documentation. Keeping track of physical changes will help you understand patterns or progressions in your menopause process. It will help you make decisions about proper exercise and nutrition, and, if necessary, treatments for prob-

lem symptoms. Likewise, writing down your feelings and ideas during this time of your life will help you make big decisions—or even
just make peace with the way your life changes.

The legendary science fiction writer Ursula K. Le Guin reflected
on her own menopause, writing, "It seems a pity to have a built in rite
of passage and to dodge it, evade it, and pretend nothing has
changed." In the next chapter we will talk about beginnings, both
physical and psychological, that can be a part of menopause. Le Guin
explained the difficulty of these new starts: "The woman who is willing to make that change must become pregnant with herself at last.
She must bear herself, her third self, her old age, with travail and
alone. Not many will help her with this birth."[24] We are here to do
just that.

2

at first glance

perimenopause, beginnings and ends

You're searching, Joe, for things that don't
exist; I mean beginnings. Ends and
beginnings — there are no such things.
There are only middles.

—Robert Frost

There will come a time when you believe
everything is finished. That will be the
beginning.

—Louis L'Amour

When author Madeline Gray wrote her influential book *The Changing Years* in 1951 after her own oophorectomy, any information on menopause was scarce and shrouded in secrecy. Gray explained that after her surgery, "I looked for books that might help me. But there were none at the time to answer all my questions satisfactorily. None at all."[1]

Appalled by the ignorance and fear she encountered among friends, Gray wanted to get women thinking differently, and preemptively about menopause. She railed against the term *change of life*, saying:

Of all the stupid phrases ever invented this is about the most stupid. And of all the misnomers this takes the prize. Certainly it is a change—and a dramatic and obvious one. But the change makes it sound like the only change. And change *of life* makes it sound as if your whole life were to be altogether different, which is far from the case. Why this change is no more the change of your entire life than all the other changes which have gone before and will come after. Living is constant change. That is its essence.[2]

Flash forward half a century to April 2002 and we are swimming in a sea of information about menopause. Oprah Winfrey was doing what she does best: trying to raise her viewers' awareness about their lives and well-being. "Are you in menopause . . . ," Oprah asked sensationally, "and don't know it?" The show was about perimenopause, and it featured a panel of experts, primarily best-selling author Dr. Christiane Northrup. The response to the show was overwhelming—Oprah's Web site was flooded by visitors and temporarily couldn't handle them all.[3] It wasn't just female viewers seeking answers to their personal health questions. Doctors were riled up, some of them taking issue with the whole concept of perimenopause, suggesting it was nothing more than a marketing scheme.

"Women's health has been phenomenally over-medicalized and commercialized, and to a large extent perimenopause is a manifestation of that," said Georgetown Medical School professor Anthony Scialli in a *New York Times* article responding to the Oprah show.[4] Dr. Adriane Fugh-Berman, a board member of the National Women's Health Network in Washington, D.C., called the term a marketing device used to encourage women to interpret natural signs of aging as premenopausal illness.[5]

Fifty-one years after Madeline Gray, the problem was the same: even the words we use to talk about menopause have the power to generate anger, frustration, fear, and controversy. They also reveal two other things. First, as menopause has moved from private euphemism—the change of life—to medical terminology—perimenopause—we are equally unable to define exactly what we are talking about. This failure of language, or in some cases success of manipulative language, is what causes these feelings of fear, confusion, or anger. Second, it shows that when we lack good, solid ways to talk about our experiences, women are the losers.

Perimenopause is a particularly poignant moment to have this conversation because it is at the supposed "beginning" of menopause. In this chapter we'll talk about getting off to a good start.

Around Menopause

The prefix "peri" means simply "around" or "about." We might even say it means "almost menopause." The term first became popular in the 1990s, during the height of HT and ET optimism. Doctors needed the word because, as we discuss in chapter 1, "menopause" in medical circles means only the time immediately following the last period. Obviously the process takes longer and is much more complicated than the simple moment when bleeding finally stops. Other major life transitions—puberty, for example—don't have this problem. We don't have to use the term *perimenarche,* because the word *puberty* implies a long transition. Older terms—both Gray's hated *change of life* and the even older *climacteric*—lack the required medical sound despite having the correct implication of a longer journey that is both physical and mental.

We believe that in the same way women use "menopause" colloquially to mean the whole process, they use "perimenopause" not to mean the entire time before the actual menopause but rather the first moments or months or years when a woman understands that her body is starting to change.

Some women don't have an "ah-ha" moment where they realize menopause is happening. When Laura asked her mom, Sue, for her first story on menopause, she stared at her resolutely and said, "I don't have one." When pressed she added, "I was in my early forties and my periods got irregular." When asked if she was surprised, Sue answered, "No, it was *supposed* to happen."

True enough, but for many of us it involves an adjustment in thinking. Our reactions, positive and negative, usually have to do with what we think menopause *means.*

If menopause, for you, means growing old, than you are going to have a very different reaction from someone who thinks the end of periods are about the greatest thing that's ever happened to her.

Most women probably start to notice when periods become irregular; their cycles start coming closer together and periods don't last as long as they used to.

When you first notice your body changing, you probably want to know for certain if it is caused by the menopause or something else. Unfortunately, there isn't really a good way to tell. Both over-the-counter menopause tests and the similar ones performed in doctor's offices rely on checking hormone levels, usually follicle-stimulating hormone (FHS) or estrogen levels. The problem is that if you *are* perimenopausal, these hormones may fluctuate so wildly that a measurement from one month to the next can create inaccurate results. Also, determining what constitutes a "normal" level of any hormone is tough because individual women vary so much. We would caution you particularly that over-the-counter tests aren't good indicators of whether you are perimenopausal, or of how far along in the transition you have come.

At this point, there really isn't a test or measure to guarantee that the menopause process has started in the same way that there is no method—besides time—for conclusively telling that it has finished. As one group of doctors explains, "No one symptom or test is accurate enough by itself to rule in or rule out perimenopause. Clinicians should diagnose perimenopause based on menstrual history and age without relying on laboratory test results."[6]

Writing down your experiences and keeping track of the ways you see your body acting differently is the most efficient method of understanding what is happening to you.

Baby Dreams: Perimenopause and Pregnancy

When menopausal symptoms begin, most people believe it means the end of fertility. For women who want children and haven't had them, believing they might be entering perimenopause can be emotionally devastating. Even if you are a woman who has all the children she wants or has decided not to have kids, this can be a difficult time.

It is totally normal to dream about babies at this time of your life, even if you've never wanted children or are quite content with the ones you have. Perhaps it is because this moment is so final, or maybe it is simply biological hardwiring to encourage you to make use of your remaining fertility. It doesn't mean you subconsciously desire a child.

If you have either never had children or would like another, there are many issues to consider with late-fertility pregnancy. Peak fertility happens in the late twenties,[7] but obviously women continue to have babies for years after this, into the mid- and late forties and even the early fifties. If you are able to conceive and want to have a child, don't let outdated opinions keep you from pursuing motherhood.

You should know that fertility declines before periods stop. Just because you are menstruating doesn't mean you are ovulating or that the other phases of your cycle are going to be right for fertilizing an egg. Natural pregnancies, however, can and do happen in perimenopausal women.[8] As more women wait to become mothers for a variety of reasons, including later coupling and marriage and a desire to build a career, older motherhood is on the rise.

If you want a baby and find that you aren't conceiving, be cautious about trying extreme measures like fertility drugs and treatments. These wildly undertested pharmaceuticals aren't very effective for older would-be mothers and are potentially dangerous. Some hormone drugs, like Lupron, may even hasten perimenopausal symptoms.[9] Talk to your doctor and don't let anyone scare you or pressure you into making a dangerous decision. Keep in mind that male fertility declines with age as well, and it may be that your partner is equally or more responsible for a lack of conception.

On the flip side, remember that just because your periods have been irregular, this doesn't mean pregnancy isn't possible. Before reliable birth control was available, perimenopausal women had what were known as "change-of-life babies," children born years and even decades after their siblings. If you don't want to get pregnant, make sure you keep using birth control until you are certain menopause has happened (a year or so after the last period).

How Soon Is Too Soon:
Early and Premature Menopause

What if you don't just *feel* too young to be in menopause; what if you are statistically too young?

Premature menopause is very rare. Only 1 to 2 percent of women will enter menopause before forty and only 10 percent by age forty-five.[10] When a woman becomes menopausal before the age of forty, we say that she has premature menopause.

It is thought that premature menopause happens when there is a problem with the immune system; the body gets confused and attacks the ovaries with antibodies the way it would attack an illness. This is an *extremely* rare condition, however, and young women who become menopausal do so much more often because of either having a hysterectomy (a total—which removes the ovaries—or a partial, which can block blood flow to the ovaries) or undergoing chemotherapy. If you have a total hysterectomy, there is no going back in terms of fertility; sometimes the damage done by chemotherapy and radiation can be reversed, and if you have a partial hysterectomy, even one that removes one ovary or part of an ovary, you can maintain some fertility, although this is certainly not guaranteed.

Don't assume that menstrual irregularities are signs of menopause. There are many things that can make periods a little erratic. Some women suffer health conditions that can make their periods temporarily irregular or render them infertile for a time (this used to be called "temporary menopause," but this terminology has fallen out of favor). Other women have health conditions, such as polycystic ovarian syndrome, that cause irregular periods throughout reproductive life.

Smoking and Early Menopause

Despite decades of public health warnings, some studies estimate that as many as 23 percent of American women were still smoking regularly at the end of the 1990s.[11] This means that nearly a quarter of American women are likely to start menopause earlier than average (and to be less fertile).[12] The link between early menopause and cigarettes was discovered several decades ago. Dr. Herschel Jick explained in 1979: "We started looking at our data for one reason or another on menopause and at the same time we were looking at our data on smoking. So we looked at the two of them combined and, lo and behold, we found that there is a striking relationship."[13]

Smokers seem to start the process about a year to two years before nonsmokers.[14] Doctors aren't sure exactly why this happens. It might be that chemicals in cigarettes cause the liver to absorb estrogen, reducing the levels of estrogen available to the body, or possibly that they increase the amount of testosterone in the body.[15] Regardless of the reason, smoking gives a signal to the ovaries that it is time to start menopause.[16] The sooner you quit smoking (which we would guess you already know you should do), the more likely it is that menopause can be delayed.

Hysterectomy and Gynecological Surgery

If you have had a hysterectomy—that means your uterus has been removed but your ovaries left intact—it has long been assumed that you will go through a normal menopause. Recently, though, doctors have been finding that women who have had the surgery often have more abrupt and severe menopauses. This is probably because scar tissue and other results of the surgery can inhibit blood flow to the ovaries[17] and cause menopause to happen faster and with more symptoms.

Similar things can happen with other surgeries, including certain types of sterilization and tubal ligation. Evelyn M. Parke was forty when side effects from birth control pills led her to get her tubes tied. When she began to have hot flashes and other menopause symptoms, she asked her doctor if it was possible she was going through the transition early. He scoffed at the idea, saying she was too young. After switching doctors, she learned that it was a possible result of her surgery. She writes, "Menopause happened to me when I was only forty years old. I didn't mean for it to happen and neither did God. It was an accident."[18]

Having a hysterectomy certainly affects how ready you feel to start or go through menopause. In a study of women in upstate New York, women who had undergone hysterectomy were far more likely to say that their menopause was early, and none of them said that it was late.[19] Compare these findings with a study of women who experienced natural menopause. Lynnette Leidy Sievert found that when asked if they were ready for periods to end, 93 percent of naturally menopausal women said they were and 98 percent said they were ready to be done with childbearing.[20]

Another problem with the idea of perimenopause is that it doesn't deal with the experience of oophorectomized women (women who have had their ovaries removed). These women technically don't go through perimenopause since it is seen as a process that ends with the last period. Unlike women going through natural menopause, who can have years to get used to what is happening to their bodies, oophorectomized women are thrown into the menopausal deep end.

Genetics

Lynnette Leidy Sievert writes that "age at menopause seems to be highly heritable."[21] That means you get more than your hair color and the shape of your hands from your mom: you may also go through menopause around the same time she did. If your mother or grandmother had an early transition, there is a chance you will as well.

Ask your mom about her menopause: How old was she? How long did the whole transition take? What was the first thing that made her think, "Maybe I'm going through menopause"? Because so many things about this experience seem to be at least somewhat related to genetics, these conversations can give you insights that may help you anticipate or understand your own change.

How closely can you expect your experience to be like your mom's? Everyone is so different, and obviously we don't always genetically resemble one parent or another; you may look just like your father or resemble a distant aunt more than your parents. And of course menopause isn't just about genes. That said, one study suggests that age at menopause is about 60 percent genes and 40 percent outside factors.[22] Another found that if a woman's mother had gone through early menopause, she was three times more likely to do so as well.[23]

Intergenerational conversations on the subject, of course, can have benefits and yield knowledge that goes far beyond whether bleeding will get irregular at the age of forty-two or fifty-two.

Portrait of Perimenopause

Very generally, some of the things commonly experienced during perimenopause include irregular periods, hot flashes, breast tenderness, insomnia, migraines, and bad symptoms of premenstrual syndrome (PMS). Sometimes vaginal changes can alter the sexual experience. If you suffered from migraines at other times in your life, you may be more likely to get them now, but you may also experience them for the first time. Both the headaches and breast tenderness are due to changing hormone levels.

The Stages of Reproductive Aging Workshop (STRAW) held in Park City, Utah, in 2001 set out to map perimenopause more firmly, creating a portrait of what it might look like for many women. STRAW divides reproductive life into five premenopausal and two postmenopausal stages. The first three premenopausal stages are the reproductive years. Around the third stage, FSH levels start to rise, and by the fourth stage menstrual cycles are getting closer together and actual periods are shorter. By the fifth premenopausal stage, women are skipping periods and may have heavy bleeding. The flooding and the missed periods usually indicate that menopause is drawing to a close.[24] Systems like this can be helpful because they can give us a general idea of what perimenopause may look like. They should always be taken with a grain of salt, however, because women's experiences are so varied.

End of the Beginning, or Beginning of the End

Winston Churchill once famously said in a speech, "This is not the end. It is not even the beginning of the end. But it is, perhaps, the end of the beginning."

In the 1990s it was still common for doctors to speak of menopause as an estrogen deficiency disease and to assume that declining estrogen was at least related to nonmenopausal problems that increased in women at midlife. In this negative view, perimenopause is the "beginning of the end." The story that women were told was one of steady decline. Now the National Institutes of Health, the North American Menopause Society, and other organizations with an interest in menopausal health have come out strongly against the "disease" model and stress how natural the process is.

In the late 1990s, a Canadian doctor named Jerilynn Prior redefined perimenopause in a way that not only clarified what we mean when we use the word, but also helped us reconsider some of the most basic aspects of this early part of the change. Like so many women, Prior, an endocrinologist from British Columbia, started to get excited about the subject of perimenopause when she went through a bad one. She writes, "Mine actually lasted over ten years! My breasts were sore, I was relentlessly hungry, and I was angry. I was angry because as a doctor, I had learned that midlife women suffered from dropping estrogen levels. What I knew was that my estrogen levels felt sky-high!" [25]

In an innovative review published in 1998,[26] Prior argued that what creates many of the common symptoms women experience during menopause is not, as previously argued, falling estrogen levels but rather the problems created by soaringly *high* estrogen and increasingly low *progesterone* levels. We think there is a crucial mental distinction here, as well as a couple of really helpful biological ones: perimenopause isn't the start of a long narrative of decline; rather, the hot flashes, headaches, and joint pains are really the menstrual cycle's "last hurrah." It is "the end of the beginning," and for many women, it is a sign of better health to come for many years after hormone levels calm down and even out.

Prior defines perimenopause as the time from the first indications of change in menstruation to a year after the last period, when it can be said with some confidence that you are postmenopausal. Although we agree with Dr. Prior's definition, for simplicity's sake we will talk about the menopause transition, a time with a beginning, middle, and end.

In the past, there have been two tendencies in approaching the situation of menopausal women. The first we have already talked about: the insistence that it is a time of physical and emotional problems, akin to an illness, that can and should be treated medically.

There is another, equally incorrect approach that says the problems women have are all in their heads, the product of an overmedicated, overdoctored culture that wants to make women sick. In this way of thinking, women are encouraged to believe that menopause is easy unless you are buying into some drug-company-authored lie. This can leave women who *do* have struggles during menopause feeling patronized, invisible, and at fault. It takes power away from the very women who most need to feel confident and assertive in meeting their health challenges. It also leaves these women vulnerable to the people who are all too eager to listen to them: product pushers. It opens them up to real drug company lies.

We know that both sets of women are out there: the ones who don't notice menopause and the ones who go through hell. We want them both to know that they are heard. Jerilynn Prior writes that the amazing unifier in menopause experience is difference: "The paths women take in perimenopause are like dozens of leaves falling into separate small rivulets up in the foothills. Each takes a different route to the ocean."[27] There simply is no "average" menopausal woman, no "normal" experience.

3

seeing red
excessive bleeding, menorrhagia, and perimenopause

There are no adequate long-term studies examining menorrhagia during the menopausal transition.
—NATIONAL INSTITUTES OF HEALTH
STATE-OF-THE-SCIENCE CONFERENCE STATEMENT[1]

LeAnn, a petite woman in her fifties sporting a blonde bob and an animated expression, shares her story:

"It was like something out of a horror movie—everywhere I looked there was blood.

"It started out of nowhere. I hadn't had a period in two months, and suddenly I was having a superperiod. I was using a pad, even two pads an hour, and barely keeping the blood from getting on my clothes. I was having trouble keeping up because I work as a receptionist and I kept having to leave the desk and run to the ladies' room."

Many women can relate to LeAnn's story. As menopause approaches and hormone levels start to shift, menstruation begins to get erratic. Some—or a lot—of bleeding at this time is normal. But how much is too much? When should a woman worry about her bleeding? And do medications such as estrogens help or hurt this common problem?

As long as people have been writing about menopause, they have been talking about perimenopausal bleeding, or "flooding." An 1837 manual suggested using opium, lead, hemlock, and a bunch of other not-so-healthy remedies to stem the tide of unwanted blood. Even these dubious cures were accompanied by the sentiment that the "mental anxiety" caused by bleeding takes a harder toll on the body than the discharge itself.[2]

When a woman experiences really heavy menstrual bleeding, either because of menopause or for another reason, doctors will sometimes call the condition "menorrhagia." "Meno" simply means "month" and "rhagia" comes from the Greek for "break" or "burst." Another term you many encounter is "hypermenorrhea," which just means bleeding excessively, in the same way that "hyperactive" means having too much energy.

Heavy bleeding is one of the most common signs of imminent menopause. It is estimated that a fourth of women (25 percent) will have at least one episode at some point. Bleeding, however, can also be caused by a lot of other things. That is why if you find that you are experiencing floods, it is important to make sure they are caused by the simple waxing and waning of hormones and not something more serious.

How many pads in a day indicate a serious problem, or how many tampons should send you running for your MD? You would be amazed by the vague answers many doctors give to this simple question. Many Web sites offer parameters in milliliters or ounces, as if a woman at home could look down and say, "Well, that's one milliliter too many! I'd better go to the doctor." Generally, it's a good idea to talk to a doctor if you find that you are soaking through more than one sanitary pad or tampon every hour for several days in a row.[3]

Dr. Jerilynn Prior explains that in a study of randomly selected premenopausal women, the average period lasted for between four and six days and women lost between 10 to 35 milliliters of blood in total. She says that if you are experiencing more than 60 milliliters of blood loss, you might want to talk to a doctor, and she adds that until a woman loses 80 milliliters, she isn't considered to be experiencing menorrhagia.[4]

So how is the average woman supposed to have any idea how much blood makes up 35 milliliters? Or 80?

Generally a normal-sized pad or tampon can hold around 5 milliliters of blood. A supersized pad can potentially hold more like 10 milliliters. So keep track of how many pads you are going through and multiply that number times 5 or 10 to find out approximately how much blood you are losing.

The Mayo Clinic cites the need to wake and change sanitary protection during the night, experiencing a period that lasts longer than seven days or is characterized by large blood clots, and constant pain in the lower abdomen during periods as "signs that you might want to check with a doctor about your cycle."[5]

This does *not* mean you need to start worrying. The chances are very good, especially if you are perimenopausal, that what you are going through is a normal—if difficult—part of the transition.

Another thing to keep track of is how you are feeling. If you become dizzy or have trouble standing, you should probably talk to your doctor. The same thing goes for heart palpitations. In the meantime, Dr. Prior recommends drinking salty fluids like bullion or vegetable juice and taking ibuprofen or Tylenol.[6]

Although no one is exactly sure why women bleed excessively around menopause, it probably comes as no surprise to you that it is most likely tied to hormone fluctuations. Specifically, it seems that when the amount of estrogen in the body is significantly disproportionate to the amount of progesterone, floods happen. Actual floods—the weather kind—happen when the atmosphere is out of balance: a low-pressure system bumps up against a high-pressure system and, *boom,* thunder and rain ensue. The same is true with the body. This may be one reason why heavy bleeding is more common at the end of the menopause transition.

Although there is no single experience or trajectory for perimenopause, it does seem that for many women the process begins with shorter, lighter periods that eventually stop coming regularly. Heavy bleeds are common after women have missed one or several periods.

On a menopause discussion board on the Internet, women described an array of experiences. Here is just a sampling of their diverse stories.[7]

One woman underwent light and heavy periods intermittently: "I had 14–21 days of non-stop bleeding, much of it of the tampon-an-hour variety, complete with clots . . . [counterbalanced with] a couple of 'was that even a period??' cycles with nothing but a few spots. . . . Before, I would spot dark blood for a day or two, then bleed red for a day or two, then spot again. Now first day I flood! All red blood."

(This woman's observation about the change in blood color is the kind of information you should share with your doctor.)

Another woman writes of having both heavy and light bleeding all in the course of the same period: "It started with a lot of spotting that would start to develop into an actual period . . . and then back down to spotting and then stop and then suddenly I'd have a little gusher a few days later and spot and stop and gush but never get all through a normal period. About three months after this started I got the first episodes of horrific flooding."

Once you have finished menopause—or think you are finished, meaning you haven't had a period for more than a year—a heavy bleed is something you should talk to a doctor about.

A recurring theme on menopause discussion boards is that periods are like bad movies—just when you think they're finally over, there is more. Many women describe the experience of a heavy period after months or years of not having one; most late or postmenopausal bleeds are nothing to be concerned about. Your body doesn't abruptly stop making hormones; it continues to produce estrogen well past menopause. Since bleeding is caused by hormone fluctuation, it remains a possibility even after you think menopause is over.

However, because bleeding could be caused by other things—some of them potentially dangerous—it is a good idea to discuss postmeno bleeding with a doctor. Be prepared for your doctor to suggest some tests, but don't be concerned that this definitely means she is worried about something; it's more likely she is just being cautious.

There are many things that can cause excessive bleeding besides hormones. Some nonmenopause causes are fibroids, polyps, infections (including common sexually transmitted diseases [STDs] such as chlamydia and gonorrhea), adenomyosis, or even pregnancy. Other serious—and infrequent—problems are cervical or uterine cancer. Cancer is obviously the most serious concern, but as Dr. Susan Love points out, it is "fortunately . . . the least common cause of abnormal nonhormonal bleeding."[8] Dr. Love adds that "to pinpoint the cause of abnormal bleeding, you'll need an endometrial biopsy."

Both fibroids and polyps are noncancerous growths that happen either on or in the uterus. We will talk much more about fibroids later in the book, but they are usually benign, sometimes annoying growths that get worse with perimenopause and then diminish or disappear after menopause.

Polyps are easy to remove with a surgical technique called hysteroscopy. This technique involves inserting a small tube into a woman's vagina and up through the cervix into the uterus; the surgeon removes the polyp through the tube. This said, don't have your polyps removed unless they are causing discomfort or other symptoms; recent studies suggest that many polyps, especially small ones, are harmless.

So you've been having bad bleeds and you've called your doctor and made an appointment. What can you expect from your visit? How can you be as prepared as possible and get the best results from your consultation?

Don't get agitated or worried ahead of time. Enter an appointment with the assumption that your bleeding is normal and healthy, and let the doctor convince you otherwise. In particular, be very skeptical if your doctor is quick to suggest a surgery or nontest medical procedure.

When you begin your visit, tell your doctor as much as you can about your menstrual cycle. What is normal for you? Describe in detail for your doctor how many days it usually goes on, what course the bleeding takes, what day is usually heaviest, how heavy the blood loss is.

Talk about your concerns and be specific about the ways that the bleeding is adversely affecting your life. Describing your particular problems is a great way to help a doctor brainstorm about nonmedical and simple solutions that might be your best option if your bleeding is, in fact, menopause related.

The doctor will probably want to start with a basic pelvic exam, during which he or she will check for infection and other basic nonmenopausal problems that could cause or aggravate bleeding. The doctor may suggest ultrasound and endometrial biopsy. In an endometrial biopsy, the doctor threads a tiny scope through the vagina and into the uterus to take a small amount of uterine tissue for testing. Like a Pap smear, it can cause cramping or a small amount of bleeding, and some women find it really uncomfortable. It is the simplest and cheapest way to rule out cancer.[9]

An ultrasound gives an image of the uterus so the doctor can get a better look at what is going on and check for obvious physical abnormalities such as a growth or tumor. Ultrasounds can be performed both from outside the body and from inside the vagina.

Even if the reasons for your bleeding are normal, if it is heavy enough, you may be in danger of becoming anemic. Because of this concern, the doctor may draw blood to perform a ferritin test, which measures the amount of iron you have stored in your bone marrow. A hematocrit test is another common procedure, usually done as part of a normal blood count, that can help check for anemia.

Another common test is a coagulation screening, which can help assess problems with blood clotting. This procedure is probably necessary only if you have a family history of bleeding disorders or clotting problems.

It's probably a good idea for the doctor to test your thyroid function, because problems with this important gland can often mimic menopause. The doctor will probably want to perform a pregnancy test just to rule out either miscarriage or ectopic pregnancy. You can still get pregnant even if you have missed several periods. For this reason it is especially important to keep using proper birth control until you are sure menopause has passed.

Some Questions to Ask Your Doctor at an Appointment to Address Heavy Bleeding

1. How much bleeding is too much? Is my bleeding heavy enough to cause concern?
2. How can I measure my bleeding at home to determine if it is too heavy?
3. If you do consider my bleeding a cause for concern, what exactly are you worried about?
4. You are recommending (fill in procedure or test). What do you hope to learn? What are the risks of this procedure? Is this procedure necessary? What are some alternative procedures and tests, and what are their respective risks?·
5. If I choose not to undergo (fill in procedure or test), what is the worst-case scenario? What is the best?
6. You are recommending (fill in surgery). Do you really think that's necessary? If so, why? What will happen if I choose not to have this surgery?
7. What nonsurgical options might you recommend to deal with my bleeding?
8. Can you give me some recent medical or scientific information on the various treatment options we are considering? What do we really know about their risks and benefits?
9. What is the likelihood that this problem will resolve itself without medical intervention?
10. If I choose to leave this problem alone, what additional problems should I be on the lookout for? What would indicate that I should come back to the doctor or seek further medical treatment?

Your doctor may recommend a number of different treatment options. First, he may tell you that your bleeding is normal, you are healthy, and you needn't do anything at all. This can be the hardest thing to do because bleeding all the time is inconvenient, to say the least, and we are trained in this culture to be proactive about things we perceive as medical problems. Remember that unnecessary medical interventions—both drugs and surgeries—can also cause unnecessary problems and pains, so if your doctor gives you a clean bill of health and you find your problem tolerable, the best plan may just be to let nature take its course and wait for what Dr. Prior calls "estrogen's storm season" to clear.

Nonsteroidal anti-inflammatory drugs (NSAIDs) like ibuprofen (Advil), taken in recommended doses over short amounts of time, can be the most basic, least dangerous way to cut down on bleeding. NSAIDs have been shown to help cut blood flow by 25 to 30 percent by changing the hormone balance in the uterus.[10] Because these drugs can have their own serious side effects (including stomach and liver damage), be careful not to take too much and don't continue taking them once bleeding has subsided.

If you are experiencing anemia, a condition where there aren't enough healthy red blood cells to carry sufficient oxygen to your heart, you should make sure you get lots of iron. You help treat and prevent it by taking an iron supplement, and also by making an effort to eat foods that are naturally rich in the mineral.

Iron-Rich Everyday Foods[11]

TYPE OF FOOD	SOURCES OF IRON
Beans, peas, and legumes	Lima beans, split peas, soy beans, kidney beans
Vegetables	Green leafy vegetables, including spinach, asparagus, green beans, peppers, tomatoes, vegetable juice
Fruits and nuts	Apricots, peaches, dates, prunes
Meats	Liver and kidney meats, beef, pork
Seafood	Clams, sardines, scallops, fish
Breakfast cereals	Cream of Wheat, Bran Flakes, All-Bran, oats, Grape-Nuts, wheat cereals
Other sources	Eggs, milk, bean soups

Anemia is, for most women approaching menopause, the only real danger with blood loss. If you opt to take supplements, you should be careful to stay on them for at least a year after your bleeding problems subside. Because taking too much iron can be as unhealthy as not getting enough, be careful not to take supplements if you don't need them and in general try to stick with food as your primary source of the nutrient.

Historically, one way doctors have treated bleeding is by prescribing birth control pills. Dr. Jerilynn Prior writes, "The evidence that they are effective is slight." That is especially true in perimenopause.[12] The same is true for hormone treatment (HT), and some women find that both make their bleeding worse. Given the additional health risks associated with both of these drugs, this is probably not your best option.

Low-dose progesterone, on the other hand, either in pill or interuterine device (IUD) form, seems to have been shown to be helpful for some.[13] In studies, a progesterone-releasing IUD called Mirena has been shown to reduce bleeding by as much as 85 to 80 percent.[14] (Remember, this is a relative, not an absolute, improvement.) Remember that any hormone drug carries serious health risks, as do IUDs.

Almost all the doctors and experts agree: if you choose hormone supplementation as a means of treating your heavy bleeding, don't plan to stay on progesterones or other hormones in the long term, which is how hormone supplements are often prescribed. Rather, you should think of it as a short-term solution, like an antibiotic. Although giving up hormones can be a shock to the system, you can do it! One mother and nurse writes of her experience, "It was so exhilarating to find that as I gradually cut out the hormones, I didn't need them anymore."

In more extreme cases—that is, when bleeding isn't responding to milder pills—a doctor may prescribe tranexamic acid, a type of drug often given to patients after surgery to prevent bleeding. It works by inhibiting chemicals in your body that dissolve proteins involved in blood clotting. In some studies this drug reduced blood flow by 50 percent over NSAIDs,[15] but there is evidence that tranexamic acid can be dangerous and can cause pulmonary embolism and deep vein thrombosis.[16]

Surgeries should always be a last resort, especially when you have a problem that will most likely go away on its own. This hasn't stopped doctors from historically and currently recommending major surgery for this problem. Excessive bleeding is a major reason for hysterectomy in the United States, and it is estimated that 50 percent of the women who experience bleeding will end up opting to have their uteruses removed.[17] Before you consider taking this step, be sure to read chapter 8. Make sure you have all the facts before you make this irreversible decision.

One of the most popular procedures for controlling excessive bleeding is dilation and curettage (D and C). It is performed under anesthesia; the doctor inserts a speculum in the vagina and opens or "dilates" the cervix, then scrapes the uterine lining with an instrument called a curette. Although this procedure is relatively safe, it is temporary, as the uterine lining grows back. Most experts today insist that it is unnecessary; we have better and less invasive options for determining the cause of bleeding and trying to deal with it.[18]

Endometrial ablation is another surgical technique that has gained popularity in recent years. Its safety and efficacy are still quite undertested, and because of some of the significant dangers it poses, we would recommend extreme caution in pursuing this option. We talk at some length about this procedure in chapter 9.

Learning to Live with It

We watched with concern as Belle, a good friend of ours still in her early forties, lay exhausted on her couch. A college professor with young children, she had never had any indication that perimenopause was about to begin until the floods started. "I feel like I can't leave the house," she told Barbara. "I'm soaking through both a tampon and a pad in half an hour." The bleeding affected every aspect of her life—her comfort in being as active at work, her energy level in keeping up with her kids, her confidence in standing before her class.

We're not going to tell you this kind of bleeding is an easy thing to deal with. In the end, however, even the National Institutes of Health has to admit that we don't have any really good solutions to offer women suffering with this problem. So in the meantime, keep in mind a few last things.

Women who are taller and have had children are more likely to have heavy flow. Losing weight can alleviate bleeding, as can cutting down your stress levels; stress always has an unpredictable effect on periods. Premenopausal women in particularly taxing situations often find that menstrual bleeding can get heavy, erratic, or even sometimes pull a disappearing act. Finally, women taking medications that can exacerbate bleeding, such as antipsychotics and certain antianxiety drugs, should be particularly aware of the effects these drugs may be having on their bodies. If you are going to see a doctor about bleeding, write down all the medications you use and ask specifically if any of them could be making the problem worse.

Periods don't want to go gently into that good night. But the good news is that they don't have a choice. All women who get old enough will stop menstruating, and the scary, frustrating, but ultimately normal heavy bleeding that can happen is something that will also end. So hang in there.

4

"is it hot in here, or is it just you?"
hot flashes, night sweats, and other things that keep you up at night

All my delight it is, and all my joy
To live, endlessly burning, and to not feel
the pain
— GASPARA STAMPA, SIXTEENTH-CENTURY POET

As a longtime first-grade teacher, Emily was used to working up a sweat running around all day after energetic students. She didn't consider that menopause might be playing a role in her overheating and would often ask the kids, "Is it hot in here, or is it just me?" One day, a student at the back of the class raised her hand. When called upon, the little girl asked sweetly, "Mrs. Josell, is it hot in here, or is it just you?" Emily explains, "It was at that moment that I realized I was starting to go through menopause."

If there is a single abiding symbol of menopause in our culture, it is probably the hot flash. Nothing is more readily identified with the menopause experience. Most of the available literature suggests that an astonishing number of American women will experience one: the

Massachusetts Women's Health study found that 75 percent of its menopausal participants had flashing.[1]

In contrast, Dr. Nancy Fugate Woods and Dr. Ellen Mitchell announced at a 2005 National Institutes of Health (NIH) meeting that while an estimated 85 percent of women report one or more menopausal symptoms, only 30 to 50 percent report hot flashing.[2] A third statistic, cited by Erica Weir in the *Canadian Medical Journal*, estimates that 75 percent of postmenopausal women and only 40 percent of perimenopausal women experience flashing.[3] We're not sure how to explain this very serious discrepancy other than to say it raises some interesting questions.

Biologically and endocrinologically, hot flashes and night sweats are the same thing. A night sweat is simply the after-hours version of the hot flash, and it is the thing that can wake and keep us up at night. Some women get night sweats who don't have hot flashes, and vice versa. Many women have both.

You may see hot flashes and night sweats referred to in professional literature as *vasomotor symptoms*. This simply means that having a hot flash has to do with the vasomotor system, a network of tiny blood vessels that exist under the skin's surface. When a hot flash happens, these blood vessels expand, flooding the skin and causing it to redden and grow warm.

Often you will hear the term *hot flush*. This is the same thing as a hot flash, although some organizations, most notably the North American Menopause Society, prefer the term *hot flash*. In Europe, the word *flush* is used more often. It probably doesn't make much of a difference, but since we are used to using the term *flash*, we will do so in this book.

As menopause expert Ramona Slupik explains, not so long ago many doctors considered hot flashes to be a function of the female imagination. This is strange because it seems that women have been experiencing the burning and chilling of the flash for a long time. As soon as there were menopause manuals, health advisers were warning women about this phenomenon. A nineteenth-century example warns of "a sinking sensation, a 'feeling of goneness' as the sufferer says, at the pit of the stomach, often accompanied by flushes of heat."[4] The nineteenth-century doctor George H. Napheys explained to patients that "the face, neck and hands are suffused at inopportune moments and greatly to the annoyance of the sufferer."

Anna M. Longshore-Potts, another nineteenth-century British writer, describes "flashes of heat followed by perspiration, then a chill, are some of the accompanying symptoms of the change of life; they may commence at any stage, from the first, before any other symptoms are noticed, or not until the catamenial flow has become irregular or more scanty than usual. These very uncomfortable flashes may continue for two years, or for ten, and they sometimes increase their severity and frequency for two or more years after the menses have ceased to appear."[5]

Modern descriptions wouldn't look very different.

Hot flashing may be one of the most symbolic menopausal experiences because it is one of the first. It is estimated that around a third of women who experience hot flashes have them before noticing any change in their periods.[6] A hot flash happens suddenly—so suddenly that by the time you notice you are having one, it can be almost over. One older woman in her mid-eighties reflected on flashing in her younger years, noting, "I never minded them because when I would realize I was sweating and flushing, I knew it was ending."

Some women say that they know when a flash is about to happen; they just get a feeling. This sense of things to come is sometimes called the "aura." When a flash happens, you suddenly notice that without any warning, you feel very hot. You may find yourself removing clothing, fumbling to find a piece of paper or other object to fan your face with, or pressing a cold soda can against your forehead. Minutes later you may start to feel cold, pulling your recently discarded sweater back around your shoulders.

If you feel like your body is confused, you're right: it is trying to adapt and compensate for all of the changes rapidly going on inside. We have to be patient—with a little time, the body *will* figure out what is going on. Like every other menopausal (and biological) experience, the hot flash is vastly different in each woman. Some flash for seconds and a rare few claim "all-night" flashes that last hours.

Hot flashes seem to follow a macro (larger) arc and a micro (smaller) arc. The larger arc has to do with how long and how frequently average women flash and sweat for. The North American

Menopause Society (NAMS) estimates that flashes increase over the course of perimenopause, reaching the highest rate of flashing during the first three years of postmenopause and then slowly happening less and less.[7] At the height of flashing, it is not uncommon for a woman to have as many as eight or more episodes a day.[8]

Of women who experience flashing during the first year of the change, only 50 percent will still be hot and bothered five years later, and then just 25 percent after the first five postmenopausal years.[9] The average duration of the menopause transition is around three to five years. NAMS reports that the median length of menopause—and by extension the length of time women get hot flashes—is 3.8 years.

The smaller, more individual arc of the flash is lived every day. Although experience varies widely, the frequency of flashes seems to crescendo in the early evening. This has to do with the body's core temperature and the way that it changes over the course of the day, reaching its highest point in the afternoon. Most hot flashes are felt, then, about three hours after the body reaches this high point.

We need to make a very important distinction between the total number of women who have hot flashes and the women who find they are unable to continue their normal lives because their symptoms are so intense. It is possible (although, as we've demonstrated, not certain) that nearly three-quarters of women who hit menopause have hot flashes. Of those women who do, only around 10 to 15 percent find that they are suffering so badly that they can't function. That means that if we estimate on the high end of available statistics, we can figure that only around 10 or 11 percent of the total population of women have hot flashes from hell. This becomes an important point when we talk about treatment. While any flashes can be a pain—coming when we least expect them or at the worst possible moments, making us uncomfortable—if we are able to get through them, they are, when all is said and done, just a hassle and not something worthy of medical or pharmaceutical intervention.

We've talked above about the similarities between menopause and puberty. Allow us to make an analogy across the gender lines: when a teenage boy begins to get erections, they come without warning, often in potentially humiliating situations. One young man, now in his twenties, describes how his would occur five minutes before the end of a school class. He knew it wouldn't be gone by the time he would have to stand and leave the room, but there was nothing he could do about it. Likewise, a hot flash strikes unexpectedly and can put us in awkward situations. Maybe we are trying to look poised while leading an important meeting at work, or a flash ruins a picture-perfect moment in the middle of a vacation we've been planning for months. However, just as no one would ever dream of medicating a young man to eliminate erratic early erections, so it seems strange that we would try to eliminate hot flashes. Both are just the body struggling to adapt to the next phase of life.

The good news about hot flashes is that they go away once the menopause transition has completed itself. A small number of women—especially those on hormone treatment—may continue to experience flashing well into their later years. In one trial of women over sixty-five, less than 10 percent continued to be bothered by hot flashes.

What Is Happening When We Start to Heat Up?

Although no one knows for sure what happens when you begin to have a hot flash, it has long been suspected that it has to do with confusion between the brain and the body. As Dr. Susan Love smartly explains, a hot flash "is misnamed: it's really an attempt by the body to cool down."[10]

A hot flash begins when the hypothalamus, a small grape-sized gland in the brain that is in charge of making sure we don't get too hot or too cold, gets a message that we are dangerously heating up. Unfortunately, this message is wrong.

Even though the air temperature has not actually changed, the hypothalamus, like a general with an incorrect battle plan, begins giving the wrong orders back to the body, telling it to start letting out heat. Seconds before you start to feel a flash, your skin temperature heats up and your heart starts to beat faster. Sweating is one of the body's most useful ways of cooling down. As sweat evaporates, it chills the skin and helps to lower the temperature of the blood near the surface. Even though your body wasn't actually exposed to hot temperatures, the sensation of heat is produced by the body's response.

After a few minutes, the brain realizes it made a big mistake and that you are actually too cold. The beleaguered General Hypothalamus turns the troops around and tries to warm the body up. One way it does this is through shivering.

Most women have hot flashes in their torsos and faces, but it's not uncommon to flush in hands, feet, and thighs as well. A typical hot flash lasts for around five minutes. Like everything else, this varies quite a lot, and a small group of women (around 7 percent) have longer flashes, while a larger group of women (around 20 percent) have shorter ones.

So how does the body get so mixed up? Here scientists are much less certain of their answers. It's possible that for reasons we can't explain, women are more sensitive to temperature change around the time of menopause. When it would normally take a drastic shift in outside temperature to cause redness and sweats, instead women respond to almost imperceptible variations around them.

For a long time scientists have believed that there is a connection between changing estrogen levels and the tendency to flash; however, this connection has never been mapped. Dr. Fredi Kronenberg often explains, "We know that estrogen plays some role," but "something else triggers a hot flash and we don't know what that is."

An article in a Harvard University women's health publication in 1997 tried to explain different "risk factors" for hot flashes. They were inundated with letters from women who said that they had none of these risks, lived healthy lifestyles and got proper health care, and were still suffering terribly. One woman explained, "I feel frustrated. I have none of the risk factors for getting them—I do not smoke, have never had PMS, and do not feel under psychological stress. However I still have drenching night sweats associated with menopause. How can this be?" The editors responded: "Although the scientists identified mathematical correlations or trends in factors that might be associated with hot flashes, it doesn't mean that a woman who has none of these factors will avoid them. It simply means that she is statistically less likely to have them. You fall into the group of women who have none of the factors but still have hot flashes, underscoring the point that there is still a lot of research to be done in this field."[11]

As a 2005 study in *Reproductive Medicine* explains, we don't even know to what extent and by what means the relationship between estrogen and hot flashes functions. Indeed, the study says, the estrogen levels in women who have hot flashes and those who don't are no different.[12]

Other hormones besides estrogen that may play a role in flashing include norepinephrine. Epinephrine is another name for adrenaline, a substance the body releases in response to stress; it increases the heart rate and raises the blood pressure and metabolic rate. Norepinephrine is similar but works on internal stressors. It's possible that menopausal women have higher norepinephrine levels. Certain studies in animals have shown that if you have more norepinephrine in the brain, your thermoneutral zone—the range of temperatures between which your body doesn't have to work to regulate—will be smaller.

Another possible culprit is gonadotropins, the hormones that cause the growth of gonads, that is, the testes and ovaries. The beginning of a flash may have to do with an increase in how much luteinizing hormone (a type of gonadotropin that tells your body to ovulate) the body is making. When your ovaries stop responding to the brain's calls for egg production, the brain makes more of the hormone.

Our Limited Tools of Prediction

The truth is that we really have no idea why certain women flash and others don't. Scientists have been trying to figure out some general correlations that can help predict which lifestyle or demographic factors may play a role. One recent study to take on some of these tough questions was the Study of Women's Health Across the Nation (SWAN).[13] This trial was designed to collect and compare the experiences of a diverse population of women.

There are small differences in hot flash statistics across ethnic lines. Black women and Latina women experience flashing in the greatest numbers, with 45.6 percent (black women) and 35.4 percent

(Latinas) of the total population studied complaining of symptoms. White women were at 31.2 percent, and Asian women experienced the fewest flashes. Researchers have long been fascinated with the low rates of flashing in Asia, particularly in Japan. It has been hypothesized, although not proven, that part of this difference may be due to the high soy content of the Japanese diet. These sorts of theories are responsible in part for the soy craze. Of course, the SWAN study was looking at Japanese-American women, and so theories about diet and lifestyle wouldn't necessarily apply to the statistics in this study.

Another risk factor for flashing seems to be socioeconomic status; poor women were more likely than their more affluent peers to struggle with sweeping heat. An earlier study conducted in the late 1990s suggested that those who were unemployed or partially employed were more likely to flash, possibly—although not certainly—due to higher stress levels.

There are other lifestyle factors that seem to have relationships with vasomotor distress. For many years, doctors believed that thin women were actually at a higher risk for hot flashes. However, a study published in January 2001 in the *Journal of Women's Health and Gender-Based Medicine* disagreed, finding heavier women more likely to have hot flashes.[14] The SWAN data also suggest that BMI (body mass index, the measure of how much of a person's body is fat)[15] is a more reliable way of predicting flashing than ethnic or class differences.

Talking about body fat brings us to the complicated question of exercise. In general, we are big fans of working out; it's good for the muscles, joints, bones, and mind. Some studies have found that working out reduces hot flashes and that being inactive increases your risk of suffering. Another study, however, found that exercise could trigger hot flashes in women who are prone to them.[16] This is because exercising rapidly raises the body temperature, and anything that makes you get much hotter much faster can exacerbate the problem. So while exercising can balance hormones and theoretically reduce flashing, the heat generated during exercise can trigger the problem.

Although there is very little evidence about the role of diet in either encouraging or curbing vasomotor problems, cigarette smoking is known to make flashing worse. This may be because smoke affects the way the body metabolizes estrogen.

Alcohol and spicy foods could be potential triggers because they cause the body to heat up; however, there is really no conclusive evidence that either is a cause of hot flashes.[17] And of course something as simple as warm air can do as much damage as any of these dietary choices.

Anecdotally, many women say that stress is a big trigger. Nita, a red-haired homemaker in her early fifties, says, "My flashes are usually started with a strong feeling of anxiety or worry about something I have been thinking about." If stress is a trigger of flashing, it is not something we have been able to show in trials. Other factors that don't seem to play a provable role include "marital status, age at menarche or menopause or having children, height, health or whether (the patient's) mother had hot flashes."[18]

Some Other Things to Think About

It is a little-known fact that women experience hot flashes throughout their reproductive lives; in fact, many women flash for nonmenopausal reasons.[19] Barbara has long spoken about her premenstrual flashing, and Laura, who is premenopausal, experienced hot flashes when she started doing Pilates.

Men can suffer hot flashes as well, particularly those taking drugs for treating prostate cancer. A Michigan State University study finds as many as two-thirds of men taking Lupron (leoprolide), Zoladex (gaserelin), and Supertact (buserelin) may experience flashing. The *Journal of the American Medical Association* reckons that figure may be as high as 80 percent.[20]

Some other conditions that have the potential to result in hot flashes include epilepsy, infection, pheochromocytoma, carcinoid syndromes, leukemia, insulinoma, and other pancreatic tumors, autoimmune disorders, and mast-cell disorders.

Thyroid disorders can also cause hot flashes. As Dr. Helena Rodbard observes, severe flashing can "actually be evidence of an underactive thyroid."[21] Yet only around 25 percent of women who talk to their doctors about menopause complaints are advised to have their thyroids screened.

Hysterectomy

One of the single greatest risk factors and one of the few proven predictors of hot flashes is hysterectomy with oophorectomy. NAMS reports that "up to 90% of women undergoing surgery-induced menopause report hot flashes."[22] Oophorectomized women go into instant menopause. At one gynecology meeting, doctors described the horror of women winding out of the haze of anesthesia after surgery, only to endure their first hot flash immediately. "They really suffer, and you just want to do *something* for them," said one young female gynecologist. Although some doctors maintain that over time, hysterectomized and oophorectomized women find that their hot flashes decline, becoming similar to rates of women going through natural menopause, this is just not borne out by the evidence, and many women continue to suffer hot flashes even into their seventies and eighties. (Menopausal symptoms after oophorectomy are probably worse if a women is premenopausal when she has the surgery.)

A Good Night's Sleep

One of the biggest problems with having hot flashes is that they can cause sleep problems. If you are continually waking up at night, are unable to fall back asleep, and are going through the day ill-rested, it compounds other stressors in your life and can make your day pretty darn unpleasant. One woman tells her story, noting, "The night sweats were the worst . . . they woke me up and I'd have trouble getting back to sleep, so I'd be tired and cranky during the day. I tried giving up coffee and wine, and I started walking two miles a day. It helped but not enough."

The problem isn't just waking up with a flash but that once roused, many women are unable to get back to sleep. A Wayne State University study found a big difference between the overall number of women who were awakened with flashing and a smaller group who were unable to return to sleep.[23] The scientists differentiated between "brief arousals" and longer "awakenings." This is very much like the experience of flashes more generally—many women get them, but a very small group of women get them severely enough to have their lives disrupted by them.

These findings were backed up by a Chicago study reported in *Behavioral Sleep Medicine* that concluded that "menopausal status plays a minimal role in sleep quality and sleep stage distribution in healthy midlife women."[24]

For a small group of women, however, this time can be hell, making them feel unwell and compromising their ability to concentrate and work during the day. So what should you do if you find yourself up at night, pacing the house, watching infomercials, and dreading the first crack of daylight? For much more information on getting a good night's sleep, read chapter 5.

Facts and Fictions about Herbs and Hot Flashes

As long as women have been struggling with menopausal symptoms, they have been trying to find simple, natural ways to deal with them. An early twentieth-century American text advised women that "baths of one part of vinegar and two parts of water often relieve these attacks of sweating."[25] Herbal medicines can seem to offer one alternative. In recent years, phytoestrogens, plant-derived compounds that are chemically similar to human hormones, have been recommended. They are found in legumes such as soy and garbanzo beans, as well as some other plants. Isoflavones, compounds found in plants that have both hormonal and nonhormonal properties, have also been used. If they have any impact on hot flashes, most likely they do so by working as an estrogen in the body, acting on estrogen receptors in a way that is similar to more traditional pharmaceuticals.

A few years ago, there was a lot of buzz about soy, and everyone was learning to cook tofu or love edamame or simply take supplement pills. We talk about soy at some length in chapter 11 (Menopause, Naturally) both in terms of the good stuff we know about it and the fact that high hopes for hot flash reduction haven't panned out. It should be mentioned here that in terms of treating hot flashes, soy has been shown to be only marginally helpful.[26] While most media attention has been focused on soy, whatever benefits it offers, although potentially slim, are also available in other beans and legumes, so if you aren't a tofu fan, fear not: you can get the same chemical compounds from kidney or garbanzo beans.

Black cohosh is a root that has been used for centuries as a menopause preparation and was one of the main ingredients in Lydia Pinkham's famous nineteenth-century cure-all potion. It is one of the more studied menopause herbs. Unfortunately, three separate trials of the herb failed to yield any or much benefit over the placebo for treating hot flashes. Still, because it is available most commonly as an over-the-counter remedy called Remifemin, it is more standardized than other herbs; it has few known side effects and no known interactions with other drugs, although there is some concern it may contribute to liver damage in a small number of people.[27]

Evening primrose oil is another very popular hot flash treatment. This herb, usually taken in capsule form, acts phytoestrogenically. A randomized, double-blind, placebo-controlled clinical trial found no benefit of using evening primrose for hot flashes over placebos. It is a common ingredient in menopause preparations available at drugstores. These products often have vague names like "women's formula" or "meno-cure." They are usually hodgepodge combinations of phytoestrogens—primrose, soy, wild yam—thrown together. In large doses evening primrose has several side effects, including nausea and diarrhea.

Because we're still unsure how these estrogenic substances interact with each other or any prescription medications you may be taking, be cautious.

Wild yam in the form of a cream is used to treat hot flashes. This Mexican plant can be used as a progesterone substitute. Although many women swear by it, the journal *Obstetrics and Gynecology* notes that the remedy has a disturbing "lack of published reports demonstrating its efficacy."[28] One 2001 study published in *Climacteric* had women keep journals of their flashes on both a real wild yam cream and a placebo cream. Women using the real yam cream decreased their symptoms. However, so did women using the placebo cream, and no statistically significant difference could be found between the two.[29]

Progesterone creams, both those called "natural" and their pharmaceutical counterparts, have shown some promise in reducing flashes. Also called bioidentical hormones, they are available by prescriptions that can be filled at a compounding pharmacy. Unfortunately, both varieties are seriously understudied. So-called natural progestin cream is particularly suspicious because it pretends to be a natural alternative to drugs when, in fact, for all intents and purposes, it functions in similar ways to prescription creams.

Look into My Eyes

Other alternative methods being investigated for treating hot flashes include magnets, acupuncture, and hypnosis. A 2004 study from Texas reported that hypnosis significantly reduced flashing and sleep disturbance in participants.[30] The only available study of acupuncture and flashing showed no real difference between test and control,[31] and no significant flash relief was shown in a randomized placebo-controlled trial of magnets.[32]

A serious problem with many of the studies on alternative practice (as with those on more traditional pharmaceuticals) is that they are often performed on a special population of women, those who have undergone chemotherapy to treat breast and other types of cancer. This is because women who have had breast cancer may have to be especially diligent about avoiding estrogens, which can accelerate tumor growth. However, the experiences of women who have had breast cancer (and often enter spontaneous menopause as a result of chemotherapy and other cancer treatments), like the experiences of women who have undergone hysterectomy, are more extreme than women undergoing traditional menopause and cannot be assumed to be the same in terms of scientific results.

Drugs

Like certain sexual difficulties, hot flashes are one of the few menopause problems that are known to be helped by estrogen. How much they are helped and what combination or form of hormone therapy is best are up for debate, and scientific studies have produced wildly different results.

A major review of oral estrogen trials that summarized ninety-nine studies sought both to look at the usefulness of oral estrogen and to compare how well estrogen alone worked when compared with combined estrogen/progestin therapy.[33] The review found that all were effective in reducing hot flashes (by up to 65 percent) and that estrogen/progestin therapy could reduce hot flashes by as much as 90 percent.

With safety concerns about HT at the forefront of many women's minds, many doctors have been pushing "lower-dose" estrogen alternatives. Although the larger safety of this option is in serious doubt, it may indeed be a better, safer hormone choice for women considering HT. It should be mentioned in this context, however, that lower doses of estrogen have been shown to relieve fewer hot flashes.

Why does estrogen cut down on flashing? We don't know. As we explained above, women with flashes and without flashes have the same estrogen levels. Another important thing to keep in mind is that selective estrogen-receptor modulators (SERMs) like raloxifene and tamoxifen have actually been shown to *worsen* hot flashes.[34] Many women who have switched from HT or estrogen treatment (ET) to SERMs don't realize that this is one side effect of the different way in which these estrogen alternatives work.

Transdermal estrogen, that is, the estrogen patch, was found to be effective in reducing hot flashes and night sweats when compared with the placebo.[35] None of the trials of this delivery system compared it with oral estrogen or progestin therapy. Side effects of the patch included headache, breast pain, leukorrhea (which is a thick, white discharge from the vaginal or cervical canal that results from vaginal or uterine inflammation), and skin reaction around the site of the patch itself. All of the patch trials were too short and involved too few participants to qualify as conclusive demonstrations of the method's safety or efficacy.

Intravaginal suppositories that deliver steady doses of estrogens, such as the vaginal E2 ring, also gave significant relief from flashing in small randomized trials.[36] Not nearly enough research has been done on this method of delivery, and anecdotal evidence surrounding similar devices—the birth control ring, for one—suggests that many women experience serious abdominal pain.

Recent evidence suggests that the addition of an androgen (testosterone) to estrogen may increase the effectiveness of the drug in treating hot flashes. Although the difference isn't that much when compared with higher-dose estrogen pills, addition of an androgen makes low-dose estrogen preparations more effective. Some of the increase in symptom relief with testosterone may be due to suppressing, or lessening, the amount of luteinizing hormone, which tells your body to ovulate. A problem with this approach is that the doses of estrogen and testosterone that are the most effective together are hard to determine.[37] Testosterone treatment carries its own serious health risks and side effects.

Nonhormonal Pharmaceuticals

When we (Barbara and Laura) attended a big menopause conference in early 2005, we waited with excitement for a lecture about emerging "nonhormonal" approaches to treating menopause symptoms. What would the doctors recommend to replace the now-disgraced HT and its relatives? Would it be a new exercise regimen? An herbal alternative? Perhaps a new breathing technique. As the young doctor spoke, it became clear that as far as he and his colleagues were concerned, the alternative to this famously failed drug was in fact . . . another drug. And not just any other variety of drug—one of the most popular and visible class of drugs in America: antidepressants.

The idea of treating hormonally related problems with antidepressants is not a new one. The drug company Eli Lilly very famously marketed a pill called Sarafem for the treatment of premenstrual dysphoric disorder (PMDD). Like many of the "sexual dysfunctions," the disease classification was a new one, but the drug marketed to treat it had the same active ingredient as another Lilly drug: Prozac. Perhaps not coincidentally, the marketing of PMDD drugs began shortly after the patent on the lucrative antidepressant was set to expire.

Just before the Women's Health Initiative (WHI) began to fall apart in 2001 (remember that although the Prempro trials weren't halted until 2002, and the Calcium and Diet trials didn't finish for several years, by 2001 indicators of problems with the hormone trials were evident), health publications began to gush over new information that suggested perhaps antidepressants and selective seratonin reuptake inhibitors (SSRIs) had the unexpected benefit of dramatically reducing hot flashing. One health newsletter explained breathlessly that a December 16th study in the journal *Lancet* found that "the anti-depressant venlafaxine [Effexor] . . . reduced hot flashes by up to 61 percent."[38]

Although it was suggested that other SSRIs might do the job, Effexor was nearly always the top recommendation. Not surprisingly, perhaps, Effexor is manufactured by Wyeth, the same company that makes Premarin and Prempro, the specific oral estrogen products taking a beating in the WHI.

Effexor, while doing wonders for some severely depressed people, is a highly addictive drug. A friend of ours in her mid-forties, a social worker, described her experience going "cold turkey." "I was shaky, disoriented, and nauseous. I felt like I was detoxing from heroin. I couldn't function." Our friend eventually had to go back on the drug and slowly taper off.

Since the findings about Effexor and hot flashes, trials have also been performed on other antidepressants. One is paroxetine, which is sold by GlaxoSmithKline under the brand name Paxil. When the study was published, reports could boast a 62.2 to 64.6 percent reduction in hot flashes; however, study participants had a significant *increase* in other side effects, including nausea, insomnia, lethargy, and constipation.[39] It seems quite strange to recommend a drug to treat a sleep-disrupting symptom with a drug that is known to cause insomnia. As a coda to this story, Paxil was removed from the market by Glaxo under orders from the Food and Drug Administration (FDA) in 2005, because of its failure to "meet manufacturing standards." Although it was returned in June 2005 after nearly a six-month hiatus,[40] serious questions remain about its safety.

Dr. Charles Loprinzi, a doctor involved in Effexor research, announced at a National Institutes of Health (NIH) conference in

March 2005 that other clinical trials of SSRIs for hot flash management included one on the "newer antidepressant fluoxetine." Fluoxetine is in fact Prozac (a.k.a. Sarafem). Again, a 45 percent
improvement was found.[41] Dr. Loprinzi participated in the trial of
Prozac as well.

Another thing worth mentioning about the trials of Paxil and
Prozac for hot flashes is that they identified smaller success rates,
that is, they eliminated fewer hot flashes, in comparison with placebo
groups than the earlier study of Effexor, although this could have
been related to dosages, not chemicals.

So are we saying that it's all a big drug company conspiracy to
switch women from estrogen to SSRIs? No. In fact, it may turn out
that these drugs can do a lot of good in managing hot flashes. We are
saying, however, that as many menopause patients started to feel uncomfortable about estrogen and began to opt not to take it, drugmakers were faced with a widening financial void. Drug development
is expensive, and one way to fill the void is to look around and say,
"Well, if that drug doesn't work, do we already have one that might?"
It is important to realize how such financial incentives drive new research into old drugs. Women deserve to understand how this system works because it influences the quality of the medical information
we receive.

Some Simple Solutions

Hot flashes always seem to come at the worst possible moment, but
there are simple things you can do—besides keeping your sense of
humor—when they strike.

Wear cotton clothing and take a bottle of water and perhaps a
handheld fan when you go out. Wear layers so that you can take some
off or put them back on according to how you are feeling. This is especially important if the weather is cold, because you may not want
to be running around in a sleeveless shirt too long but there may
come a moment when you are very glad that you're wearing one.

Deep breathing has been found to be very effective for many
women. If you feel a flash coming on, focus on your breath and try to
keep deliberately breathing in and out as your heart begins to race.

Talk to your doctor about paced relaxation programs and try a yoga class at your local gym.

Keep a record of when you flash. This can tell you a lot about what triggers your particular problems—perhaps a glass of wine, or the time of day. Write down when you experience a flash, how long

Other Nonhormonal Drugs Tested for Use in Hot Flash Treatment

DRUG NAME	MANUFACTURER	TRADITIONAL USE/STUDIES	SIDE EFFECTS
Neurontin (gabapentin)	Pfizer	Treatment of seizures, intense nerve pain (such as shingles). Two randomized, double-blind, placebo-controlled trials have shown a 46% reduction in flashing versus 19% in the placebo group.[42]	Nausea, dizziness, trouble operating machinery. May also cause certain kinds of depression. Interacts with several types of drugs, including naproxyn (the main ingredient in the painkiller Aleve) and phenobarbital. A very serious drug, often given to women who have had cancer and can't consider estrogen.

(continued)

DRUG NAME	MANUFACTURER	TRADITIONAL USE/STUDIES	SIDE EFFECTS
Bellergal	Novartis	Sedative containing phenobarbital and bella-donna, among other things. Used to treat cluster headaches. Very little testing.	Nausea, blurred vision, sensitivity to temperatures. Pregnant women and people who smoke shouldn't take this drug. Can interact adversely with a host of other drugs, particu-larly antacids and antidepressants.
Catapres (clonidine)	Boehringer Ingelheim	Treatment of high blood pressure; alcohol or nicotine withdrawal. Testing has shown that the drug reduces hot flashes, but not by enough to make it worth the extensive side effects.	Agitation, constipation, nausea, loss of sex drive, abdominal pain, change in heartbeat, among many others. As one doctor says, "Toxicity from this agent limits its utility in the clinic."

Aldomet (methyldopa)	Merck	Treatment of high blood pressure. Very little study, but what has been performed suggests that it doesn't work very well for treating hot flashes. A very powerful drug.	Drowsiness, headache, muscle weakness, swollen ankles or feet, upset stomach, vomiting, rash, among others.

each one lasts, what you were eating, wearing, or doing at the time it came on, and any other information that might be useful.

In general, avoid alcohol and caffeine on days when you are particularly concerned about flashes, and also avoid big or spicy meals.

In very real ways, hot flashes are a rite of passage. They won't last in most women, and they are a shared experience we can talk about with others going through the transition.

5

the science of sleep
night sweats, wakefulness, and getting some shut-eye

*Life is something that happens when you
can't get to sleep.*

—Fran Lebowitz

i really wouldn't have noticed menopause at all. Except for the
sleep." Laura is driving with her friend Marilyn, a woman in her
mid-fifties, who is describing her experiences in the past four years.

Every night is the same. I fall asleep around ten-thirty or
eleven PM without a problem. Then around two or three in
the morning I am suddenly wide awake. I try to fall back
asleep, but eventually I get worried about waking up my husband. I go in the other room and watch TV until around five
or six. Then I'm usually able to get another hour of rest before I have to get up and get ready to go to work. I've seen
every bad TV show you can get on DVD and I'm sick of
spending my days exhausted. What can I do to change this?

A lot of women feel like Marilyn: worn out and with no good
night of sleep in sight. In Marilyn's case, her sleep problems started
with menopause but persisted long after she was finished with the
transition. She took over-the-counter sleep aids but didn't like the
idea of needing medication to get rest. She tried tapering off and

found that it didn't work. Frustrated, she reluctantly started popping the pills again.

Why does sleep become so difficult just around the time in your life when you need it the most? And how does it relate to menopause?

As we discussed above, one of the main things that wakes women up at night during midlife are night sweats—late-night hot flashes. For some reason, some women are able to cool off, roll over, and doze right back to dreamland. Others will spend countless hours wide awake and tired as hell. Some women find that they wake up and are unable to get back to sleep even without night sweats. Clearly there's some connection between sleep and midlife, whether or not it's connected to menopause.

Catch a Wave: From Waking to Sleeping

Falling asleep happens in several stages. Scientists break sleep into two broad categories—rapid eye movement (REM) sleep and nonrapid eye movement (NREM) sleep. NREM sleep can be broken into four more categories as you travel from those groggy moments on your pillow to deep, sound sleep. When you are awake, your brain waves move quickly: your brain makes what are called alpha waves (when you are relaxed) and beta waves (when you are more alert). Think of these choppy waves as being like the ocean on a windy day. Alpha waves are longer than beta waves.

During the first stage of NREM, when you begin to drift off, you may find random images passing through your head and your muscles begin to relax. This is the time when it is possible to start out of your sleep with a sudden jerk of your leg. The second stage of NREM sleep is the longest, accounting for between 45 percent and 55 percent of the total sleep cycle. Your body cools down and your breathing and heart rates slow. By the third stage, your brain begins to generate superslow delta waves, like the ocean on a peaceful day. In the last stage of NREM sleep, you are sleeping so deeply that you become nearly impossible to wake. If you have ever sleepwalked, had night terrors, or talked in your sleep, you did it in this stage.

REM sleep is dream sleep (although we now know that dreaming occurs in other phases as well).[1] It has long been theorized by scientists to be important to memory, overall health, and functioning. When it begins, your brain waves speed up to waking levels and your heart and breathing speed up again.

The total sleep cycle takes about 90 minutes to complete (allowing for individual variations); approximately 25 percent of that time is spent in REM sleep.

What Does Sleep Do for Us?

Marcos G. Frank writes, "The notion that a good night of sleep improves memory is widely accepted by the general public. Among scientists, however, the idea has been hotly debated for decades . . . despite a steady accumulation of positive findings over the past decade, the precise role of sleep in memory and brain plasticity remains elusive."[2]

Although we think of memories as things we make during our waking hours, in reality it may well be that the actual biological process of forming a long-term memory happens in our sleep; an increasing number of scientists believe this is the primary function of slumber. One theory of how this might work is that during the day we very briefly store information in our working memories before moving it more permanently and safely to our long-term memories.[3] Evidence for the association of sleep and memory has been found in studies of animals, which have observed a correlation between type and amount of sleep and meaningful experiences. In other words, when you have things you need to remember, your body sleeps differently.[4] A study at the University of Pennsylvania in 2003 found that when people failed to get the generally recommended eight hours of sleep, they started to perform poorly on cognitive tests.[5] Christine Gorman writes, "Perhaps that what sleep really is—a series of repeated cycles of pruning and strengthening of neural connections that enables you to learn new tricks without forgetting old ones."[6]

It's possible that sleep helps to repair neurons; important chemicals like growth hormone are released in deep sleep. As we get older, we have less slow-wave sleep.[7] As a result, we have different amounts of certain hormones and can have trouble moving important information into long-term storage. Cathryn Jakobson Ramin writes, "No one knows why slow-wave sleep disappears, but one thing's for sure: everyone wants it back." [8]

These changes are obviously partly biological, but they may have a psychosocial component as well. How much stress you carry around and how healthy you are may have more of an impact on your ability to get your z's than your age. A poll conducted by the National Sleep Foundation (NSF) found that pain and discomfort accounted for most of the sleep problems experienced at midlife and beyond. Those who were healthy at mid- and late life were actually more likely to get their regular eight hours than their younger counterparts. The NSF president James K. Walsh concluded, "In spite of the emerging science linking sleep quality and health status, most people believe that poor sleep is an inevitable consequence of getting older. But NSF's poll findings reinforce the relationship between good sleep and good overall health." [9] Another thing that can affect slumber is hormone levels, making it harder to fall—and stay—asleep. Then the stress, mood swings, and night sweats of menopause can create roadblocks to a good night's rest.

Many women experience trouble sleeping as part of their menstrual cycles. Some women with premenstrual syndrome (PMS) find it nearly impossible to drop off until their period comes, after which their sleep patterns return to normal. Like mood swings, menopausal sleep problems are much worse when a woman is in the throes of perimenopause and will usually (although not always) abate when she finishes the transition. No one knows why this might be, but some scientists theorize that the hormone fluctuations of the change alter circadian rhythms. Yet the number of women who have some sleep problems during PMS may be larger than the number who struggle with menopausal sleep.

Why does sleeplessness stick around for some women for years after their last period? The answer is, in part, that bad sleep habits die hard. If, like Marilyn, you've come to rely on some sort of sleep aid, it can be even harder to get back to healthy sleep.

Just how much sleep we really need is up for debate. Although a good body of research supports the common belief that eight hours (actually seven to nine) is the gold standard, other research has suggested that too much sleep is equally unhealthy: a study published in 2002 in the *Archives of General Psychiatry* found that people who slept more than eight hours a night had shorter life spans than those getting between six and seven hours.[10] This study was very controversial, and other doctors were quick to point out that depression is associated with sleeping more and might have influenced the data. Still, lead study author Dr. Daniel Kripke concluded, "This is a happy message for five, six, seven hour sleepers and insomniacs that there's nothing to worry about."[11]

While we wouldn't steer anyone who is able to get it away from a good eight or nine hours, we would say that this diversity of results regarding how much sleep is healthy shows that there probably isn't actually an exact amount that is optimum. Everyone is different, and probably a combination of your own biology and lifestyle will determine the amount that is right for you. Still, there is a good body of evidence that being sleep deprived—no matter how much sleep you actually need—makes you less likely to remember information and lowers your immune-system response.

While you may or may not have more trouble getting sleep as you age, it is a myth that you simply need less sleep.

The Way We Sleep

We are very particular about our sleep in Western culture. We want our bedrooms quiet and secluded. We want darkness and a state-of-the-art mattress with high-thread-count sheets. We want eight hours of sleep at a time.

Sleep is very different for people living in other cultures and places. Catherine M. Worthman and Melissa K. Melby write about some big differences in how, when, and why people sleep, noting that the incredible diversity around the world suggests a need for us Westerners to "reconsider definitions of 'normal' rest and sleep patterns."[12]

The ways we construct our sleeping environments is often a direct response to the world around us. If we have young children, we may be far more sensitive to the small night noises around us for fear our children might need us. Similarly, if we have teenagers we may sleep lightly, listening for their comings and goings, concerned about curfews missed and late hours spent studying. When we sleep and for how long are as culturally dependent as our down comforters, and sleep choices are often determined by physical factors in the environment. Many foraging cultures don't have the idea of a "bedtime"; instead people choose to fall asleep when they feel like it. Because of this fluidity of sleep and waking activity, people learn to sleep through loud music and conversation. Among herding peoples in hot climates, it's typical to rise early and then nap at midday, staying out of the harsh rays of the sun while they are strongest. Among certain African and South American foraging peoples, it's common to sleep on a hard surface with minimal bedding. These peoples often sleep with fires burning and monitor the fire's changes subconsciously, the way a mother might listen for a baby's cry.

How we organize our work and social lives has a big impact on when we want to sleep and when it's socially acceptable to do so. People living in New York City may have a very different feeling about the noises inherent in urban environments and may rely on them to fall asleep, while people from rural places may need more quiet or, at least, different kinds of noise. Laura grew up in a family with three younger children and she learned at an early age to tune out loud noises and activity around her. The Gebusi people of Papua, New Guinea, avoid deep sleep because they believe it is when humans are susceptible to harm from evil spirits.[13]

What we believe culturally about sleep will have a big impact on how we experience it individually. If we are convinced that we are incapable of performing properly at work without exactly eight hours of sleep, then we are more likely to doubt ourselves and to struggle in those instances where we don't attain that goal. If we believe that not sleeping makes us more productive, we may be more likely to ignore important signs that we aren't getting enough rest.

When we are stressed or worried, it can affect our ability to sleep. We've all had the experience: we are exhausted and desperately trying to doze off, but instead the thought of things undone or problems unsolved carries us further away from dreamland. In Western culture, our response to fear is wakefulness. Compare this with the

Balinese people of northern Bali, whose socially conditioned response to fear is sleep. They even have a term *tadoet poeles*, which roughly translated means "fear sleep."[14]

We, who have the most control over our sleep environments, expect the most from them. We're not wrong about these preferences—and we're not right either. Whether behaviors are learned or born, in the end they are how we understand a good night's rest, and they dictate conditions under which many of us are able to find sleep.

Watching the Clock: Different Ways of Looking at Insomnia

Hannah was worried about a big presentation that she was giving for work the next day, and even though all she wanted was to be well rested, she found herself unable to drop off to sleep. After an hour or two of tossing and turning, she went to the living room to watch TV. By 4:30 in the morning, slumber was no closer, her fridge was a lot emptier, and that phone-order closet-condensing kit was starting to sound like a really good deal.

Insomnia can look very different from person to person. If you have *sleep-onset insomnia*, you struggle to fall asleep initially. Although many things can cause this problem, the most common are stress and anxiety.

Sleep-maintenance insomnia happens when you have trouble staying asleep. This may mean that your night's rest feels broken into pieces, or it may be that you wake at unreasonably early hours—say 2 to 4 AM—and just can't get back to sleep. Fragmentary sleep can be caused by a number of things, but one of the most serious is a disorder called *sleep apnea*. A less serious but frustrating and uncomfortable problem is called *restless legs syndrome*.

Getting up in the small hours of the morning and being unable to sleep through the night are often signs of an underlying source of anxiety or depression. If these patterns persist, doctors will often check for a potential psychological cause. You may have gotten into a certain habit during menopause and are having trouble breaking it, or sometimes it just happens.

If you are struggling to get to sleep, don't toss and turn for more than fifteen or twenty minutes. Instead, go to another room, dim the lighting, and do something relaxing. Although some people find television restful, it may not be your best bet for falling asleep. Try reading a book instead, or doing a crossword puzzle. Take a warm bath, or meditate. Anything that helps you to calm down and begin to clear your brain of all the thoughts that keep you up.

If you find that you are waking up a lot at night, try thinking about what might have woken you. If you feel it's a noise that's waking you (unfortunately, that may include your beloved partner's snoring), try taking steps to eliminate it. Perhaps wear earplugs or shut your bedroom window at night to limit noises from outside.

Chronic pain is also a sleep thief. During menopause many women find that they have more aches and pains than they used to. In fact, internationally, aches are a more frequently reported "menopause symptom" than hot flashes.[15] The good news is that treating the source of your discomfort, whether it's aching joints, heartburn, or a headache, will often help evasive slumber return.

If your comforter makes you too hot or your sweetie keeps the bedroom toasty, it may be difficult for you to relax. Have a conversation with anyone you share a sleeping space with about what makes the space sleep-ready for you. Try to find compromises where desires conflict.

Another way of talking about insomnia is as acute (temporary) or chronic (long-term). If there's something stressful going on in your life—perhaps a family member died or you are working for a big promotion—you may find yourself temporarily unable to sleep. If this goes away after a few weeks or at the most a month or two, you don't need to worry about it. Sometimes, though, acute insomnia becomes something longer-term.

Did Someone Call Me "Snorer"? The Truth about Sleep Apnea and Other Breathing Problems during Sleep

According to the National Sleep Foundation, 90 million people in America snore, and 37 million of them do it regularly.[16] Usually it's only a problem to someone trying to catch sleep in the vicinity of the snorer—in other words, it's not too serious. Once in a while, though, it can be a sign of the very dangerous condition sleep apnea.

Sleep apnea happens when you temporarily stop breathing at night. There are three types of sleep apneas. Obstructive is the most common. It happens when something—usually tissue in the back of the throat—blocks the airways. Central sleep apnea occurs when the brain doesn't tell the muscles to breathe. Mixed apnea is a combination of the other two disorders.[17]

Sufferers may wake up gasping for air. Although men are more likely to have the problem for much of their adult lives, women are more likely to develop it during menopause. Like heart disease, sleep apnea appears differently in menopausal women from in men of the same age. Generally symptoms are milder, perhaps because progesterone acts on muscles to relax them.

Around 18 million Americans have sleep apnea, and potentially one in four postmenopausal women. If undiagnosed, sleep apnea is associated with heart attacks, strokes, heart disease, and other very serious problems. Symptoms include being really sleepy during the day and waking up with a massive headache. The most common treatment is use of a device that helps you keep breathing through the night.

Besides sleep apnea, snoring can be caused by a number of things including obesity, nasal congestion, and allergies. Drinking alcohol may increase your chances of snoring as well. What happens when you snore is that your soft palate, or uvula, vibrates with the back of your throat, making the noise we associate with the condition. Besides keeping you or your loved ones up at night, it can give you headaches and generally leave you feeling tired.[18]

One of the best things you can do to curb snoring is to lose weight, which can eliminate or reduce some of the fatty deposits that stand in the way of smooth breathing. You can also try breathing strips that help open up your airways.

And keep in mind that the National Sleep Foundation estimates snoring leads partners to lose about forty-nine minutes of sleep each night: "300 hours a year."[19] That's no small thing.

Other Sleeping Problems

Restless legs syndrome is a condition in which a person has an uncontrollable urge to move his or her legs, often accompanied by unpleasant sensations sometimes described as prickling, or like pins and needles. It makes it hard to hold still and it is more likely to happen at night. Recently there has been a lot of advertising for pharmaceuticals to treat this problem. We would really advise you against taking them. These drugs are new and have far-reaching effects out of proportion to the problem. Laura has suffered from restless legs syndrome since puberty. It's very frustrating and can happen at the worst moments—when she is sitting in a conference at an important lecture or when she is trying to relax and watch a movie. The only thing that really helps is to get up and walk around. Sometimes that's not possible, and it can be torture. Still, in most circumstances, walking around for a few minutes is an option, and a better one than enduring under-tested medications and powerful, unpleasant side effects, including, strangely, a propensity to gamble or other reckless behaviors.[20]

Recently some doctors have theorized the condition may be due to a lack of foliate and iron. If that is the case, it would explain why some women experience this problem in perimenopause when heavy bleeding can deplete iron stores. Try taking a supplement or just eating iron- and foliate-rich foods and see if this makes a difference for you.

Narcolepsy is a rare condition characterized by excessive sleepiness and an inability to transition into sleep properly. It is not directly associated with menopause. Sufferers may go from being wide awake to deep sleep without warning or at inappropriate times (although many won't, as movies would have us believe, drop into sleep suddenly or lose muscle control due to the common side effect of cataplexy). Narcolepsy happens, it's believed, because sufferers lack a chemical in their brain and spine called hypocretin.[21] Doctors usually treat this problem—which affects around 550 people out of a million—with alertness drugs such as Provigil.

Active Sleep: What You Can Do to Get a Better Night's Rest

Knowing why you can't sleep may be all well and good, but you are probably asking "What can I do! I'm sitting up at three in the morning and I'm reading this book instead of getting much-needed rest!" So you'll be relieved to learn that there are changes you can make during the day and in your nighttime environment that can make a big difference in how many z's you're catching.

Lets start with nighttime preparations. If you are waking up each night drenched in sweat, you should make sure you have a quick way of cooling off. Keep a fan near the bed, or a remote control for an air-conditioning unit. If you aren't sleeping in cotton bedding, it's probably time to buy some soft, absorbent, cotton sheets that can handle it if you start dropping gallons of sweat. The same thing goes for your sleepwear: make sure you are wearing pajamas or nightshirts made of cotton or fabrics that absorb moisture or dry quickly. Keep a spare pair of pj's right next to the bed so that if you wake up wet and uncomfortable, you can make a switch without having to turn on a light or get out of bed. Keep a pitcher of ice near the bed; either you can use the ice itself or it will have become refreshing, cool water by the time you need it.

If insomnia is your problem, start by making sure your bedroom environment is conducive to sleep. If you know that the sun will stream in every morning at an early hour, buy heavier curtains or shutters that will help keep the daytime out until you are ready for it. Keep a pair of earplugs next to the bed and consider using a white-noise machine (fans can serve the same purpose). Make sure the temperature in the bedroom is set to your liking.

We should mention that many scientists believe keeping the room a little cooler promotes better sleep. This may be because the air lowers your body temperature, mimicking the body's slow internal drops as you drift off.

Daytime Plan for a Great Night's Sleep

First Half of the Day

- Wake at the same time each morning, even on weekends.
- Exercise. Physical exertion helps to regulate circadian rhythms and is especially helpful for menopausal women. One study found that overweight postmenopausal women who engaged in moderate exercise found it easier to fall asleep than their inactive counterparts.[22] Unfortunately, exercising late at night can get your heart racing and can actually keep you up, so get your exercise in early.
- If you are going to drink caffeinated beverages, the earlier the better. Try to set an hour after which you won't have coffee or caffeinated soft drinks or any chemicals that might promote wakefulness.
- Try not to use the bedroom for anything except sleep and sex. (This can be impossible if, like many urban dwellers, you are living in a tiny one-bedroom apartment or studio space.)
- We often focus on the importance of shutting out light at night, but it may be equally important to get some sun during the day. This will help to adjust your body rhythms.

In the Evening

- Finish eating several hours before going to sleep. The only exception to this is if you suffer from bad dreams; some nightmares may actually be the result of hunger. In general, though, a full belly doesn't go well with a full night of sleep. The same thing goes for alcohol: if you are going to have that glass of red wine (for your heart, of course . . .) be sure to drink it several hours before hitting the hay. While alcohol is a depressant and can make you sleepy at first, eventually it speeds up the heart and can encourage early-morning waking and choppy sleep patterns.
- Engage in a relaxing activity for about an hour before bed. Read, talk with family, anything that helps you let go of the events of the day and move closer to bed.
- Try to go to sleep at the same time each night. Hold yourself to a "bedtime" in the same way you would a little kid.

If you are busy with work duties all day and caring for family all night, you may find that you didn't make space to think about or do the things you wanted to during the day. This is a problem because it shoves all your concerns into that space of time when you are supposed to be resting. Teenagers will often stay up late because, among other reasons, it gives them time alone away from parents or friends, when they can relax, think, and be themselves. As adults we aren't too different: our brains want a little freedom each day just to be by themselves. Make sure you give that to yourself before trying to close up shop for the night.

If you work on shifts (like nearly 20 percent of Americans), your work/sleep schedule may differ considerably from the traditional model. You may have to adjust your body clock to deal with being up when it's dark out and snoozing through broad daylight. Your biological impulses are working against you on this, and it makes you more likely to suffer from daytime sleepiness. Likewise, if you travel internationally a lot, for either work or pleasure, changing time zones and jet lag can cause some big complications in sleep schedule.

What about napping? For some people who sleep erratically—many seniors in particular—it is a lifesaver. If you are having trouble sleeping through the night, though, don't nap. Let the tiredness build up so that your body is forced to sleep in the time you give it. Napping on weekends, however enjoyable, can be bad because it gets the body accustomed to resting more sporadically. The result can be that when you are back at your desk on Monday, 2 PM rolls around, and your body is ready for its afternoon siesta. If you struggle with sleep problems, try not to keep significantly different hours on the weekend and during the week.

Finally, don't be shy about keeping pets out of the bedroom. It can be hard to say no to an animal you love, but trust us, they will be fine, and you will be a better pet parent if you are rested.

Sleep in a Bottle

We've all see the ads: the happy butterfly or the soothing music notes travel down into quiet, peaceful homes, kissing happily sleeping people. It looks so nice, so calm, so easy. *U.S. News and World Report* notes that "current sleep medications aren't as miraculous as their marketing suggests,"[23] but are better than their predecessors. That's not saying very much when your points of comparison are the barbiturates that caused many an overdose by Hollywood starlets in the 1950s and '60s and more recent drugs like Halcion and Restoril, whose side effects include disorientation, dizziness, and problems functioning.

The new prescription drugs for sleep—hypnotics with lovely names like Lunesta and Sonata and Ambien—essentially slow the brain's activity. The biggest problem with these sleep "remedies" may be the way that people use them, not the drugs themselves.

All of these drugs are designed to treat *acute* insomnia—they are for short-term use. They aren't meant to be taken day after day for months or years. If you're experiencing a period of stress that is preventing you from sleeping, this might be a solution for you. On the other hand, if you haven't been sleeping well for years, you should consider other options. Most FDA approvals on these drugs suggest use of three weeks or less. In the case of Ambien CR—a slow-releasing tablet designed to prevent waking prematurely—there were initially no safety data for use beyond three weeks, and an assessment of side effects was performed only two weeks after the drugs were discontinued.[24] In the summer of 2006, the maker of Ambien CR announced breathlessly that the drug had been approved safe for "long-term use."[25] The study this new information was based on lasted only six months. Certain trials of other pills, such as Sonata (zaleplon),[26] have lasted up to a year.

The problem with a lack of long-term safety data is that we don't really know what side effects (besides addiction) might occur with more extended use. Reports have begun to emerge that, for example, the drug Ambien, which is prescribed to around 24 million Americans a year, has been linked to cases of sleepwalking. Some of these cases were benign, but others involved driving while asleep, shoplifting, and eating thousands of calories without being aware of the behavior.[27] One Florida woman went from a size 1 to a size 12, eating raw eggs and whole loaves of bread in her sleep. Safoni-Aventis, the manufacturer, can reasonably claim that its drug won't cause this kind of problem when properly used, because "proper use" implies taking the drug for only a very limited time. Unfortunately, most people, once they start using sleep medications, have trouble stopping.

Amber, a therapist in her mid-forties, began taking a hypnotic sleeping aid temporarily after her middle son had some serious health problems. She was so worried about her three boys that she found it impossible to get rest. Her doctor prescribed a a popular sleep aid, and she slept like a baby for the first time in months. The problem was that two years later, though her son had recovered completely, she was still popping a pill several times a week to sleep. When Amber tried to discontinue taking the drug, her sleep troubles returned.

One of the problems with taking hypnotics is that they are addictive—not as addictive as older drugs, but dependency-forming, nonetheless. So much of sleep is about routine; if taking a pill becomes part of how you fall asleep, from both a chemical and a psychological perspective it can be difficult to make changes. The same thing is true of over-the-counter sleep aids, including Benadryl, Tylenol, and Advil PM. If you get used to the sensation of a drug lulling you to sleep, you will be at a loss when you set out to do it on your own.

Another consideration is that many sleep medications can alter your ability to get REM sleep or to complete your sleep cycles. So while you may be sleeping for longer periods of time, the quality of your sleep may not be very high. All sleep drugs—prescription and over-the-counter—can adversely affect your memory and cognition.

A final note about drugs: watch out for medications you are taking for other health problems that might affect sleep. These can include antidepressants, decongestants, and blood-pressure drugs. Ask your doctor for more information about this if you are concerned.

Cognitive Behavioral Therapy

Some professionals recommend a nonmedical approach to sleep problems using cognitive behavioral therapy, a strategy used to treat other serious problems including depression. Scientists at the Stanford University Sleep Disorder Clinic are among those who use this therapy to teach patients to modify their lifestyles to achieve health goals. When sleep-deprived journalist and author Cathryn Jakobson Ramin attended the clinic, hoping to improve her sleep, psychologist Tracy Kuo prescribed Ramin a late bedtime and had her set her alarm clock for exactly six hours later. When the alarm rang, whether she had slept or tossed the whole time, she had to get up. Only when she was able to successfully sleep for six hours straight could she sleep another fifteen minutes later. The idea was to create a routine in Ramin's preparation for sleep and sleep patterns and slowly build up her ability to snooze for longer stretches.[28]

When to Go to the Doctor

You may not need to talk to a doctor about your sleep problems. Because so many cases of insomnia are caused by temporary stresses, they tend to resolve on their own. For women, perimenopause may be a time when it is better to be tired, disruptive though it may be, than to start a potentially addictive or dangerous drug regimen. But if your sleep problems persist for more than six months to a year, or if they are making your life unpleasant, by all means talk to your doctor.

Before you go in for your doctor's visit, keep a sleep journal for two or three weeks. You can download a sleep journal from the Internet by Googling "sleep journal." There is one available as a PDF from the University of Washington at http://faculty.washington.edu/chudler/pdf/sleepjj.pdf. The journal will help you and your doctor identify external factors that can be changed to make your sleep easier as well as help her see if there are any medical issues that need to be addressed.

Tell your doctor about your family history. Did anyone else in your family tree suffer from serious sleep problems? Since most sleep problems aren't genetic, this sort of information could point the doctor in the direction of a disorder like narcolepsy.

Mention any medicines you take that could be contributing to your problem and bring any information you may have read or any questions you want to ask.

The doctor will probably assess your general appearance to see if you've gained or lost weight, if you are maintaining hygiene, and other things that could point to illness or depression. A blood-pressure check is useful because certain disorders—in particular sleep apnea—are associated with increased blood pressure.

The doctor will check your head and neck to see if a thyroid disorder, which can cause sleep trouble, might be an issue, or a condition such as a deviated septum, which could challenge nighttime breathing. Your doctor may choose to perform some cognitive tests to assess how your brain is working. Certain kinds of dementia and other brain disorders can disrupt sleep.

If you and your doctor are unable to find lifestyle changes that work, he may suggest a test called a polysomnogram. This is essentially an overnight sleep study that monitors your brain activity to check when and how soundly you are sleeping at different points in the night. A daytime test that follows a polysomnogram, called a "multiple sleep latency test," is performed once in a while when a doctor is trying to measure daytime sleepiness to determine if a patient has narcolepsy.

If you know your sleep problem is caused by something specific, treat that thing: if your partner snores, you don't need a sleeping pill. Don't try general solutions to fix a specific problem.

6

getting it on as you get on

menopause, aging, and sexuality

Young love is from the earth,
and late love from Heaven.

— TURKISH PROVERB

he year was 1929, and Dr. Marie Stopes was fighting mad. No one was going to tell Stopes, England's answer to Margaret Sanger,[1] that older women couldn't enjoy sex. She had already caused a scandal in England when she published the popular *Married Love*, a frank treatise on sexuality that resulted, at least in part, from research done after a troubled (and unconsummated) first marriage.[2] In 1929, at the age of forty-nine, she wrote a new book in which she counseled aging women not to listen to stereotypical cultural images of older women and sex.

In that book, *Enduring Passion*, she gave practical information on hormone compounds, having a good body image, and dealing with minor menopausal complaints, and took on the massive task of responding to a culture that suggested the idea of sexually active older women was not just distasteful but potentially immoral. Nineteenth-century conventional wisdom held that sex after conception was no longer possible was sinful.

Stopes railed against "the opinions of crudely material and base-minded men," mostly doctors, who suggest that only "young and attractive" women exist. Other women, including "artists, social workers, home-builders, [and] wise old women ... [those] whose lives reveal thoughtfulness," were automatically excluded from sexual consideration.[3]

In taking upon herself the role of opposition leader, Marie Stopes had volunteered for a big job. She was determined, however, to convince women that although they might find menopause to be disruptive, if they would just relax and hold tight for a few years, they would find themselves in the midst of their sexual primes. *Enduring Passion* shares the stories of woman after woman who, after passing through the "change of life," are able to enjoy sex spontaneously and happily. In one example, a sixty-year-old begins "for the first time at that age to enjoy sex union." An added bonus: "Her husband's passion and delight in her increased after that age." Such enthusiasm didn't need to end at sixty: "It is recorded that an old lady when asked at the age of 80, at what time a woman ceased to enjoy union with her spouse replied: you must ask someone older than I; I do not yet know."

It is amazing to realize that nearly eighty years later, many social attitudes regarding menopausal women and sex have changed very little. Certainly the images we see on television and in popular culture can be discouraging. Aging actors continue to be cast opposite women decades their juniors, and most magazines not directly geared at middle-aged or senior women hardly show pictures of anyone over thirty-five.

This has begun to change slightly. With the popularity of shows like *Desperate Housewives* and the prominence of celebrities like Michelle Pfeiffer, Demi Moore, and Diane Keaton, it is becoming more common to think of women at midlife as being not only sexually active but sexually desirable. This progress, however, can seem slow, and images of young women still dominate when setting the boundaries of desirability. Not that every woman sees this as a problem; one woman writes, "It has been a great relief to me to not have to maintain the public image of being a sex object as I did in my twenties or thirties. This is one menopausal change that I have found to be pleasant."[4] Images of sexual older women are still very rare.

Sexual problems some women experience at menopause are the second biggest reason for deciding to take hormone treatment (HT), so obviously a lot of women are apprehensive about the ways their bodies are changing and the implications this can have for their sexuality and relationships.

We have to be careful: we don't want to discount real problems women experience as a result of hormonal or bodily change, but at the same time, we don't want to assume too quickly that all women will have sexual difficulties with menopause. In fact the majority of women will have no problems at all, and many women will experience an *increase* in desire. This latter fact horrified one nineteenth-century gynecologist, who wrote in a scandalized tone that women "desired men more than ever." As one author astutely notes, "Many women head straight into menopause believing that their sex life will suffer and they act accordingly." The brain is a powerful thing, and if we become convinced in advance that we will struggle sexually, we are in danger of becoming self-fulfilling prophecies.[5]

What Happens to Our Bodies When We Are Aroused?

What happens to the female body when it becomes aroused? Science has yet to provide a satisfactory model of women's arousal. Here is one guess:

As you start to get aroused, through touching, visual images, or other stimuli, cells in your vagina begin to make moisture that wets the vagina and vulva. You may begin to feel your breathing get fast, and your heart rate and blood pressure increase. The clitoris swells as it fills with blood, and the nipples can become erect. The vagina changes size and shape, growing longer. Some 75 percent of women develop a flush that starts near their stomach and spreads upward toward the breasts.

As arousal continues, the labia may actually change color, darkening, and the clitoris begins to react to folds of tissue that surround it. After sex (whether the end result is orgasm or simply pleasure), swelling decreases and the heart rate and blood pressure slowly begin to return to normal.[6] This model is based on Master and Johnson's original 1960s theory; however, sexologists such as Leonore Tiefer have critiqued it at some length for ignoring the diversity of female experience and for trying to imagine that women's bodies work sexually in the same way men's do.

How Does the Body Change as We Age?

How does this (no pun intended) rosy picture alter when the body hits "the change"? As a woman's reproductive cycles wind down, her hormone levels drop—sometimes slowly, sometimes dramatically. It depends on the individual. As this happens, the walls of the vagina grow thin and can become less elastic.[7] Thinning occurs in part when fibrous connective tissues replace muscle cells. The surface of the vagina flattens; at first, this is just a few cell layers, but eventually capillaries can become visible and the surface grows smooth, shiny, and pale.[8] This lack of flexibility makes it harder for blood to flow through the area. This means, among other things, that it is harder for the body to make moisture. Less moisture and thinner walls mean that the whole area is more likely to be injured during sex and is more prone to infection and irritation, including annoying but treatable problems like urinary tract infection and vaginitis. When a woman experiences this kind of tearing and increased irritation, doctors say that she has "vaginal atrophy."

This is one reason why it is important to be diligent about lubrication. As the vagina gets smaller, it may feel tighter during intercourse, and a woman may feel the friction of sex more acutely. This can make the whole area more sensitive to the touch.[9]

The hood of the clitoris—the drooping bit of tissue that guards our most sensitive bits—may recede, leaving this tiny bundle of nerve endings in more direct contact with our partners. The result can be like walking barefoot—it can be pleasurable if we are walking carefully on smooth surfaces but can be a shock if we come in contact with a rougher one. For many women, though, increased clitoral sensitivity is a good thing and can actually increase pleasure.

Other potential changes include a weakening of the pelvic muscles. This can cause two problems. First, it can allow small amounts of urine to leak out during day-to-day life and also during sex. While this is something you would probably want to discuss with your doctor, it is nothing to get too upset about; this happens throughout a woman's entire life (female ejaculate is thought to be at least significantly made of urine).

One way to strengthen the vaginal and pelvic region is to exercise the muscles. Kegel exercises are a simple way to do this. Kegels involve tightening and toning the pubococcygeus muscles, which are located between the pubic bone and the tailbone.[10]

To perform a Kegel, tighten the muscles in the vaginal area as you would do to stop the flow of urine or pull up a slipping tampon,[11] and keep them tightened for ten seconds. Try repeating this ten to fifteen times at three points in the day.[12] If you work on this, you should see some improvement within two or three months. Sex expert Betty Dodson created a small metal barbell that can be used to strengthen vaginal muscles. An added bonus of the barbell is that it can double as a highly durable sex toy. (You can purchase the barbell at www.bettydodson.com.)

As a woman ages, the number of vaginal contractions during orgasm may decrease, and contractions in the rectum may cease entirely. This change happens in men as well and has nothing to do with menopause. In rare cases, the uterus may actually descend into the vagina, or the bladder or rectum may begin pushing on the vaginal wall. One way doctors have traditionally dealt with this more serious sexual complication is by performing a hysterectomy, an extreme and unnecessary solution to this problem.

All of this sounds a lot scarier than it is. The truth is that as long as sex feels good, you aren't experiencing unnecessary pain, and these changes aren't interfering with your day-to-day life, then none of these things are worth worrying about. Like the rest of your body, your vagina looks different as you age, but just as beautiful. If you feel good about your body and realize that change is not necessarily a bad thing, you will be in great shape to enjoy yourself and your partner(s) as you age.

What Are the Big Problems Women Have?

You might be surprised to find out how many medical classifications there are for female sexual problems. Low libido? You may be suffering from hypoactive sexual desire.[13] Trouble having an orgasm? You could have either female orgasmic disorder or female sexual arousal disorder. Among other things, this is an interesting illustration of how common physical experiences are repackaged as diseases in need of pharmaceutical cures.

Most of the new ways of classifying women's "sexual problems" have been created in the past decade by doctors who are interested in solving them almost exclusively with drugs. These so-called diseases aren't like a strep virus or the chicken pox, something you can test and see definitively in a lab. Instead, they are a collection of vague, ill-understood symptoms that have been organized together to make them seem medically quantifiable and containable.

A lack of desire can be caused by many things. Stress, for example, can really put you out of the mood. This is true in younger women as well as their menopausal counterparts. One forty-nine-year-old lawyer notes, "It seems like hormones aren't so much a factor in libido as touch and mental preparation. If I've been concentrating hard on some topic or job and suddenly am presented with the opportunity of having sex, it's really hard to get interested or aroused. But if I've been thinking about it ahead of time, with lots of kissing and cuddling thrown in, I get interested, regardless of how bad I formerly thought I would feel." Both possible causes, physical and psychological, have to be carefully considered, and the answer is often a mix of the two. But the moment we stick a fancy medical name on what we are feeling, it seems only right that we would try to fix it with drugs.

After nearly a century of treating female sexual problems almost completely with psychology, scientists and drug company executives realized they were letting a potentially lucrative market go untapped. The new system of classifying "female sexual dysfunction" came about through a series of drug company–funded conferences on female sexuality that have taken place since the approval and massive success of the drug Viagra. Viagra made clear in the pharmaceutical context what prostitutes have always known: that people are willing to pay for good sex. Since more women supposedly experience sexual problems than men, it seemed logical that there should be a drug for them as well, and a flurry of dubious research into women's sexual health got under way. So far, many of the proposed drugs and cures are unproven, ill-researched, and potentially dangerous. As one women's health advocate puts it, "Women must be skeptical when they hear about a new scientific breakthrough and a magic pill every five minutes . . . it may not be very sexy, but consumer awareness must become part of sex education in the 21st century."[14]

How many women experience sexual problems?[15] It's tough to find statistics that aren't tied to scientists with a financial stake in sex drugs.

Part of the problem is that there is really no reliable way to test for problems. Sex isn't easy to measure, and desire is nearly impossible to chart in a lab. Attempts to measure female arousal have reached the extreme: one of the only medical tests involves something called a vaginal plethysmograph.[16] This device has a small electronic unit that emits light and a small electric current, and a photocell detector, which is a thing that detects and measures light and other kinds of radiation. Both of these are encased in a clear acrylic probe that is inserted into the vagina.[17] The female patient stimulates herself, and the device measures changes in the color of the vagina and then calculates blood flow.

This is not a particularly effective way of gauging sexual problems and it is obviously not something that all women would feel comfortable with. It also ignores the basic problem that sex for men and women is cultural and psychological as well as physical and biological.

What Can Drugs Do for Us?

There are two major camps in the world of research on sexual problems in women: those who focus primarily on the psychological and social causes of sex disturbance and those who believe the issues are medical and more adequately addressed by pharmaceuticals. These two sides often come to blows.

American sex changed forever at the end of the 1990s with the introduction of a small blue pill called Viagra. Jokes proliferated, but within a year sales topped $1 billion, making its producer, Pfizer, the second biggest drugmaker in the world.[18] These sales leveled out, but the sea change in looking at sex problems as medical conditions continued to gain momentum. Smart drug company executives (as well as doctors who had honestly and earnestly been converted to the medical sex camp) began to understand Viagra as the tip (pun intended) of an enormous and profitable iceberg. An intense race to find the female Viagra is still being waged, and for both men and women sex has gotten a little more, well, clinical. A March 2001 *Consumer Reports* article notes, "The pill's effectiveness clearly demonstrates that many sexual problems stem from physical rather than psychological causes."[19] Of course, the flip side of this is that many people have come to believe that every sexual problem can be solved by popping a pill, which is clearly not the case.

At first many doctors thought, "If Viagra will work for men, why not women as well?" On the surface it made sense. When men are aroused, their bodies create a chemical that relaxes smooth muscle tissue, allowing greater blood flow to the genitals. Another chemical comes along later and counteracts the first, letting blood drain out and the penis resume a flaccid state. Viagra works by inhibiting the second chemical and allowing the first to keep a man erect longer. The same chemicals exist and work in women's bodies as well. Clitoral tissue also becomes erect when a woman is aroused, so there is logic to the idea that Viagra could ease sex for gals as well as guys.

Unfortunately, trials of Viagra in women have failed to yield the desired results.

One thing we can take away from the failure of Viagra in females is the danger of making hasty sexual analogies between men and women. Indeed, a huge problem with sex research is that findings from studies performed only on men are often applied to women.

The dearth of research on women and sex goes far beyond Viagra. As Dr. Irwin Goldstein, formerly of Boston University, points out, this research is still "in its embryonic stage. There are no medical textbooks of female sexual health. It's odd to think about drugs when we don't even know how the vagina works."[20]

Dr. Goldstein has become a very visible presence in the camp of doctors and scientists who believe in the potential of drugs to cure most sexual struggles. In fact, he was a primary organizer of the Boston conference that kicked off the "women's sexual dysfunction" frenzy. In a *New York Times Magazine* cover story in 2000, Dr. Goldstein said that without discounting "psychological aspects ... at a certain point all sex is mechanical."[21]

The quest to know how the vagina works is an unusual one. In the past decade, doctors like Goldstein and Jennifer Berman have been busy watching sexual response in laboratory animals and culturing clumps of animal genital tissue to see how they contract and relax.[22]

On the other side of the sex research divide are those who believe female sex problems to be largely products of culture and individual experience. One of the most visible voices in this movement is the psychologist Leonore Tiefer, who takes a hard line against "doctors, managed care organizations and pharmaceutical companies [who] would prefer the quick fix" of a little blue pill and ignore the complexities of sexual psychology.[23] Dr. Carol Tavris, a behavioral scientist based in Los Angeles, explains, "Most of what passes for science on the new female sexual dysfunction is really product testing controlled by business." She explains that research into drugs often happens at the expense of other types of learning: "Today, sex research can get thousands of dollars to study, say, blood flow to the rabbit clitoris, but not a dime to look at variations in sexual responses in diverse groups of women. They're happy to tell you what's normal and what's abnormal, but in fact no one knows."[24]

This conflict over funding has many aspects. Many scientists and doctors hoping to do sex research get funding through drug companies that hope to develop new products and markets. If you aren't performing research that will enable drug sales, it can be very hard to secure monies.

The *British Medical Journal* noted in 2003 that while "the corporate sponsored creation of a disease is not a new phenomenon, ... the making of female sexual dysfunction is the freshest, clearest example we have."[25] The article points out that while doctors such as Goldstein and Berman may well believe that drugs are the answer, they are squarely in the pockets of companies like Pfizer. Indeed, Pfizer was the sponsor of the series of conferences organized by Goldstein in which various aspects of female sexuality were reclassified as "dysfunction" and "disorders."

Tiefer, who saw these meetings as part of a drug company plan to "promote the medicalization of women's sexuality,"[26] notes that the new definitions were in some ways "another item on the growing list of so-called sexual dysfunctions associated with women through the ages, including hysteria, nymphomania and frigidity." It is a compelling argument; while we would certainly hope that there will be new solutions for women who are sexually struggling, the new terminologies do bring to mind the bizarre pathologizing of female sexuality used by conservative Victorians to keep women in their place.

Drug company dollars have become even more central to sex research in the current political environment, where, as a 2005 *Psychology Today* article notes, public funding for sex studies has increasingly come under attack.[27] In 2003, conservative congressmen forced an audit of sex studies receiving public dollars. In an age when Senator Bob Dole became the face of Viagra, even conservative forces are comfortable with research that confines itself to looking at sex in a laboratory context. It is less comfortable with studies that look at actual sex histories of various people, and again this creates a bias against certain types of research.

Leonore Tiefer and her colleagues have taken on the role of the loyal opposition, working to reinforce the importance of various psychosocial factors in female sexuality. They argue that focusing too exclusively on medical explanations "ignores the implications of inequalities related to gender, social class, ethnicity, sexual orientation, and socio-economic condition."[28]

A recent and profound example of the danger of rushing sex-drug research is the FDA rejection of a testosterone patch for women designed to treat flagging libidos. The patch, made by Procter & Gamble, would have been the first "FDA sanctioned drug designed to address women's sexual problems."[29] The testosterone patch is a hormone treatment (HT) designed to release hormones slowly and steadily into the body. Even if the patch works, it is unclear what the safety hazards of taking testosterone over longer periods of time might be; it would need long-term studies to prove it is safe for use over decades.

Procter & Gamble justified its bid for approval by presenting two trials that suggested the drug increased desire. On the surface, these trials looked good: they were performed on 1,100 women and they demonstrated a significant improvement over the placebo. One thing, however, pointed to the possibility that the company was not being entirely rigorous in their science: the trials were performed entirely on women who had had complete hysterectomies and oophorectomies.[30] As we have mentioned, women who have undergone these major medical procedures experience very different and often very extreme menopauses. Studies performed on this population of women cannot and should not be used to draw conclusions about women experiencing natural menopause. When a company tries to justify hasty approval by manipulating research studies, it is right and wise that it should fail.

In this case the FDA did the right thing. FDA panel members voted against approving the patch and said their reasons for doing so included "discomfort" with the clinical trials and a lack of information on long-term health effects.[31] Among those distraught about the decision was Dr. Irwin Goldstein, who said he believed the drug would "empower women to ask their doctors about care and finally motivate researchers to better understand the physiology of what happens when a woman has sexual dysfunction."[32] While acknowledging a lack of solid information about the patch, Dr. Goldstein argued that if the FDA had waited for such knowledge about Viagra, countless men would have been denied a much-needed sexual aid.

The Role of Hormone Therapy

It has been a very bad couple of years for HT. One by one, claims of its health benefits have been discredited. Most of these claims, such as its protective effects against heart disease, were never affirmed by the FDA. One thing, however, that HT *was always* approved to do, since the original FDA approval of DES, the first synthetic oral estrogen approved for menopause in the Unied States, in 1941, was to treat certain types of sexual problems. Specifically, hormone preparations containing estrogen help to prevent vaginal dryness and dyspareunia, that is, painful intercourse. This is because there is a correlation between these sexual problems and low estradiol levels.[33] HT has been shown to restore muscular elasticity and increase lubrication and sexual sensation.[34]

Several studies suggest that estrogen is equally effective for this purpose when taken orally (systemically) and used as a cream (topically). A recent trial performed as part of the Women's Health, Osteoporosis, Progestin, Estrogen (HOPE) Trial found relief from atrophy with lower doses of estrogen (Premarin).[35] The vaginal ring, a circular device that is inserted into the vagina and releases hormones, has also been shown to be effective, and in one study, women preferred it to cream;[36] however, as the *Journal of Obstetrics and Gynecology* concluded in a massive Fall 2004 review of hormone therapy, there is really no solid evidence that taking a specific type of estrogen, in any specific dose or for any period of time, is more effective than another.

Also, and this is an important distinction, HT has *not* been shown to be useful in treating a declining libido.[37]

What Psychological Factors Can Play a Role?

Study after study insists that sexual desire and the loss of it have to do less with hormones than with other lifestyle factors, most notably psychological considerations.[38] At a recent National Institutes of Health conference, field experts concluded that menopausal status is an inadequate basis for assessing sexual problems at midlife, which have as much to do with "life stressors, contextual factors, past sexuality and mental health concerns."[39] Dr. John Bancroft, director of the Kinsey Institute at Indiana University, found in a private study that "the two biggest factors determining whether a woman reported distress were the emotion she felt during sex and whether she was depressed or tired."[40] As Dr. Steven R. Goldstein (not to be confused with Irwin Goldstein), a professor of gynecology at New York University, is quick to point out, "Changes in midlife sexual function are not a simple case of 'take away hormones, take away the desire.'"[41] Another expert observes, "You can have a woman with low testosterone switch to a new partner and suddenly her libido is just fine."[42]

A dramatic example of this scenario is erotic pioneer Betty Dodson. The author of several books on sex, Dodson was determined not to let the changes incurred at midlife interfere with enjoying a healthy, pleasurable sex life. When she discovered in her mid-fifties that she was beginning to experience pain with intercourse, she gave up penetrative sex and explored other pleasures. When joint pain began to interfere, Dodson tried to focus on writing about sex rather than having so much of it. When this proved unsatisfying, she began exploring estrogen replacement. This offered relief and replenishment for her vagina, but the thing that ultimately solved her sex dilemmas was the appearance of a new partner, Eric Wilkinson. In his early thirties, Wilkinson is decades Dodson's junior, and their passion became the subject of the recent book *Orgasms for Two*. Explaining her now ten-year relationship, she writes, "I encourage older women not to buy into society's negative messages about sex fading as we grow older. More and more of us need to push aside all of those self-image problems with the monster of vanity whispering, 'you're too fat, too wrinkled, or too old.'"[43]

Of course, we're not suggesting that women ditch their husbands and partners and start shopping for younger lovers. What this example demonstrates is the power of the mind in rejuvenating us sexually.

Marital Stress

The effect of marital stress on activities in the bedroom can be profound. As the sexologist Laura Berman (Jennifer's sister) bluntly puts it, if a woman hates her husband, there is no drug in the world that is going to help her have good sex.[44] An Ohio State study designed to look at the results of marital fighting found that when couples argue, it wreaks havoc on their hormone levels and hurts their immune systems.[45]

The health effects of a bad relationship go far beyond the bedroom. A 1997 report in *Psychosomatic Medicine* notes that "abrasive marriages may make some older people more vulnerable to infections and slower to heal." A study published in the *Journal of the American Medical Association* in 2000 found that women in high-stress marriages were three times more likely to suffer repeat heart attacks when compared with women in happier relationships.[46] So it is not just good sex in the balance when we talk about what is at stake in a broken or wounded relationship.

Menopause is an opportune moment for working on problems that have been developing over the years because it represents such a clear transition; it gives us the chance to decide: "Before I go on to this next part of my life, I want to work on [fill in the blank]."

Another major change in our lives around menopause that can have a big impact on our relationships with romantic partners is the impending independence and adulthood of children. This has sexual implications for several reasons. First and most basically, it has to do with how you and your partner view each other. If for decades you have seen each other as "Mom and Dad" or "Mom and Mommy," it can be disorienting suddenly to see each other as individual people again. Also, couples regain time that was spent raising children. This can be a scary thing because it means that you have more time to spend with each other. And of course it can be a wonderful thing for the same reason, giving people a chance to remember why they loved each other before the kids came along.

Laura's mother, Sue, struggled with the departure of each of her four children for college and beyond. At first she was very sad, and she and Laura's father argued over what their new roles and responsibilities were. Now, however, Sue is a dedicated hospice social worker who recently went back to school for a postgraduate certificate in her field. She is also involved in nonpastoral counseling through her church and works for other volunteer organizations that serve the senior population in her area. She and Laura's father are able to enjoy activities that they never had time or money for when they were busy raising a family and they are really enjoying this new chapter in their lives and relationship.

If you are divorced, widowed, or have always been single and are involved in new or emerging relationships, you face your own challenges at this point in your life. Unlike your teens and twenties, when all of your peers were dating and experimenting with newly understood sexual selves, when you are starting to see yourselves sexually again at midlife it can feel like you are all alone. With many friends in long-term partnerships, there is less cultural reinforcement or information to tell you what it is like to deal with new partners and a new and changing body at the same time. Luckily, as more women find themselves in (or choose to be in) this situation, there are great Internet and print resources to help along the way.

One young widow in her fifties humorously describes her experiances dating at midlife: "I can't imagine why a man would want to date a younger woman—with hot flashes and things like that, women my age can't wait to get their clothes off!"

So When You Have Problems, What Can You Do about It?

One bit of simple but sound advice can be just to relax and slow things down in the bedroom. Take longer with foreplay; this will give you more time to increase your natural lubrication and to get yourself ready for sex. This may be a really good thing for your partner as well. Mount Sinai School of Medicine explains that "men, too, experience an increase in the time it takes to reach erection, and the orgasm will feel different and can occur with less warning time."[47]

Sometimes the simplest solutions are the best. A basic lubricant such as Astroglide or KY can solve a lot of problems. These come in a variety of compositions, from water-based to those that have glycerine, to those that are silicon-based, to plain old massage oils. Lubricants can be purchased at any drugstore, but many female-friendly sex shops sell them in trial sizes for around fifty cents a package. One such shop, New York's Toys in Babeland, has a Web site where supplies can be purchased (www.babeland.com) from the privacy of home.

Try buying several varieties and experiment with your partner to find out which is right for you. Some doctors advise against oil-based lubricants like Vaseline or baby oil. These can damage condoms and they are also more likely to cause irritation in many women.[48] Replens is a long-acting lubricant that lasts three days and can be reapplied several times a week. It provides moisture on an ongoing basis and doesn't need to be applied right before or during sex. An interesting side fact about both Replens and Astroglide is that they are slightly acidic and can help prevent bacteria that can cause vaginal infections from flourishing.[49]

Communicating with your partner is always important. Studies suggest that feeling "emotional closeness" with a partner is as important as proper functioning in the creation of good sexual experiences. Take the changes your body is going through as an opportunity to experiment and communicate with your partner in new ways.

What We Talk about When We Talk about Sex:

Tips for Better Partner Communication
1. Try to bring up your concerns outside the bedroom. If you try to talk about problems you are having during intimate moments, it can create an overly pressured emotional dynamic. Wait for a less loaded setting to voice your worries. Try to avoid arguing in bed.[50]
2. Try to avoid using critical language when you phrase your concerns.
3. Don't be overly sensitive to your partner's comments in response.
4. Be specific with suggestions and complaints. Doctors at the Mayo Clinic suggest, "Don't say hazy, unclear things like 'we need to be more romantic.' Instead offer concrete ideas such as holding hands more often."[51]
5. Be positive—focus on solutions rather than problems.
6. Be hands-on when in the bedroom—show your partner what sort of touching feels good; tell your partner when you find something pleasurable or arousing.
7. Learn to become more comfortable with your body. As sex therapist Dagmar O'Connor explains, "If you are self-conscious about your physical appearance, you won't get much pleasure out of sex."[52] Find nonsexual opportunities to be naked together.
8. Learn to share fantasies and desires with your partner. Learn to focus on your own sexual pleasure as well as your partner's.
9. Take turns initiating sex.
10. Try new positions. This not only adds to sexual excitement by creating novelty, it can have the very practical outcome of helping you find ways to make love that are physically more comfortable. Some of the most common (and nonmenopausal) sexual

difficulties in midlife have to do with aching joints and muscles. One women writes that having sex lying side by side eased joint pain that was making it hard for her to enjoy herself in bed.[53]

For women having intense irritation and pain with intercourse, part of the solution may lie in reprioritizing penetration as a measure of sex. If penetrative intercourse is too painful, do it less often and make other activities—intimate touching, oral sex, mutual masturbation—more central in sexual encounters. Guide your partner as he or she touches you, explaining how your pleasures have changed, and have your partner do the same. This can be an exciting process, as both partners realize that to some extent they have new lovers.

Read up on sex together: learning can itself be a turn-on and, more important, it can help you understand your body better. On one Internet site, a woman in her mid-fifties explained that as a result of studying up on her menopausal sex problems, she learned how to have orgasms for the first time. This may be an extreme example but it makes the point that we are never too wise or too experienced to learn something new.

Most basically, continuing to have sex on a frequent basis helps to keep us sexually healthy. Many sexual complications in the second half of life are the result of neglect and infrequent use. Our bodies can be a little like vintage cars: if properly maintained, they are far superior to anything new; if ignored, they can become less useable. Intercourse can help keep vaginal walls more elastic and responsive.[54] Even if we don't have a regular partner, masturbation can help keep us functioning sexually because it keeps blood flowing in the genital area and helps maintain vaginal acidity that prevents infection. Masturbation is also a good way to better understand your own body, what kind of touching feels good, and what helps you reach orgasm.[55]

We've said it before in this book, and we will say it again: exercise is one of the best things you can do for yourself. In terms of sex, it can increase your stamina and keep your bones and muscles in better shape. It also helps to keep fluctuating hormones on a more even keel.

It is important not to get discouraged. One doctor explains, "If you set impossibly high standards for each sexual encounter, you're setting yourself up for disappointment. Repeated letdowns lead eventually to diminished desire. . . . If a particular encounter is a flop, don't assume that all future encounters will turn out bad, too. Remind yourself of other encounters that did turn out well."[56] Start to keep a record of sexual experiences, ideas, and fantasies, always being mindful of the physical feelings that come with them. Keep a record of how often you have sex, which partner initiated it, and what you liked or disliked about it. This will help you to see patterns: for example, something that makes you less likely to be in the mood, or a particular thing that makes sex appealing.

Devices and Desire

In the absence of any really efficacious drugs, there is one medical device approved for the treatment of sexual problems in women. According to its advertising, the Eros is the "first clinically proven and FDA-cleared treatment on the market."[57] It's a small plastic cup that is placed over the clitoris and "attached to a small, battery-operated pump." The cup creates a light sucking that leads to increased blood flow in the area, and thereby, erection and increased sensation. In trials, 80 percent of women experienced more sexual satisfaction when using the device. It is a prescription item—and a really expensive one, costing around $350.

A much less expensive alternative is a small vibrator, which costs more like $30. Some women don't like the idea of the vibrator, associating it negatively with other "off-limits" sexual devices, pornography, or other items that they don't see as part of their more traditional sex practices. While this is understandable, it is important to consider all solutions (and their relative costs and benefits) when trying to solve a real medical issue. As a doctor at the Mayo Clinic notes, "Although this idea might make you uncertain at first, try using a vibrator to help you discover your erogenous zones. Don't let old ideas keep you from using something that specialists in sex therapy often recommend to help women find their pleasure points."[58] The truth is that many women have benefited from experimenting with vibrators or incorporating them into their sex play.

The Role of Chronic Disease in Midlife and Late-Life Sex Problems

Several illnesses, chronic and otherwise, can put a dent in desire and sexual performance. And of course, if you are suffering from something treatable or manageable, libido will return when the illness is addressed.

In the bedroom, an underactive thyroid gland can cause low energy, sluggishness, and weight gain,[59] as well as low androgen (testosterone) production. Other chronic problems that can interfere with sex include iron deficiency, depression, and heart disease. Heart disease is one example, but anything that interferes with blood flow can make it difficult to get turned on. Some other troublesome conditions include osteoporosis and diabetes.

While you should be careful, always being sure to engage in practices and positions that don't put too much strain on muscles, joints, and bones, Dr. Robert Butler offers the good news that "sex is not only safe for most patients, it can be beneficial. . . . The physical exertion associated with sexual intercourse is about the same as walking up two flights of stairs. Thus sex is even possible for most people with heart disease, cancer, stroke or hypertension."[60] So next time you are enjoying some "alone" time with your partner (or partners), remember that you are doing something that is not only good for you emotionally but has physical benefits as well.

Hysterectomy and gynecological surgery can have a huge impact on sexual functioning *and* desire. For more information on this important subject (hysterectomy) check out chapter 8.

When Drugs Are Part of the Problem

Drugs taken to treat chronic illness can often contribute to sexual problems. Whenever you are taking more than one drug, but particularly when you are taking several, it is important to be aware of the potential interactions and side effects.

This is one instance where the patient has to be proactive and self-educating. Read up on your medications, particularly those you are taking on a long-term basis or to treat or prevent a chronic illness, and see if they are known to have side effects, including sexual complications. When you have this information, you are better prepared to explore options. Is there a drug you could be taking instead that doesn't have sexual consequences? Are you taking unnecessary drugs with side effects that outweigh benefits?

The *Journal of the American Medical Association* estimates that 25 percent of sexual problems in men are either caused or complicated by medication.[61] Some prime culprits include antihypertensive drugs, which reduce blood flow to the groin, and antidepressants, whose role in decreasing desire has been well documented. Others include anti-Parkinson's drugs, antipsychotics, corticosteroids (taken for arthritis), and pain medications, as well as beta-blockers and diuretics used to treat heart disease.

It has long been known that estrogen therapy's close cousin, the birth control pill, can cause problems with libido. While HT and ET can help with physical problems by increasing lubrication or thickening the vaginal wall, it can actually cause problems by dampening desire.

Some Really Good News

So now that we've talked about all the potential problems associated with sex at midlife, we want to leave you with some positive thoughts. First, menopause doesn't necessarily lower libido. Many women actually experience an increase rather than a decrease in desire at menopause. In 1910, one stuffy male doctor wrote with terror that many women experienced "the horrors of retained libido" that tormented women in their middle years as "summer is sometimes prolonged into autumn."[62] We can laugh about such attitudes now, but many women who feel new longings and desires worry that they are abnormal when they aren't; one study from Hanover Medical School in Germany reports that 41 percent of women over the age of forty-five in one trial reported having orgasms "often," while a mere 29 percent of younger women could say the same.[63]

Although certain hormones such as progesterone stop production nearly entirely during menopause, it turns out that testosterone drops much less significantly, by only about 29 percent.[64] And as estrogen levels plummet, having more testosterone may be what causes an increase in the sex drive.[65]

How long can we hope to keep having sex? Well, as Marie Stopes's eighty-year-old friend says, if we are lucky, we may never get old enough to find out. A report in the *Archives of Sexuality* published in 1988 found that in a sample group of people between the ages of eighty and one hundred two, 60 percent of men and more than 30 percent of women reported still having penetrative sex, and (are you ready for this?) 83 percent of men and 64 percent of women said that they still engaged in other sexual behavior, like touching and caressing. A 2007 *New England Journal of Medicine* study found that 73 percent of 57- to 64-year-olds were still enjoying sexual activity, as well as 53 percent of 65- to 74-year-olds and 26 percent of 75- to 85-year-olds.[66] It seems that a woman's capacity for multiple orgasms is not affected by age. So let's hope that with the right care and attention to these most intimate parts of our bodies and lives, we can all be enjoying happy, healthy sex lives into our second centuries.

7

the swing versus the slump

menopause, mood, and depression

The word happy *would lose its meaning if it were not balanced by sadness.*

—CARL JUNG

You've got to talk to my mom," a young friend of Laura's said hurriedly over the phone in the summer of 2005. "She hasn't slept in a week, and we were out at dinner last night and out of nowhere she burst into tears. It's been happening a lot lately, but every time we try to speak to her she just says she can't talk about it. I think it might be . . . you know . . . related to your book."

Sure enough, when Laura spoke to her friend's mom, Leora, opened up about night sweats and bursts of emotion that came and went like so many thunderclouds over a mountain. "I'm fine . . . perfectly happy . . . even energetic," she explained, "and then suddenly I feel so overwhelmed—like my life is totally out of control and I don't know what to do about it. And then I'm back to fine.

"The worst part is," she added, "I don't know which to trust—the ups or downs."

As women, we get used to having our moods associated, sometimes rightly but mostly wrongly, with our menstrual cycles. We spend years fighting cultural assumptions that when we get upset it's because "it's that time of the month." We try hard not to deny the annoying and disruptive ways premenstrual syndrome (PMS) can affect us without giving in to sexist assessments of female mood. It's pretty common for menstruating women to stand up for themselves and say, "I'm not upset because I'm getting my period, it's because something has happened to make me angry."

As menopausal women, we have to face these challenges anew. Laura was walking down the street in her Brooklyn neighborhood recently when she heard two women talking. "I think she was going through something else . . . she was out of control," the one said to the other. "I know," her friend answered. "I bet she's menopausal."

But is there actually a connection between menopause and mood? Does being menopausal make you more prone to suffer from depression? And if so, what can you do about it? These questions are very complicated, and even the experts disagree on the answers.

Before we can even get to the role of menopause in our psychological well-being, we need to make a distinction between depression and mood swings. These two very different experiences are often conflated, both consciously and unconsciously, when it comes to talking about women's health.

A mood swing is a fast-moving change between good and bad moods that doesn't last very long; it is what Laura's friend's mom, Leora, was going through. A mood swing is a lot like PMS. They are both caused in part by hormonal shifts. In perimenopause, estrogen levels fluctuate pretty dramatically, and that can have an effect on how you feel. In fact, graphs charting estrogen in perimenopausal women literally resemble a roller coaster with numerous ups and down, dips and rises.

Over the years, drug companies have worked hard to blur the distinction between a mood swing and a depression. A dramatic example of this in premenopausal women is the creation of premenstrual disphoric disorder (PMDD). This disease, essentially bad PMS, was "discovered" by the drug company Eli Lilly just as its blockbuster drug Prozac was about to go off patent. Shortly after announcing the discovery of PMDD, Eli Lilly proudly touted the cure: a drug that was chemically the same as Prozac but marketed under the pretty new name "Sarafem."

The description of the new "disorder" at the Lilly Web site asks,

"Does the following sound familiar? Month after month, a week or so before your period, you experience intense mood and physical symptoms. Irritability, mood swings, tension as well as breast tenderness and bloating can be part of the picture."[1] While insisting that PMS and PMDD are distinct, the Lilly folks don't really explain *how* they are different medically. Rather, they play on female patients' insecurities, noting that when this problem strikes, "you don't feel like the woman you usually are the rest of the month," and adding that PMDD sufferers have more problems with husbands and children.

In general, the makers of antidepressants would prefer you not make a distinction between mood swings and depression because their products have never been shown to help mood swings.

So what do we actually know about depression and menopause? Or mood swings and menopause, for that matter?

It has become very normal in American life to say things like, "I'm so depressed—my team didn't make it to the World Series," or "That movie made me feel depressed for *days*." When we say things like this, we don't mean to suggest that we have a serious medical condition. We mean simply that something disappointed us or made us feel sad.

Lots of people do, unfortunately, suffer from a major depression at some point in their lives. A major depression can be the result of something big happening to us—the death of a loved one, trouble at work, or some other stressful life event—or it can develop out of nowhere, seemingly without cause. It can happen only once in a lifetime or be something that a person struggles with over decades.

Estimates about exactly how many Americans suffer from major depression vary widely. Generally it is thought that around 17 percent of Americans will suffer from a major depressive episode during their lives. That's almost one in five people.[2]

We have gotten used to certain messages about depression. For example, most people know that depression happens because of a chemical imbalance in the brain caused by a lack of certain chemicals like serotonin and norepinephrine. And there are drugs that have become very popular, like Prozac, which help restore the chemical balance in the brain—right?

Well, maybe. The truth is that no one knows what causes depression or why certain people are more likely to suffer from it than others. Imbalance in serotonin and other neurotransmitters (chemicals that help brain cells communicate) has been one theory about why people get depressed. And in recent years, many scientists and doctors have come to seriously doubt that it is the right one. Journalists Ray Moynihan and Alan Cassels write, "Specialists in mental illness remind us the idea that depression is caused by a deficiency of the brain chemical serotonin is in fact just one scientific view among many—and a simplistic and outdated one at that. But it is a theory kept very much alive by the massive marketing machinery"[3] of drug companies.

The "serotonin hypothesis," as it is too infrequently called, was first put forth by a Harvard University psychiatrist named Joseph Schildkraut, who in his research in the 1960s came to believe that depression was associated with low levels of norepinephrine. His work was later used to suggest serotonin, another brain chemical, as the likely culprit in depressive illness.

In a startling 2005 review of the history of the serotonin hypothesis, authors Jeffrey R. Lacasse and Jonathan Leo argue that to "identify a chemical imbalance at the molecular level is not compatible with the extant science."[4] Not only is there little solid clinical evidence to support the science behind selective serotonin reuptake inhibitors (SSRIs), they say that science "has provided significant counterevidence" to "the explanation of a simple neurotransmitter deficiency."

Why the confusion? First, the existing studies aren't very good. They are often too small to give any real information and have to contend with too many variables. Many of the trials are industry-funded, and those that are performed at universities and in medical schools often receive money either directly (through grants and contracts) or indirectly (through financial ties with scientists) from the pharmaceutical companies. This makes it very difficult to trust the data that do make it to publication.

Another problem is that in arguing for "chemical balance" in the brain, scientists have failed to establish what would constitute a *good* serotonin or norepinephrine level. This is essentially like sending someone on a treasure hunt without a map. It also makes it nearly impossible to say what a bad chemical balance would be.

Finally, Lacasse and Leo explain, scientific attempts have been mounted to try to create depression by lowering serotonin levels, but "these experiments reaped no consistent results." They note, "Likewise, researchers found that huge increases in brain serotonin . . . were ineffective in stemming depression."[5] Author Jacky Law adds, "While on the average depressed patients may have low levels of serotonin activity, about one half of these patients have normal levels of serotonin and a few may even have levels that are unusually high."[6]

We're not saying that chemicals in the brain may not be behind depression; on the contrary, it seems very likely that they are. The relationship at this time, however, is so little understood as to require further explanation before it can be responsibly put forth as justifications for drug marketing.

Looking at the case of estrogen and heart disease, we can see that it is dangerous to jump to conclusions about how to treat chronic illness based on an undertested model. We certainly aren't suggesting that SSRIs don't work for some people. There is compelling evidence that for many folks these drugs are lifesavers; they have allowed many people we know and love to return to normal life. We are saying, though, that they aren't a panacea. They won't work for everyone or for every psychological problem. And they certainly won't prevent (nor should they) the human reality of sadness and periodic emotional struggle that is part of making a life in this world.

Perhaps most important, they won't treat menopausal mood swings.

Women experience depression at significantly higher percentages than men. Understanding what the condition looks like goes a long way to helping make the sometimes muddled distinction between illness and natural mood fluctuation, between something that needs medical attention and something that needs patience, communication, and time.

Harvard psychiatrist and anthropologist Dr. Arthur Kleinman explains, "There is no question in my mind that severe clinical depression is a real disease . . . but mild depression is a totally different kettle of fish. It allows us to re-label as depression an enormous number of things."[7] Edward Shorter, author of *A History of Psychiatry*, adds that the boundaries of depression are being pushed "relentlessly outward," noting that what was before the 1960s a familiar but less common problem has become "tantamount to dysphoria, meaning unhappiness."[8]

Contrary to those little quizzes you see in magazines and in doctors' offices—many of which are designed and distributed by drugmakers—you can have one or several depressive symptoms without being clinically depressed. Depression is classified as either major or minor, depending on how many symptoms are present and how long they last. Peter J. Schmidt, a doctor who has studied menopausal and perimenopausal mood, notes that "major depression has an estimated lifetime prevalence of 17 percent and affects approximately twice as many women as men."[9] Minor depression's prevalence is about the same as major.

In major depression, also called "clinical depression," a person suffers multiple symptoms for a long period of time in a way that starts interfering with her life. This can mean fighting symptoms for just a couple of months or for many years. If someone has a history of major depression, they may recognize the onset of a new bout in a matter of days. If you have never suffered a major depression, it may take you much longer to understand what you are going through.

Symptoms of depression include enduring sad or anxious mood, loss of interest in things that used to be pleasurable, frequent tears, feelings of worthlessness, helplessness, and hopelessness, eating and/or sleeping too much or too little, exhaustion, restlessness, agitation, and even, potentially, thoughts of violence or suicide. It can also cause a host of mysterious physical ailments, including joint pain, headaches, and stomach and digestive problems that are often misdiagnosed.

Dysthymia is a word we use to describe serious depression that causes milder symptoms than a classic major depression but is ongoing for a longer amount of time. Dysthymic people are often tired and generally lacking in enthusiasm for life.

Depression is a huge public health issue. One major study on the subject estimates that after heart disease, depression is the "leading source of disease-related disability in developed countries."[10]

People enter clinical depression for any number of reasons. As with so many chronic illnesses, genetics seem to play a role. People in families where depression is common are often at a greater risk for developing the problem themselves. Of course, it should be noted that not everybody with a family history develops the illness. And major depression can occur in people who do not have family members with the problem: "This suggests that additional factors, possibly biochemistry, environmental stressors and other psychosocial factors, are involved."[11]

It has been shown again and again that there is a relationship between substance abuse and depression. This becomes a "chicken and egg" question: Do stress and depression lead to greater drinking or drug use, or do the use and abuse of these substances lead to depression? The truth is probably a complicated tangle of the two, with one problem feeding and exacerbating the other.

There can be significant differences in the ways that ethnic and racial groups exhibit depression. African Americans are more likely to express somatic symptoms like aches and pains and/or headaches, when compared with whites or Latinas. This might be one reason why black Americans tend to be diagnosed less frequently than Americans in other racial groups.

Also, although the ratio of men to women equals out with age, one of the biggest undiagnosed depressed populations can be found among the elderly. People in this age group have unique challenges, including being widowed and dealing with health problems, isolation, and financial worries that younger working adults are less likely to be faced with.

Women and Depression

It is estimated that somewhere between 10 and 23 percent of women will experience a major depressive episode during their lives.[12]

Doctors observe that until puberty, depression rates among boys and girls are about the same, whereas after hormones begin kicking in, the rates among girls skyrocket.[13] This difference virtually disappears again after menopause, although female rates do remain higher than male rates into old age. These two things—the onset of higher rates of female depression at puberty and declining rates following menopause—have led some to theorize that perhaps fluctuating hor-

mones play a role in making women more susceptible to psychological problems. However, as the Mayo Clinic articulates, "Puberty is
also often associated with other changes that could play a role in depression, such as emerging sexuality and identity issues, parental
conflicts and evolving social expectations."[14]

So is it nature, nurture, or some indefinable combination of the
two? As in the case of women's sexual issues, it is very hard to separate the two and even harder to draw any conclusions about treatment based on such distinctions. We know, however, that women
across national, ethnic, and economic lines experience depression at
higher rates then men.

Let's travel down this road for a minute and ask how little ovaries
could cause such big sadnesses.

We know that the hormones we make in our reproductive organs
have an effect on our minds because scientists have found estrogen
receptors in the brain in places such as the pituitary and hypothalamus.[15] So it's at least possible that we have menopause "on the brain"
literally as well as figuratively, and hormones like estrogen, progestin,
and androgens have effects on the processes in the brain.[16]

However, the vast majority of scientific data suggests that there
is a limited connection between reproductive transitions—that is,
menarche, menstruation, and menopause—and the onset of depression. The majority of women not only do not become depressed at
menopause, they "don't experience significant mood changes."[17] So
whether or not female biology plays a role in increased rates of depression over a lifetime, it doesn't seem to be true that menopause
causes depression.

Peter J. Schmidt writes, "The majority of women do not develop
depression during the menopausal transition. . . . Studies report no
increased prevalence of major depression in women at midlife (age
range approximately 45–55 years)."[18] The National Institutes of
Health (NIH) makes no bones about it: "Menopause, in general, is
not associated with an increased risk of depression. In fact, . . . research has shown that depressive illness at menopause is no different
than at other ages. The more vulnerable to change-of-life depression
are those with a history of past depressive episodes."[19]

The *American Journal of Public Health* notes that while psychological distress (different from depression) is "associated" with irregular menses at midlife, it is impossible to tell which part of this is biological, environmental, or a combination of the two. It concludes that it is likely that "midlife stresses influence mood more than does menopausal status."[20]

So why do so many people, including doctors, assume that blue moods and menopause come hand in hand? And why do studies vary so wildly in their statistics and conclusions involving the numbers of menopausal women who experience depressive incidents? One reason, Schmidt points out, is that many studies don't differentiate between populations of women who already have histories of depression and those who do not.

Women who experienced major depressions as young women may be more likely to have another onset during the menopause transition.[21] This seems to be particularly true at the beginning of perimenopause, when estrogen levels are unusually high, and right after menopause, when levels are consistently much lower for the first time.[22]

If you are a woman who has struggled either at one time in your life or consistently over the years with depression, you should be aware that at menopause you are at a point of potential increased vulnerability. If you go to see a doctor about your menopause, this is part of your medical history that you should mention.

A recent study published in *Archives of General Psychiatry* found that women who had not experienced depression before menopause were more likely to undergo "new onset depressive symptoms and disorders."[23] Study authors observed that these symptoms were correlated with hormonal shifts. This may mean that some women do have depressions for the first time during menopause. However, it may also simply point to mood swings, which are in many ways like "depressive symptoms." A related Massachusetts General Hospital study found that women who go into menopause at younger ages were more likely to suffer from depression for the first time.[24]

Barbara would like to add to this that studies rarely if ever differentiate between women going through normal menopause and women who have had hysterectomies and/or oophorectomies. One Scandinavian study found that among women who had hysterectomies, those who chose to have their ovaries taken out had "higher anxiety . . . and poorer emotional partner relationships."[25] If you are thinking about having or have had a hysterectomy, before you get, well, sad about this, take note that other studies have emphasized the importance of education before the surgery in counteracting depression afterwards[26]—and also the importance of "partner support and knowledge."[27] That means making sure your partner, friends, children, or whoever comprises your support system understand what you are going through and can be there in an informed way to offer you emotional support.

Another nonmenopausal cause of midlife depression are thyroid problems. Research suggests that "anxiety and depressive symptoms were more severe in patients with overt hypo- and hyperthyroidism."[28]

Dr. Joyce T. Bromberger points out that "reproductive transitions are also times of psychological and social changes. Primary care physicians need to be sensitive to the potential effects of reproductive hormone changes, but not to assume that hormones are necessarily symptom inducing." She makes two important points here.

The first is that doctors may assume that menopause lies behind a woman's mood problems. This mistaken notion could lead to incorrect treatment and the overlooking of crucial life factors that are impacting a female patient.

The second point is that life transitions aren't just physical, they are often psychological. Although the evidence correlating menopause and depression is not good, there are excellent data to support a connection between stress and depression. Unfortunately, the time of life when women go through menopause can also be the time when careers are changing, children are growing up and moving away, romantic relationships are adjusting to middle age, and many other major stressors are occurring.

In addition to age-specific stresses, women across the world face additional pressure from a host of factors throughout their lives. The Mayo Clinic notes, "Women are more likely than men to shoulder the burden of both work and family responsibilities. . . . They're also more likely to have lower incomes, be single parents and have a history of sexual or physical abuse, all of which can contribute to depression."[29]

So what about mood swings? It seems pretty clear that they have some relationship to menopause and hormones, but what exactly is that relationship? "Researchers have confirmed that hormones have an effect on the brain chemistry that controls emotions and mood; a specific biological mechanism explaining hormonal involvement is not known."[30] This has a lot of implications. It's like saying, "We know that this man and this woman are related, but we're not sure how." And what you can know about the two people and how they relate to each other has everything to do with first knowing how they are connected. The same thing is true with trying to establish medical relationships, or causality.

So does menopause make our moods worse? Or does this transition simply allow us to vent long-pent-up feelings about people and events we have been dealing with for years?

On a great menopause online message board a woman writes, "I do feel that some of my own moodiness during peri—including phases of wanting to bite people's heads off for things I would have ignored earlier in life—has had a hormonal component. But in almost every specific case I can think of, the irritability didn't come out of thin air. There's always been something . . . word or deed, someone else's or my own—that truly bugged me. The hormonal element just sort of cranked up the volume of my reaction."[31]

Menopause, like PMS, puts a yellow highlighter on anything that's bothering us. The issues are real; but that said, our reactions can be more dramatic than they would have been previously—things we might have let go, we choose to tackle head-on.

In the Study of Women's Health Across the Nation (SWAN), researchers learned that perimenopausal women report more "psychological distress" than either pre- or postmenopausal women. Dr. Schmidt identifies late peri- and early postmenopause as the time where this "vulnerability" is most expressed. He writes that estradiol seemed to improve mood in perimenopausal women[32] but not in postmenopausal women, those five to ten years past menopause.[33] In other words, at a time when hormones could cut down on hot flashes or help you sleep through the night, they could help control your mood swings as well.

Prescribing ET and HT for women with mood problems during

menopause is complicated. While some women seem to benefit for one reason or another, others can actually become depressed when using hormone products (the same thing is true with birth control pills).

Lauren, a family counselor in Ohio, had bad experiences on birth control, at one point becoming seriously depressed and switching to another contraceptive method. The mood problems abated when the pills went away. When she became perimenopausal in the 1980s, her doctor put her on Prempro. She describes her experience: "Within five months I was walking along the river with my dog (a daily outing we loved). It was late December and the river was flowing rapidly. I looked at it and thought, 'If I jump in, all this depression will be over.' I knew these thoughts were not healthy. I went home and stopped the medication immediately."

The doctor switched Lauren to another HT preparation: "In September I was walking through an open field. I knew the asters were a beautiful blue, the Joe-pie was purple, goldenrod was yellow, and the sky should be brilliant blue, but everything looked grey and sad. I knew this had to be the medication depressing me again. That was the end of any HT medication, and my life rebounded in about three months. I have been very angry to learn that for many years the doctors have known the side effect of depression came to fifteen percent of Prempro medication users. I most certainly was one of them."

If you had a bad experience on birth control, you probably shouldn't try to manage menopause symptoms like hot flashes using HT. Regardless of your history with hormone products, you shouldn't take hormone products for primary prevention of depression.

St. John's Wort

St. John's wort, or *Hypericum perforatum,* is a very popular herb that is used to treat a variety of problems, including anxiety, insomnia, wound healing, kidney and lung problems, and burn recovery.

In Germany the herb is generally accepted as an alternative to prescription drugs for depression. In the United States it is a popular over-the-counter supplement. As with so many herbs, the exact mechanisms through which it works aren't understood. As Jerry Cott explains, "St. John's wort is one of the best known yet least understood of the modern herbals."[34] Originally a European plant, St. John's wort can now be found growing wild across the United States, but most people come into contact with it in the form of capsules, tinctures, and teas.

During the 1990s, St. John's wort's popularity rose alongside pharmaceutical antidepressants like Prozac and other SSRIs. Initial clinical data looked promising: an overview of twenty-three studies of the herb in the *British Medical Journal* found that it was more effective than the placebo and had fewer side effects than doctor-prescribed antidepressants.[35]

Suddenly St. John's wort was in everything: lip balm, tea, energy drinks, even cough drops. Especially at a moment when so many people were discovering the downsides of prescription antidepressants, the idea of a natural alternative made many feel there was hope. In the euphoria, few people slowed down to ask the important questions we must always face with herbal medicines: about supply, quality, dosage, drug interactions, and, most important, the lack of good placebo-controlled clinical trials.

Two major studies published in the *Journal of the American Medical Association* (*JAMA*) threw some cold water on the St. John's wort enthusiasm. The first, conducted by Richard Shelton and his colleagues, compared St. John's wort with a placebo and found no greater relief from the herb than from the sugar pill.[36] When the results of this trial were published, they drew a flood of criticism from natural medicine proponents and alternative practitioners, who pointed out methodological flaws as well as the fact that it was funded by Pfizer, the makers of Zoloft. Against this last charge, defenders of the trial pointed out that Pfizer was itself trying to develop a St. John's wort preparation and so had a financial stake in the study's success as well as its failure.

Another trial a year later—this one conducted by the National Institutes of Health—also concluded that St. John's wort was no better for major depression than the placebo. In their results, also published in *JAMA*, the scientists concluded that while some of the results might be due to problems with their study methods, "the complete absence of trends suggestive of efficacy for *H. perforatum* is noteworthy." [37]

While St. John's wort can boast multiple trials of varying length and quality (most herbals lack even tests of suspect quality), it has to contend with the fact that it has been tested in different quantities and forms in different places, which leads to inconsistent trial results. [38] Particularly in placebo-controlled trials, the benefit for major depression seems to be minimal. The jury is still out, but many people find benefits from supplements despite the serious questions raised by these two major studies. Whether this is the product of the placebo effect or an as-yet-unproven clinical benefit remains to be seen.

If you decide to try St. John's wort, you should know that it can interact with a number of drugs: chemotherapy and anticancer drugs (such as irinotecan), drugs to treat HIV/AIDS, and birth control pills. This last one is particularly significant for perimenopausal women because it is thought that it has something to do with the way the herb interacts with estrogen and its receptors. If this is true, there are obviously unexplored implications for women whose estrogen levels may be dramatically high at times, not to mention perimenopausal women who are still ovulating, because there may be a potential for St. John's wort to allow unintended pregnancies. In particular, use of St. John's wort with birth control pills has been shown to cause "intermenstrual bleeding," [39] bleeding between periods that perimenopausal women may already be contending with. Until the exact reasons why the herb causes this reaction are better understood, menopausal women should at least be thoughtful when considering it as a depression remedy.

Side effects of St. John's wort include dry mouth, dizziness, diarrhea, nausea, increased sensitivity to light, and tiredness.

Cognitive Therapy

Time and again, both some form of psychotherapy alone and the combination of drugs and therapy have been shown to be effective treatments for many depressions.

A particularly popular method is called "cognitive behavioral therapy," which focuses on getting patients to recognize and restructure negative thinking. The idea is that our thoughts determine our feelings and behavior. Unlike traditional therapy, which can go on indefinitely, CBT can be done in a shorter amount of time.

Employers are increasingly recognizing the benefits of counseling and therapy sessions, and many insurance companies will provide some—if not complete—coverage for sessions. If you are depressed, don't be afraid to seek counseling or ask your doctor to refer you.

Exercise

Another fantastic remedy for mood is exercise. James Blumenthal, a professor of medical psychology at Duke University, explains, "What the studies are showing is that exercise, at least when performed in a group setting, seems to be at least as effective as standard antidepressant medication in reducing symptoms in patients with major depression."[40] A study published in the *American Journal of Preventive Medicine* concluded that aerobic exercise (running, biking, or working on the elliptical machine—anything that gets your heart moving) could help treat mild to moderate depression.[41] Even though working out has been shown to be good for treating this problem, it's hard for people who are in a depressive state to motivate themselves to hit the gym.

Good Communication

One thing that will most certainly make your life better is if you can communicate how you are feeling and the things you are dealing with to your family and friends. Trying to keep bad feelings inside will make those who love you feel alienated. You may want to spare them the burden of your sorrow, but in the end they will feel you are distancing yourself from them and keeping something from them. Try to articulate what you are feeling and don't let anyone tell you that your feelings are just the result of menopause.

8

the secret hystery
the truth about hysterectomy and oophorectomy

madeline Gray was not a woman accustomed to helplessness. A journalist and author of several books, Gray was
still in her early forties when she underwent a total hysterectomy.
Later, in 1951, she would describe her experiences in a landmark
book about menopause, *The Changing Years*: "A few years ago I had
what is known as a surgical menopause—a change brought on by an
operation. That means I was thrown into the midst of this thing
headlong. I had no time even to get mentally 'set.'"[1]

Like most people in the 1940s and 1950s, Gray turned with
deeply engrained trust to her doctor for information. She was disappointed when he responded with dismissal: "While he . . . had done
an excellent job, he was both far too busy and too abrupt to bother
with me. . . . As to my future worries, he curtly dismissed them by
telling me to go home and forget about the whole thing. Besides, the
worries were all imaginary anyway."

Next Gray turned to her friends—and met profound ignorance
on all sides. Her qualms were answered with urban myths, horror
stories, and more questions; but Gray wasn't one to take this lack of
information sitting down. Instead she wrote a book that was one of
the first patient-to-patient guides to speak frankly about menopause.

If we asked you to guess what physical commonality one in three
American women have in common by the time they die, what would

you say? Perhaps you would guess cholesterol that exceeds a certain level or bones that have thinned. Would you be surprised to find out the answer is that they don't have a uterus?

It is estimated that around one-third of American women will undergo surgical removal of their uteruses and often their ovaries as well. That adds up to around six hundred thousand procedures a year and a $5 billion industry.[2] Many of these procedures are performed on women who are still getting periods, plunging them instantaneously into the discomforts of the change. The younger the woman at the time of ovary removal, the greater her suffering is likely to be.

Even experts are often astounded to find out that hysterectomy rates in the United States are still so high, assuming the days of routine uterine removal to have passed along with girdles and crinolines. How many of these surgeries are really necessary? If, scientifically speaking, we know so much more about women's bodies, why has so little changed?

If you take away one message from this chapter (if not this book), it should be that a menopause that happens surgically is not the same as one that happens naturally. A study performed on women who've undergone hysterectomy and oophorectomy just isn't applicable to women whose hormones have ebbed as the result of time and aging. So no matter which category you fall into, your first question when you hear about a new study on some type of menopause medicine should be: Did the women who were studied go through menopause naturally or surgically?

If we could get you to take away a second message, it's that many of the problems associated with hysterectomy are actually caused by oophorectomy.

It's no secret that if you and your ovaries part ways while you're still menstruating, you should brace yourself for a tough premature menopause and rapidly thinning bones. Less well understood is the fact that after menopause, your ovaries continue to make small amounts of estrogen for years, as well as testosterone and other androgens responsible for lust and desire. The removal of the ovaries also removes these hormones, which directly results in less vaginal lubrication and a thinning of the vaginal walls. This not only decreases a woman's sex drive but can make sex just plain uncomfortable.

Problems in the bedroom, unfortunately, are just the beginning of the concerns raised by unnecessarily cutting out our ovaries.

When a woman opts to have her uterus removed—for whatever reason—it is extremely common for the surgeon to take out her perfectly healthy ovaries as well.

"Most women consent to removal because they are led to believe that the ovaries cease functioning at menopause," says Nora Coffey, founder of the Hysterectomy Educational Resources and Service (HERS) Foundation. "They may not know that ovaries are the female gonads equivalent to a man's testes, and that the operation can diminish female sexual desire and responsiveness."

What Coffey is suggesting is that oophorectomy functions like castration. That's a scary word, and our intention isn't to get you upset (especially if you've already undergone the procedure). For some women in some circumstances, it's the best decision. We want to be honest with you, though. We want to have a frank conversation that has been left far too long to the silent, fear-plagued corners from which Madeline Gray fought fiercely to free herself. Far too many unnecessary procedures have been going on, and until we all start talking—and getting educated—this won't change.

The Missing Piece Meets the Big O

In the early 1970s, a freelance writer, editor, and mother of two daughters named Edith Sunley had a total hysterectomy.[3] After the surgery, she found that she experienced a "drastic libido loss." Among other things, Edith lost orgasmic sensation after the removal of her cervix. When she sought medical help for her troubles, her sex therapist encouraged her to do her own research and find out what other patients and their doctors had to say on the subject. After all, some women felt fine after surgery, while others were miserable.

At that point in time there were a lot of misconceptions among both doctors and patients about what happened to your sex life after total hysterectomy. Many male doctors claiming expertise on sexuality were almost sadistic in their views. For example, in an article called "Castration in the Female" in 1969, Dr. William Filler wrote that hysterectomy "triggers a neurotic reaction, guilt feelings related to masturbation, extramarital activities, or a previous criminal abortion." He added that for women, "hysterectomy is perceived as punishment for real or fancied sins." Doctors assumed that problems were all in women's minds. On the other side of the debate were women who insisted that all orgasms were clitoral and therefore removing internal organs wouldn't affect them.

Edith fought back, collecting studies and interviewing the most serious scientists in the field. What she found was that many women experienced serious sexual difficulties after hysterectomy. Before the operation, 76 percent of married women were having normal intercourse. After surgery, 45 percent gave up sex altogether, and another 35 percent were unhappy with their sex lives. Although she was never able to get her groundbreaking work on the subject published, she insured that we now have a record of the fact that women have known for some time that total hysterectomy greatly impacts and potentially damages sexual functioning.

In 1990, Maryann Napoli researched a total of fourteen studies that had been conducted to measure the sexual responsiveness of women following their hysterectomies. While the majority of women cited no change in their sexual responsiveness, a very significant minority, 35 percent, reported either a decrease in their sexual desire or an inability to orgasm.

The extent to which hysterectomy affects one's sex life is still a topic of intense debate. A 2004 study and a 2000 meta-analysis (a statistical analysis of a group of studies) found no significant change in either responsiveness or desire.[4] Larger trials, however, have come to the opposite conclusion. A British study of more than 8,900 women found that a significantly higher number of those who had undergone surgery experienced problems with sex, more still of those who had also had their ovaries out.[5] Others have found reduced vaginal and clitoral sensitivity.[6]

While the conversation stays open, it's interesting to note that during the nineteenth century, hysterectomies were used as a fix for "excessive female desire."[7]

Beverly Whipple, sex researcher and the author of *The Science of Orgasm*,[8] notes that "there are at least four different nerve pathways involved in sexual responses. If these nerves are cut or damaged, sexual response will change."[9] With the uterus and the cervix being key elements in many women's abilities to orgasm, is it surprising that the removal of such organs would make sex less enjoyable?

A Brief Hystery

Taking out a woman's uterus for medical reasons is an ancient procedure. Christopher Sutton notes that "the first operation was reputedly performed by Soranus in the Greek city of Ephesus in AD 120, although there is an even more vague reference to the procedure having been performed fifty years before the Common Era by Themison of Athens."[10] Hysterectomies continued to be performed occasionally in Europe throughout the Middle Ages and early modern years. These surgeries usually happened when the uterus prolapsed—pushed forward and out of the body. They usually ended tragically, because in addition to the problems of infection, sepsis, and blood loss, the bladder was often accidentally removed as well. All of these early procedures were performed through the vagina.

Modern gynecological surgery began in 1809 when Ephraim McDowell set out to remove a ten-pound ovarian tumor from the abdomen of a Kentuckian named Jane Todd Crawford. Sutton notes, "In these litigious times surgeons are naturally apprehensive of the outcome of their work, but pity poor Ephraim McDowell who had to contend with the knowledge that several of his townsfolk were erecting a gallows for him, should the patient die at the hands of 'the dreadful doctor.'"[11] Luckily for both Crawford and McDowell, the operation was a success, and the first abdominal gynecological procedure had taken place. Crawford went on to live another thirty-two years, and a memorial hospital in Greensburg, Kentucky, is named for her.

The path from cyst removal to intentionally taking out the uterus happened because of misdiagnoses. Doctors would cut into the abdomen hoping to remove a cyst, only to have a fibroid emerge. Unsure of how to put the fibroid back, doctors opted to try removing the whole organ. Charles Clay, a British physician, was the first to try this intentionally in 1843, and sadly lost several patients to hemorrhage shortly following the procedure. Twenty years later Clay would become the first to successfully perform the operation in Europe, but not before the original honor went to an American, Ellis Burnham, in 1853. In the earliest years, women had the common dangers of medical procedures before the twentieth century to contend with. They also had the trauma of surgeries performed without the benefit of the anesthesia that would become increasingly available only as the nineteenth century drew to a close.

The earliest modern oophorectomy occurred in November 1856 in Tennessee. A young African-American woman named Matilda was suffering bleeding and a tumor following a failed pregnancy. Dr. William J. Baker and several colleagues etherized the young woman and then removed her uterus, fallopian tubes, and ovaries. Matilda lived on for thirty-four more years.[12] While Matilda's hysterectomy, if not her oophorectomy, were necessary, women in the black community are still far more likely than their white counterparts to undergo this surgery without good cause.

As the years passed and mortality declined, due in part to changes in surgical technique and better attention to instrument sterilization, hysterectomy changed from being an emergency procedure and a last resort to being a first-line defense against gynecological ailments and cancer. Sutton adds, "Almost inevitably, the increased safety of the operation led to an explosive increase in the number of hysterectomies performed."[13]

The Elephant (Egg) in the Room

The issue patients and doctors alike have been most concerned about, quite understandably, is the specter of ovarian cancer, which is extremely difficult to detect, especially in its early stages when the five-year survival rate is a high 90 percent. The overall five-year survival rate—only 37 percent—is a testament to how rarely the disease is caught in time. "What I see often enough are women who had hysterectomies at forty-nine, and then at fifty-nine they have ovarian cancer, and I feel bad that this was a missed opportunity to prevent disease," says Michael Prefontaine, MD, at Baystate Hospital in Springfield, Massachusetts, reflecting the long-held consensus of the medical community. "Of course I don't see all of the other women who keep their ovaries and do well."[14]

If ovarian cancer is the justification for taking the ovaries along with the uterus, the rationales for hysterectomy are far more numerous. Among them are heavy bleeding, uterine fibroids, endometriosis, uterine prolapse, pelvic pain, and, of course, uterine or cervical cancer[15] (we'll talk more about these various problems in chapter 9). It seems worth noting that fibroids—one of the most common reasons for hysterectomy in the United States—usually significantly improve and disappear after menopause.

For some patients, though, hysterectomy is absolutely the right answer. Some critics have insisted that if only 10 percent of procedures are performed because of cancer, that means that 90 percent of hysterectomies can be avoided. Different paths are right for different people; in the end, patients must decide for themselves if the benefits of surgery outweigh the costs. The answer for some women is a resounding yes. There are, however, many less drastic—and even nonsurgical—alternatives for many of these very serious gynecological problems.

Consider this: "American women are twice as likely to have a hysterectomy as women in England and four times as likely as Swedish women. French doctors almost never perform a hysterectomy for fibroids, which is the most common reason for hysterectomy in this country."[16] Such big differences from country to country suggest, among other things, that a certain amount of subjectivity is involved in making the decision to perform the surgery. If the operation were clearly the best or only option, you simply wouldn't have such significant international variance.

Hysterectomies Are Not All Alike

If you were surprised to hear that so many women are still undergoing surgery, you may be further amazed to find out that the most common form of hysterectomy is still the one that carries the most risks and adverse affects and has the longest recovery time.

There are several types of operations, but all hysterectomies involve the removal of the uterus, and most require hospitaliza-tion as well as a significant recovery time lasting at least four to six weeks.

Total Hysterectomy The most common form of hysterectomy. It in-volves removing the entire uterus as well as the cervix.

Subtotal or Supracervical Hysterectomy Removal of only the upper body of the uterus. The cervix is left in place.

Radical Hysterectomy A procedure in which the uterus, cervix, and upper vagina are removed.

Oophorectomy Removal of one or both ovaries.

Bilateral Salpingo-Oophorectomy Both fallopian tubes and both ova-ries are removed.

(Madeline Gray objected to this overly technical terminology, pre-ferring to call removal of the uterus and ovaries together a "total" or "Pan-Hysterectomy."[17])

There are several methods by which these various procedures are performed. The most common is called an "abdominal hysterec-tomy." To do this, a surgeon cuts into the abdominal wall. It is similar to what happens when a woman has a cesarean section (which is, in-cidentally, the only surgery more common in female patients). The recovery time is estimated at four to eight weeks or longer.

Another technique involves going through the vagina, and in-creasingly, doctors are performing laparoscopic surgery to remove the uterus. This minimally invasive technique uses small incisions to insert medical equipment and conduct the surgery internally. Both vaginal and laparoscopic surgeries leave patients with recovery times that are measured in days, not weeks or months.

So why would doctors push a more invasive and potentially risky method? We can think of two big reasons: in the short term, a surgeon requires specialized, more intensive training to perform laparoscopy, and if a doctor can make the same amount of money by sticking with the simpler, old-fashioned method, she has little incentive to move outside her comfort zone. In addition, each lapa-roscopy takes longer to perform than traditional abdominal hysterectomy. If a doctor is trying to maximize the surgeries he can perform in a week, recommending a laparoscopic procedure is not his best bet.

If you are considering having a hysterectomy, make sure you explore all your options. Ask your doctor questions about potential adverse effects, recovery times, fatality rates, and anything else that is relevant or of concern to you. Don't let your questions be dismissed; you deserve to have all the facts before you make such an important choice.

If you are having a hysterectomy, don't be pressured into "having it all out." Even though many women retain more sexual sensation and sustain less damage to the bladder and intestines by having less of their uterus removed, leaving the lower part of the uterus and the cervix in place, many doctors are hesitant to go with a more moderate approach because of concerns that it leaves patients more vulnerable to cancer. This is a very serious concern, but it is worth considering that tests like the Pap smear and genetic screening for vulnerabilities to cancer have made it less necessary for many patients to take drastic measures to prevent gynecological cancer.

Parker's "Aha!" Moment

For many years, William Parker, a California-based gynecologist and medical school professor, believed that it was "good prevention" for women forty-five and older to relinquish their ovaries when they went for a hysterectomy and that after menopause these once-productive little glands turned into ticking cancer time bombs that were better out than in.

What changed Parker's mind was not a doctor nor a scientist, but a layperson who had her own thoughts about women's health. In 1984, Janine O'Leary Cobb, a Canadian mother of five and professor of humanities and sociology at Vanier College in Montreal, started *A Friend Indeed,* the grandmother of menopause newsletters. Parker says it was her review of his book, *A Gynecologist's Second Opinion*, published in 1996, that got him thinking. She'd liked it, except for his position on removal of the ovaries during hysterectomy. She'd heard from too many newsletter readers who complained about loss of energy, concentration, interest in sex, and even interest in living after having their ovaries removed. "I never forgot your comments," he wrote to her years later. "I want to thank you for putting some doubt in my mind that what I had been taught may not have been well thought out or true."

Parker understood how many of the ovaries removed each year were perfectly healthy and at low risk of becoming cancerous. He wanted to find out what the result of all this potentially unnecessary cutting was. He knew that an ideal scientific trial would involve about 10,000 women scheduled to have hysterectomies. They'd be randomly divided into two groups—one group would have their ovaries removed, the other would keep them—and monitored for decades. But what sane woman would give up her right to keep her ovaries or not? Clearly this was not going to happen.

So Parker got in touch with his former student Michael Broder, MD, a gynecologist and an expert on health outcomes research, who had longed to contribute to changing ideas about oophorectomy ever since he was a third-year medical student in 1989 at Case Western Reserve University. "I was on rotation in surgery," Broder recalls. "A youngish woman was being wheeled into the operating room. She cried out to her surgeon, 'I don't want my ovaries out.' The doctor scolded her, 'What if you get ovarian cancer some day, and I would have been the one who left the ovaries in. That could be malpractice.'" As a student, Broder felt he couldn't say anything, "but I wanted to tell the woman to jump off the operating table and run," he says.

Parker and Broder decided to take data from two hundred quality studies and use a mathematical model to estimate the survival impact of leaving the ovaries in versus taking them out. Broder introduced Parker to Zhimei Liu, PhD, a native of China who was an authority on bringing modeling techniques to clinical medicine.

Parker invited Jonathan Berek, MD, an eminent gynecologic oncologist, surgeon, and chair of Obstetrics & Gynecology at Stanford University School of Medicine, and the editor of widely used textbooks on the field, to join them, along with Donna Shoupe, MD, a gynecologist and endocrinologist at the University of Southern California Medical Center who'd been pleading with her colleagues to go easy on the ovaries for twenty years. "I saw that the practice of taking out healthy ovaries continued in the face of huge information on negative consequences to heart and bones," she tells us. "The gynecologists only know half the story because they don't take care of heart disease."

Cindy Farquhar, MD, a New Zealand–based world-class epidemiologist who studies hysterectomies, completed the team.

The Results

The findings were far more dramatic than any of the researchers expected. Based on their model, if 10,000 women between the ages of fifty and fifty-four undergo a hysterectomy with oophorectomy, they will have forty-seven fewer cases of ovarian cancer by the time they reach eighty than a similar group who keep their ovaries. The oophorectomy group, however, will suffer 838 additional deaths from coronary heart disease as well as 158 more deaths from hip fractures. (These numbers reflect women who do not have estrogen therapy; with estrogen, women without ovaries live longer, but that assumes staying on the drug forever.) "Forty-seven women are spared ovarian cancer but at a cost of almost nine hundred women's lives whose hearts and bones failed without the normal hormone support made by the ovaries," says Parker. Unless a woman is at high risk of developing ovarian cancer based on genetic testing or family history, the study showed, there is no real advantage of removing the ovaries.[18]

In 1990, Maryann Napoli stated that unless there is a history of ovarian cancer in the family, a woman's chances of getting the cancer are only one in one hundred. Fortunately, the most recent studies show the risk of ovarian cancer to be even less common than previously thought—one in two hundred for those without a genetic predisposition. Compare that to heart disease, which kills one out of two women.

Educating both women and doctors about the symptoms of ovarian cancer could save many a woman's ovaries: according to Dr. Jonathan Berek, these include unexplained change in bowel or bladder habits, gastrointestinal upset (gas, indigestion, nausea), unexplained weight loss or gain, pelvic or abdominal pain or discomfort,

bloating or swelling, a constant feeling of fullness, fatigue, and abnormal bleeding.

A Sad Hystery: The Press, Hormone Therapy, and Science by Press Release

While Dr. Parker is fighting to keep women's ovaries in place, a separate but related battle is currently emerging that also relates deeply to
oophorectomy. Since the Women's Health Initiative (WHI) cast
doubt on the effects that hormone therapy (HT) and estrogen therapy (ET) had on cardiovascular health, doctors and scientists have
been scrambling to recast the "estrogen and heart" conversation in
terms that aren't so negative. Since the WHI findings about HT, ET,
and the heart, a slew of headlines have been speculating on the benefits that estrogen has for younger women's cardiac health. The most
recent "shot across the bow" is a study published in the *New England
Journal of Medicine* that argues that younger women can have healthier hearts if they pop their hormone pills.[19] Particularly alluring is the
fact that this trial uses WHI data to make its point.

What might not jump out from the findings but is absolutely
crucial is that the data used was from the estrogen-only arm of the
trial. That means that all the women being analyzed had already undergone surgery and had either a partial or total hysterectomy before
joining WHI.[20] Even more significant: their younger ages at the time
of hysterectomy (average age was in the early to mid forties) suggest
that many of them did so while still menstruating.

Throughout the past several decades, again and again, data involving hysterectomized and oophorectomized women is presented
as though it is about natural menopause. This simply isn't true.
Women who have had a surgical menopause are actually more likely
to benefit from estrogen and will react to hormone therapy in dramatically different ways from their sisters who have had natural
menopauses. This absolutely crucial nuance is lost in seductive but
simplistic headlines that proclaim, "Estrogen Shows Benefit for
Heart Health," "When HRT Helps the Heart," and "Doctors
Change Course Again on Estrogen Therapy." It is incredibly misleading to imply that *most women* would benefit from taking estrogen

and, in fact, the authors of the original article never implied such. Amazingly, this article wasn't even looking at actual heart attacks: it was measuring coronary artery calcification, just one risk factor in a heart attack.

For Barbara, this is eerily familiar. In her 2003 book, *The Greatest Experiment Ever Performed on Women*, she described how, in 1982, a radiologist named Harry Genant conducted an experiment on thirty-seven women who had had their ovaries removed. Importantly, these women had all been menstruating at the time their ovaries were taken out and thus their bodies were quickly thrown into a state of surgical menopause. Genant wanted to discover if giving these women Premarin would prevent them from losing bone mass. He discovered that the women in the trial who had received Premarin each day were much more able to retain bone mass than the women on the placebo. He published his results in an excellent *Annals of Internal Medicine* paper called "Quantitative Computed Tomography of Vertebral Spongiosa: A Sensitive Method of Detecting Early Bone Loss after Oophorectomy."

Genant's very important find was very soon distorted. As Barbara stated, "Something got lost in translation—the truth." The fact that the women in the trial had all had their ovaries removed was completely omitted from most reports of Genant's study in the popular media, and women were soon being advised to take HT in order to keep their bones healthy. It appears that the same thing is happening now, only it is the health of the heart that is being promoted.

If you have had an oophorectomy—particularly if you did so as a young woman while you were still menstruating—you may need to take ET. A study from the Mayo Clinic in 2005 confirmed the findings of the Parker study about oophorectomy and increased mortality.[21] Led by Dr. Walter Rocca, the Mayo doctors found that women who had one or more ovaries removed before menopause were at greater risk for serious neurological illnesses, particularly Parkinson's and Alzheimer's disease. It seems—although it's not certain—that for this small group of women (that is, premenopausal women under forty-five who have had ovaries removed) taking ET may help prevent certain health problems.[22]

A hard-hitting *Time* magazine piece asks, "Too Many Hysterectomies?" and concludes that this "drastic procedure," which upsets "a woman's hormonal balance and was a possible danger to her emotional balance as well" should be curtailed and used only in necessary situations.[23] This piece could have been written last week, but it wasn't. Instead, it graced the magazine's pages in 1969. Let's not take another forty years to start asking important questions about the real consequences of gynecological surgery and insisting on better alternatives. Like Madeline Gray, let's keep pushing when we aren't satisfied, and be a part of locating the solutions the future has the potential to bring.

9

down under
vaginal and reproductive health as you age

I would encourage women to be reluctant to give up any of their organs until someone can prove to them it is in their health's interest.

—Dr. William Parker

Stephanie, a forty-two-year-old African-American woman and a busy college professor at a small New England liberal arts school, was shocked when her doctor discovered fibroids during a routine gynecological exam. He told her that they were causing her belly to protrude a little—she thought she had just put on weight—and that they could cause other health problems as well, including the bleeding she had come to believe was the onset of perimenopause. Her doctor suggested she consider hysterectomy.

Stephanie still harbored the hope of having children someday, but she had put so much effort and love into her career that she just hadn't found the time. Now, tenured and in a committed relationship with another academic, a family seemed like a real possibility, a possibility that hysterectomy would eliminate. And what if she chose not to have the surgery? What problems could she expect?

Some estimates say that 40 percent of American women develop uterine fibroids at some point in their lives,[1] making fibroids more common than blue eyes.[2] Other estimates are much higher: Dr. William Parker writes that "more than 75 percent of women can be found to have small fibroids" when examined with high-tech imaging equipment.[3] Any woman can develop fibroids, although we do know that among African-American women the instance is higher. Although fibroids are almost always benign, meaning they won't start as or become cancer, these small masses are the leading cause of hysterectomies in the United States, becoming the rationale for one out of every three of the 600,000 surgeries performed each year.[4]

As with so many other aspects of gynecological medicine, no one knows why fibroids happen. They begin as irregular cells in or on the uterine wall. They grow, forming small mounds of uterine tissue that look, depending on the type of fibroid, like new potatoes, tulip bulbs, or a ginger root. They can be pink, yellow, or light blue in color. They can vary in size as well, ranging from nearly imperceptibly small growths to something around the size of a basketball; the largest reported fibroid weighed 140 pounds.[5] Most will be somewhere between the size of a chestnut and a tennis ball.

Fibroids pose almost no serious health risks, but inconveniences can range from none at all to more frustrating or painful problems. The most common side effects associated with fibroids are worsened periods, bleeding, and abdominal pain and pressure. Occasionally, women also suffer from difficulty with urination, and very rarely fibroids can cause problems with pregnancy or miscarriage. According to Dr. Susan Love, the most common side effect of fibroids is excess bleeding, sometimes bad enough to make anemia a danger.[6]

Some of the biggest problems with fibroids are cosmetic: the really big ones can make the belly protrude, creating a physical resemblance to a pregnancy. Perhaps because of this, some gynecologists will refer to the size of a fibroid in gestational terms—a "twelve-weeker," for example, being about the size of a three-month-old fetus.[7] Even these larger fibroids are often not dangerous but just unattractive or at worst uncomfortable.

There are three major types of uterine fibroids: *submucosal*, which grow from the inside of the uterine wall into the uterus; *intramural*, which actually grow in the wall itself; and *subserosal*, which grow on the outside of the uterus. Instead of growing directly on the uterine wall, some fibroids will develop a branch or an arm called a "pedicle" that anchors them. Fibroids with pedicles can create more serious problems. As experts at the Harvard Medical School explain, "The stalk remains attached to the uterine wall, allowing the tumor to swing inside the uterus or into the abdominal cavity. As the uterus contracts in an effort to rid itself of this 'foreign body,' the pedicle may become twisted, causing bleeding, pain and sometimes infection."[8] In rare instances, the pedicle may become long enough that the fibroid may actually stick through the vagina.

It has been suggested that fibroids have to do with the body's response to estrogen and possibly progesterone.[9] Dr. William Parker explains that "each individual fibroid starts from a single cell growing the wrong way."[10] We know that estrogen plays a role, because "fibroids do not occur before puberty, when estrogen and progesterone production begins, and once a woman has a fibroid, it will shrink after menopause." What this means is that if you have fibroids and you can hang in there for a few years, the problem will most likely get much better. For some women, however, that is a difficult "if."

The relationship between fibroid growth and estrogen and progesterone is not straightforward. Although there is a burst of hormones at puberty, fibroids rarely develop until later in the reproductive years. Dr. Parker writes that "you might expect that women with fibroids are making too much estrogen or progesterone. . . . However, if we measure hormone levels in the blood, these women have absolutely normal amounts."[11] Instead it seems likely that the cells that become fibroids metabolize estrogen and progesterone differently.

In recent decades, some gynecologists have begun to question hysterectomy as a response to fibroids. As doctors at Cornell Medical School explain, "Fibroid removal is almost always an elective procedure—if they are not causing you a problem, you don't need to treat them."[12] Dr. Parker is even more explicit:

> Surgery is only reasonable if you have symptoms that truly warrant the risk, time, stress and money that an operation entails. Remember, most patients with uterine fibroids need no treatment. If you have fibroids, the odds are you will not need to do anything about them. . . . I consider careful observation to be the primary treatment option.[13]

Many women choose to live with fibroids—why wouldn't you if they're small enough that they can't be seen and aren't causing problems? That said, let's assume you have fibroids that are disrupting your life because of heavy bleeding or discomfort, or you're concerned about the (extremely rare) risk of cancer, or the bleeding is beginning to interfere with your daily life. Maybe you have one of the more serious problems caused by overgrown fibroids—like the blocking of blood flow to the legs and heart, causing swelling and potentially putting you at risk for blood clots. What are your options for dealing with the fibroids besides hysterectomy?

One of the most long-standing surgical procedures to deal with fibroids is called *myomectomy*. Unlike hysterectomy, this option helps women like Stephanie retain their fertility. It involves entering the abdominal cavity and individually removing each fibroid. It can be done by actually opening the abdominal cavity (abdominal myomectomy) or by inserting high-tech surgical equipment in through the belly button or vagina (laparoscopic or hysteroscopic myomectomy). Compared with hysterectomies—at 200,000 fibroid-justified surgeries a year—the procedure is rare. It is estimated that around 18,000 myomectomies are done in the United States each year.

If you decide to have an abdominal myomectomy, the doctor will inject the uterus with Pitressin (vasopressin, a chemical that slows bleeding).[14] After making an incision just above the pubic line, the doctor cuts the uterine tissue, pulling it aside. The fibroids are then separated from the uterus, and the organ is sewn back up. Because it is an invasive procedure, the recovery period for an abdominal myomectomy is about as long as for a hysterectomy, four to eight weeks. While the other types of myomectomy are far less traumatic for the body, they sometimes cannot be used for either particularly large or numerous fibroids or for certain growths on the outside of the uterus.[15]

Laparoscopic myomectomy involves inserting a tiny camera containing surgical equipment into the abdominal cavity through the navel. It works best for dealing with small growths on the outside of the uterus, while hysteroscopic myomectomy, which uses a small camera inserted directly into the uterus through the vagina, is better for treating tumors inside the uterus.[16] Both of these options cause relatively little physical trauma and have short healing times—around a week. While doctors are removing increasingly large fibroids with these tools, there are still some that are too big for laparoscopic or hysteroscopic surgeries.

All three procedures are most probably temporary solutions, with studies suggesting that somewhere between 25 and 50 percent of patients experience a recurrence of fibroids.[17] In a study of 145 women with a medium age of thirty-eight, 27 percent were able to give birth after having the surgery.

Another increasingly common surgical intervention is called *uterine fibroid embolization* (UFE). Unlike most uterine surgeries, this procedure is performed by a specialist called an interventional radiologist. This doctor inserts a catheter into the main artery of one of the legs and threads it through to the uterine artery. While myomectomy is a removal procedure, UFE injects tiny plastic particles into the uterus. These pellets act as a plug, blocking the flow of blood to the fibroids. Starved of blood, the fibroids soon shrink or even disappear. After embolization, most women experience cramping and abdominal pain, and some women have far more severe side effects.

UFE is a new, undertested, and fairly controversial surgery; the first procedures were performed around 1995.[18] Carla Dionne, the executive director of the National Uterine Fibroid Foundation and an advocate of the procedure, sees the small number of embolizations performed and the dearth of information on it as the result of a power struggle between different types of care providers, namely the interventional radiologists on the one hand and the gynecologists and surgeons, on the other. She suggests that gynecologists are protecting their interests by limiting the number of surgeries performed by alternative providers.

There are other very serious concerns about UFE, and we feel that such an optimistic view of it is unwise while it remains undertested. For example, it's not conclusively known what effect the procedure has on fertility. UFE is not a good way to deal with either large fibroids or subserosal growths with pedicles. While some pamphlets advocating the procedure rave that it is "minimally invasive" with few side effects except mild cramping, that is not the experience of every woman. The authors of this book know women who have experienced such terrible pain following UFE that they were forced to go back and undergo hysterectomy.

More distressing problems include developing increasing pelvic pain and fever. This can stem from several causes, including free-floating fibroids that occur when their pedicles deteriorate, and a condition called postembolization syndrome. The latter can involve serious infection (sepsis) that must be treated with heavy doses of antibiotics and has a long recovery period; it can, in fact, be fatal. Misembolization happens when the plastic pellets end up where they don't belong. One particularly frightening example: "One patient reported in the medical literature, the particles went to the wrong blood vessel and caused the breakdown of her buttocks."[19] Another more frequent complication involves the loss of clitoral sensation.

When you are considering a new procedure you must decide, first, if you really need any surgical procedure at all; and second, if you are ready to bear the responsibility of trying something new that may come with unanticipated or more serious side effects than you expected. "New" is rarely a favorable adjective in medicine for surgery as well as drugs; it often simply means "unproven."

On the monetary side of things, because UFE is considered a new procedure, it isn't covered by many insurance companies and can end up costing around $15,000 if you are paying for it out-of-pocket. Dionne argues that this is another problem between the gynecologists and the interventional radiologists—in order to get the surgery approved by many insurance companies, you have to get approval from a gynecologist.

Myolysis is a procedure that uses laproscopic electrical currents to shrink blood vessels. Like UFE, the impact of this procedure on fertility is dubious. Both the scar tissue that may form as a result of this intervention and its potentially adverse influence on the uterine wall are thought to be potential dangers to future childbearing. Whenever blood flow to the ovaries is blocked, early menopause also becomes a risk.

Another experimental technique is *endometrial ablation*, used primarily to treat women who are experiencing heavy bleeding with their fibroids. It does this by using lasers and heat or a balloon with hot liquid to destroy the uterine lining. Obviously this is not a good option for women who are still hoping to have children because in many cases it permanently destroys the cells that produce menstrual blood and provide the physical environment for a fetus to grow.

If you decide you don't want surgery but find that you want to take action to reduce your fibroids, your doctor may suggest some pharmaceutical options. Unfortunately, none of the drug alternatives are very good.

GnRH (gonadotropin-releasing hormone, the messenger the brain sends to trigger hormone release and ovulation) is used by doctors to shrink fibroids. In this case the chemical is manipulated to prevent ovulation instead of trigger it. This happens when the hormone is manipulated in a lab to change its duration in the bloodstream. The result is that instead of causing the body to release estrogen and progesterone to cause menstruation, production of estrogen and progestin is suspended by the ovaries. Without the chemicals serving as food, fibroids starve and grow smaller. As soon as you stop taking the drug, fibroids start absorbing hormones again and begin to grow. Because of this, GnRH is used primarily to make fibroids smaller so that they can be more easily removed with surgery. Two common GnRH drugs used for this purpose are Synarel and Lupron. These are very serious drugs, and there is a lot we don't know about their dangers, particularly about their cancer risks. At the very least they can cause side effects that resemble more severe menopause symptoms. And the cost can be prohibitive: up to $2,000 a year, often uncovered by insurers.

Birth control pills have been used to shrink fibroids, although some women find that they have the opposite effect. For years it was thought that lots of women experienced fibroid growth taking oral contraceptives, but now it seems more likely that this is a rare side effect.

Because of the unpredictable effect of estrogen and progesterone drugs on fibroids, women going through the menopause transition who suffer from fibroids should think twice about taking HT for the symptoms of perimenopause. It has long been suggested that HT aggravates fibroids. A study published in the December 2001 *Obstetrics and Gynecology* found that women with fibroids were able to use the birth control patch without growth enlargement, but much more research is still needed to justify the recommendation.[20]

Given that fibroids tend to shrink after menopause, the reduction and elimination of fibroids are one of the many benefits of getting through the change. When other aspects of the transition are getting you down, keep some of these positive things in mind.

Endometriosis

Endometrial tissue makes up the lining of the uterus. It is the thing that thickens each month and then breaks down and becomes menstrual blood. Sometimes this tissue grows on the outside of the uterus, the ovaries, pelvic area, or bladder, and still breaks down in accordance with monthly cycles. The blood has nowhere to go and becomes trapped in the body, leading to scar tissue and cysts. This process can be painful and can lead to fertility problems. It doesn't, however, cause cancer.

Like fibroids, endometriosis usually resolves itself after menopause. The diagnosis is often made during a pelvic exam or with a sonogram, although, as Ingrid A. Rodi explains, "the diagnosis of endometriosis can only be confirmed by looking at the pelvic organs at the time of surgery."[21] Doctors often treat this problem hormonally with either birth control pills or progestin treatment. Two other drugs, danazol (Danocrine) and GnRH, are used as well.

Danazol is a synthetic steroid that acts like testosterone in the body, and like testosterone therapy, it has masculinizing effects, including facial hair, deepening of the voice, shrinking of the breasts, weight gain, and acne. GnRH drugs include Lupron, Zoladex, and Synarel. Besides being powerful medications with a host of unanswered questions swirling around them, including cancer concerns, they are a poor choice for perimenopausal women because they cause menopause symptoms and aggravate bone thinning. Although they act through different mechanisms, all of the drugs used to treat endometriosis work by reducing estrogen in the body and starving the errant tissue of its nutrients.

Endometriosis was (and to some extent remains) a cause for hysterectomies. While many women with this problem may not require any treatment, let alone a pharmaceutical or surgical alternative, so-called conservative surgery can be used in severe cases as an alternative to hysterectomy and oophorectomy. This procedure removes endometrial tissue and scar tissue from the outside of the reproductive organs. It can be temporary, and women who pursue this option often find that endometriosis recurs.

Adenomyosis

Adenomyosis is a noncancerous condition that is often mistaken for fibroids. This problem occurs in few women—less than 10 percent and can cause pain and bleeding. It happens when cells that line the uterus grow directly onto its muscle. When the cells bleed each month as part of the menstrual cycle, they irritate surrounding muscles. The condition is considered harmless but causes severe cramping, menstrual periods, and pain. Adenomyosis tends to develop after childbirth, and there is some belief it is associated with it—particularly if you have a caesarean. The bad news is that there is no effective treatment for adenomyosis except hysterectomy. The good news is that like fibroids, the problem often resolves after menopause when the hormones that trigger menstrual bleeding dip.[22]

Ovarian Cysts

The ovary is a particularly striking organ to look at. White and full of waves and ridges, ovaries resemble little seashells or miniature brains on either side of the uterus. For something so small, the ovaries do quite a lot. Not only do they make reproduction possible, but they continue to manufacture hormones long after the reproductive years.

Ovaries can cause a lot of problems too.

A common problem is benign cysts. Ovarian cysts come, like families, in functional and dysfunctional varieties. Many noncancerous ovarian growths are called *functional cysts*. They are fluid-filled pouches that develop on the side of the ovary, usually as a by-product of ovulation.[23] They form, remain for several months (typically one to three) and then shrink and disappear. Like fibroids, functional cysts tend not to occur after menopause, but they can be much worse when you are perimenopausal.

There are several ways functional cysts occur. When the body is getting ready to ovulate, it produces a follicle, a cystlike cellular structure that makes hormones and eventually ruptures to release an egg. A follicular cyst happens when luteinizing hormone doesn't cause ovulation and the follicle never releases an egg. About the size of an almond or a small grape, follicular cysts are rarely dangerous, rarely cause pain, and often disappear on their own within a couple months.[24]

If the body does manage to ovulate, and the follicle keeps growing, it can turn into something called a *corpus luteum cyst*. (*Corpus luteum* is a term used to describe the follicle once it has released an egg.) Sometimes, as the egg bursts from the follicle and heads down the fallopian tube, it seals off the follicle, trapping fluid inside. The follicle may continue to grow and become a cyst. Corpus luteum cysts usually go away on their own in a short amount of time, perhaps as little as several weeks.[25] Once in a while, more serious complications can develop, including the cyst growing to four inches in diameter, bleeding, and even twisting the ovary.[26] If you are taking certain drugs, including the fertility drug Clomid, you may be at a higher risk for developing this kind of problem. Make sure you share this sort of information with your doctor when assessing potential causes of pain or discomfort.

After menopause, the possibility of having a *dysfunctional cyst* is higher. A dermoid cyst forms from the same material as a human egg. They are rarely cancerous but can get very large and be painful. The Mayo Clinic explains that because they grow from egg materials, dermoid cysts may "contain tissue such as hair, skin or teeth." Like corpus luteum cysts, they can grow in a way that twists the ovary and causes lots of pelvic pain. Cystadenomas can also cause ovarian twisting. They are very large cysts—up to 12 inches—that are filled with a thick, mucuslike fluid. Endometriomas happens because of endometriosis (a condition where tissue that usually grows on the inside of the uterus grows on the exterior), and has something in common with subserosal fibroids. Endometriomas grow on the outside of the uterus and can attach to your ovaries.

Cysts can be discovered in a number of ways, but the most common is through a pelvic exam. If the doctor discovers cysts, he will probably suggest a sonogram. The doctor will want to consider the size and shape of the cyst, if it is filled with fluid, and a number of other factors to determine whether treatment is necessary. As long as you're not having terrible pain, most functional cysts can be left alone and periodically monitored. If your doctor is concerned, he might suggest having a laparoscopy. This procedure helps establish how big the cyst is and whether it should be removed.

A laparotomy is a slightly more invasive procedure designed to remove the cyst. Be very clear if you opt for laparotomy that you are not agreeing to oophorectomy. Be very firm with your doctor on this subject; you might want to put your wishes in writing for your records. A laparotomy allows the doctor to test for ovarian cancer. Another important reason to be sure about what sort of procedure you are having is that if cancer is discovered, the doctor may decide to take out the ovaries, uterus, and possibly the lymph nodes and omentum. These decisions can be made while you are still under anesthesia, so you need to understand exactly what the surgery involves and discuss all possibilities with your doctor prior to the surgery.

Most cysts require no treatment. Don't be unnecessarily pressured by health care professionals into treating cysts if you don't want to.

Uterine Prolapse

Another common cause of hysterectomy is *uterine prolapse.* This happens when the stress of having children, or just of aging, weakens the muscles in the pelvic region. In particular, the muscles that hold the uterus lose strength, and it drops down or lowers its position in the pelvis. As Dr. Christine K. Cassel explains, the uterus "can sag down into the vagina, or it can actually protrude outside the vagina. In either case it is uncomfortable." When the uterus shifts position, it can cause problems for the bladder and bowels. Unfortunately, as with so many urogenital problems, the major symptom is aching and pain in the abdominal area, and it can be very difficult to tell what sort of problem you are suffering from because so many of these conditions start with light to moderate pelvic pain.

For years, doctors didn't hesitate to remove the uterus when this problem presented itself. We think women should be very careful about pursuing this option too quickly, especially when there are other things that can be done first.

You are much more likely to develop uterine prolapse if you have vaginally delivered children, because the process of giving birth can really stretch or damage the muscles in that region. Women who have never had children may experience prolapse as well, though it's much less common. Some doctors think that this might mean that some women are genetically predisposed to the condition.[27] Other things that can contribute to developing prolapse include chronic coughing (here is yet another good reason not to smoke!), intensive lifting of heavy objects (either with work or with your exercise routine if it is too intense), and various kinds of pelvic tumors.[28] Whatever the primary cause of your uterine prolapse, it sometimes becomes evident around or after menopause. One reason for this is that either as a result of hormone decline or just from more general aging, the muscles of the pelvic region can lose stretchiness and the urogenital tissues can thin. Loss of pelvic strength partners with earlier damage to create the condition of prolapse.

Some women choose to leave the problem alone particularly if it isn't causing significant discomfort or inconvenience. We always want to encourage you to think about whether your current pain or discomfort is worse than the treatment you are considering for it.

Keep in mind that there are other surgical options besides hysterectomy. In the most common, the muscles of the region are tightened and the bladder is lifted back into position.[29] If a woman wants to pursue nonsurgical options, Kegel exercises are a good start, and devices such as pessaries (a small plastic or silicone device) are excellent nonsurgical treatment options.

Two last things to consider: a very small group of women may develop as part of uterine prolapse a more serious problem called a *fistula*. A fistula happens when the rectum or bladder begins leaking into the vagina; this can cause serious infections. Women with this problem should receive surgical attention. A less serious problem, called a *cytocele*, can cause confusion by seemingly ending urinary incontinence while actually signaling prolapse.

Pruritus Vulvae and Vulvodynia

Sometimes doctors and scientists can't resist giving fancy medical names to common problems. Many general books on menopause will talk about a problem called *pruritus vulvae*. Before you get too worried, you should know that this complicated name simply means "itchy vulva." Many women suffer from vulval itching throughout their lives, but some find it gets worse around menopause.

There are many causes of this problem. It can happen because of skin disorders such as eczema, dermatitis, lichen simplex, and psoriasis, or it can be the result of an infection such as thrush, trichomoniasis, and some sexually transmitted infections. It can even happen simply because of an allergic reaction to perfumes.

Although the vast number of cases of vulval itching are annoying but not serious, in rare instances they can be the result of skin cancers or even the extremely rare vulvar cancer. Because of this, it is never a bad idea to talk to your doctor or gynecologist if you find the problem persistent.

Most of the time, the solution can be as simple as wearing loose-fitting cotton clothing, avoiding excessive scratching of the area, and washing properly. Some other suggestions include avoiding friction in the area that accompanies activities like bicycling and horseback riding, and giving up nylon pantyhose and tampons.

Vulvodynia is a condition that is similar to pruritus vulvae but characterized by burning instead of itching. The tissue thinning that occurs around and after the time of menopause seems possibly to aggravate both conditions.

Changes in the vaginal and reproductive parts of the body happen for all of us as we age. Our faces don't stay the same, so why would other parts of our bodies? The challenge is to accept the ways our bodies change and to be realistic about it. Don't let fear prompt you into making decisions for surgery unless it is truly necessary. Always consider that time is often the best cure for both physical problems and the anxiety that accompanies any period of great transition.

menopausal approaches

10

the world is flat

the new and changing role
of hormone therapy in
menopause

*I cannot be awake for nothing looks to me
like it did before. Or else I am awake for
the first time, and all before has been a
mean sleep.*

— WALT WHITMAN

a barely contained sense of disbelief, frustration, and utter confusion ran throughout the marbled-floored halls in Bethesda at the National Institutes of Health (NIH) meeting one early spring morning in 2002.

When a prominent doctor who had spent years touting the benefits of hormone therapy (HT) took the podium to speak, her voice sounded strained, and her words summarized what so many in the audience were feeling. "It turns out," the doctor admitted, "that the world is indeed flat."

What this respected physician and her colleagues were meeting about, and what women around the world would soon struggle to understand and believe, were early results from the Women's Health Initiative (WHI).

When the massive WHI was organized in the early 1990s, it was conventional wisdom among many doctors that a lot of time, money, and womanpower were being spent to prove what everyone already knew: HT and estrogen therapy (ET) would prevent heart disease. When early trial results concluded that *more* women on hormones had heart attacks, the result in the medical community was palpable shock and a halt to the estrogen-plus-progestin wing of the huge federal trial.

For decades, HT had been prescribed for every conceivable ailment, from treating depression problems to alleviating wrinkling skin to preventing chronic diseases like Alzheimer's. One doctor, in zealous worship at the estrogen temple, declared that it should be placed along with fluoride in the drinking water supply. Most were less extreme than this, but it was pretty standard by the late 1990s to believe that menopause might be an estrogen deficiency disease and that *not* giving it to every female patient of a certain age was probably akin to malpractice. One doctor friend of Barbara's insisted that the WHI was a waste of money. "Obviously, the women on the hormones will be living longer," she said. "It's unethical to leave volunteers on the placebos for the full eight and a half years of the trial. At some point they'll have to stop the study and offer hormones to everyone." The vast proportion of her colleagues concurred.

So now to be told that HT not only hurt the heart but was responsible for a panoply of other problems, including an increased risk of certain cancers, strokes, blood clots, and Alzheimer's, created a paradigm shift of epic proportions in menopause medicine.

Not everyone was surprised by this turn of events. Barbara was chief among them.

In 1975 the *New England Journal of Medicine* reported in a series of articles that the risk of endometrial cancer in estrogen users was five to fourteen times higher than in nonusers, and the Food and Drug Administration (FDA) responded by ordering label changes that warned of the potentially lethal effects of the drugs. In 1977, Barbara wrote a best-selling book called *Women and the Crisis in Sex Hormones*,[1] in which she outlined the dangers of estrogen drugs, including birth control pills, diethylstilbestrol (DES), and hormone and estrogen treatments for menopause. Years of lies and false claims on the part of salesmen cloaked in physician's dress—the most

notorious being Dr. Robert Wilson and his book *Feminine Forever*[2]—
had catapulted HT to the status of a menopause must-have. All that
had changed by the 1970s, as women began to get angry about dangers they hadn't been warned about and began to be empowered as
patients.

How did HT come back? And now that we find ourselves at another watershed moment, how do we know what to believe?

Hormone History

The story of how estrogen drugs became the biggest sellers in the
Western world at times resembles an epic movie more than scientific
history. For centuries the sex glands of animals were employed (often
controversially) as aphrodisiacs, youth tonics, fertility boosters, and
to ease the symptoms of menopause in various cultures.

When Merck, a German drug company, began to publish its famous *Merck Manual* in 1899, it already listed primitive estrogen
preparations. One drug, called Ovariin, was derived from the dried
and pulverized ovaries of a cow. The product was flavored with things
like vanilla and was recommended, along with belladonna, cannabis,
and opium, for treating "climacterica" (menopause) and other female
reproductive ills.

Although these preparations would have had a mild effect, the
real holy grail of this maturing field—an estrogen that could be taken
by mouth and absorbed easily and actively in the body—had yet to
be found.

In the 1920s, the anatomist Edgar Allen described the hormone
cycle in a female mouse. With biochemist Edward Doisy, he developed the Allen-Doisy test to measure estrogen content. This was a
big step forward in hormone medicine.

A race began among major drugmakers to recruit promising scientists to develop new drugs. James Bertram Collip, a young Canadian pharmaceutical star who had helped create insulin, was recruited
by the Ayerst company. His first drug, a product called Emmenin,
was derived from the urine of Canadian women in late pregnancy
and it hit the market in 1930. Eventually, the company and its scientist would settle on using mares' urine, and the drug bearing the name

of its key ingredients—PreMarIn (pregnant mares' urine)—was born.

In 1937, just before the start of World War II, a medical race involving estrogen was coming to a head. Nazi chemists, including a young scientist named Johann Butenandt, developed and patented ethinyl estradiol, an oral estrogen that is still a component in nine out of ten twenty-first-century birth control pills. Afraid the Nazis would corner the world market on this potentially lucrative drug, British scientists struck back. Edward Charles Dodds and his associates created the estrogen DES, which could be taken in liquid form or as a pill and would cost only $2 a gram, compared to estradiol's $300. To make sure that the Nazis would make little money off their estrogen, British scientists published their formula, making it public property.

In the months right after he synthesized DES, Dodds was already worrying about a cancer link. On occasion, stilbestrol powder blew around in his lab, and he noticed that the men on his staff who handled it were growing breasts. Dodds rushed out samples, meticulously packaged, to a young researcher at the National Cancer Institute, which was just being established in the United States. The chemist's concern didn't come out of the blue: the German lab's estrogen, given to mice, induced mammary cancer.

In the October 1940 issue of the *Journal of the National Cancer Institute*, it was reported that DES produced breast cancers in both male and female mice. There were other papers providing similar warnings about the new drug, but by the time they were published, a marketing behemoth was already underway to use DES for every imaginable problem. It was originally approved for menopause symptoms (as well as senile vaginitis, lactation suppression in women who had recently given birth, and treating gonorrhea), but DES would become notorious several decades later when its use for miscarriage prevention led to cancers in the mothers and reproductive abnormalities and cancers in their offspring.

At the same time that warnings about estrogen drugs were being published, the *Journal of the American Medical Association (JAMA)* was spreading some good news: along with the journal *Endocrinology*, *JAMA* published a report confirming the benefits of the hormones in curbing hot flashes. *JAMA* acknowledged the drugs might cause cancer, and never suggested any other benefits such as antiaging properties.[3]

This history is so important because it reminds us that, among other things, doctors were aware of the serious health implications of ET and HT products since their creation; no one should have been surprised when the WHI showed higher breast cancer rates among participants taking Prempro.

On May 23, 1940, Eli Lilly asked the FDA for permission to market DES. Lilly's application papers included a report by Drs. K. K. Chen and P. N. Harris listing studies in mice and rats showing that males as well as females might develop breast cancer when given the drug. Intersexuality appeared in male rats, mice, and chickens; milk production in animals was reduced, and miscarriage in cows was observed. Lilly withdrew its application, along with other drugmakers, on November 11, 1940, when they were advised that they would be rejected.

Before long, Lilly and the other drugmakers recovered from the sting of their unsuccessful first approval bid. The regrouping that followed was a first blueprint for joint spin-doctoring by the drug companies, and it laid down the basis for the formation of Big Pharma, the powerful industry lobby that would officially start business in 1951. Lilly and their associates hired Carson P. Frailey, the vice president of the American Drug Makers Association, who designed a massive campaign to collect positive science and get doctors to write pressuring favorable letters to the FDA. On September 19, 1941, the FDA officially approved the use of DES for the treatment of menopause symptoms.

Following Lilly's example, the makers of Premarin soon had their drug approved as well. Approval for hot flashes was all well and good, but some drugmakers had grander notions about the possibilities of estrogen for the menopausal woman. Some doctors agreed. Among them were Dr. Fuller Albright in 1940, who first proposed ET as a bone strengthener for oophorectomized women, and Dr. Robert Greenblatt, who in 1943 suggested testosterone pellets (with estrogen) could be a long-term drug for sexual problems. Dr. William Masters, later to coauthor the best-seller *Human Sexuality*, published his first article, followed by a dozen more, on the effects of HT on aging women. The historian Elizabeth Siegel Watkins has called Masters "one of the architects of the campaign to expand the use of sex hormones from short-term remedy . . . to long-term therapy."[4] Among other things, Masters suggested that menopause is responsible for failing bones, cardiovascular disease, and senility.

Such ideas may have been in the air, or even in the water, but it was a Brooklyn doctor named Robert Wilson who brought them into the public consciousness in a startling fashion. In 1966, Wilson published a notorious best-seller called *Feminine Forever*. It was no surprise that Wilson's book was a hit: it raised women's fears by comparing menopause to "living decay" and insisting that the postmenopausal woman was essentially sexless or, worse, a man. Menopause wasn't just part of every woman's life; Wilson compared it with diabetes and suggested that like that dreaded illness, menopause needed constant and vigilant pharmaceutical management.

Wilson lacked the credentials and medical evidence to support his claims. The support he did have, and that was in spades, was financial assistance from several powerful drugmakers.

Another doctor fueling women's fears was the psychiatrist David Reuben, who in 1969 would gain fame as the author of *Everything You Always Wanted to Know About Sex*. In that book, he claimed, "As the estrogen is shut off a woman comes as close as she can to being a man."[5] Perhaps because of snake-oil salesmen like Wilson and Reuben, and perhaps because of smart marketing and dubious science, estrogen sales doubled and tripled in the mid-1960s through the mid-'70s.

However, by the late 1970s, revelations about endometrial cancer, persistent consciousness-raising by the women's movement and new FDA warning labels on estrogen products had resulted in a dramatic drop-off in prescriptions. Could this dwindling market be revived, or was estrogen to go the way of peace signs and Pucci-print jumpsuits? How could HT and ET be made relevant and even essential to the new, empowered woman of the 1980s?

The answer came in 1982 when Dr. Harry Genant published what is now a classic paper in the *Annals of Internal Medicine*.[6] Genant recruited twenty-seven volunteers, all of whom were still menstruating when their ovaries were removed. In a randomized, double-blind clinical trial he showed that patients who received an intermediate dose of Premarin retained bone mass far better than those on lower doses or placebos. When Genant's findings were summarized and published in the mass media, the take-home message was loud and clear: ET and HT will save your bones from the ravages of osteoporosis. While Genant's trial never tried to hide the fact that it was conducted on oophorectomized women, nearly every article covering his work failed to make this crucial distinction clear.

The genie was out of the bottle. Drugmakers saw their salvation in raising fears about crumbling bones. And they began to think: If concerns about one chronic illness could generate a market for hormone drugs, what about heart disease? Alzheimer's disease?

Whose News?

One reason that the WHI results were so shocking is that, over several decades, the news media failed to report negative findings about estrogen. The *New York Times,* for example, published the positive results about estrogen and heart disease from the Nurses Health Study on the front page. Only a short while before, bad news from the massive Framington Heart Trial was buried in the back pages. A study comparing HT coverage before and after the WHI found striking results. When the results of the Heart and Estrogen-Progestin Replacement Study (HERS) Trial were published in 1998, giving some of the first bad news about HT and the heart, only half of the articles published even mentioned a potential risk to taking the drugs.[7] After the WHI, these numbers were up to almost 75 percent. Study authors noted that before the WHI, "the majority of these articles presented information about the potential benefits of HT," and also observed that news outlets practiced "selective disclosure," failing to explore the dangers of the drugs."[8]

While we are against sensationalizing the WHI results, the truth is that, as antiageism activist Margaret Morganroth Gullette notes:

> Before 2002, Americans could read about menopause and not discover that women's health advocates thought hormone treatment dangerous. Far from teaching the controversy, the

media acted as if it didn't exist. Since 2002, despite clear evidence of estrogen carcinogenesis, many in the media are in effect promoting the hormone comeback that Big Pharma wants.[9]

By the late 1990s the claims for estrogen had grown so outrageous that we had to start a separate file for "HRT—Weird" to have enough space to save the articles that were flooding our in-boxes and desks. Although the language had changed since Robert Wilson wrote his book, the claims remained essentially the same—and if anything, had inflated. In addition to preventing heart disease, Alzheimer's, and osteoporosis, HT would iron out your wrinkles, take fat off your thighs, hydrate your eyes, improve the quality of your fingernails, and clean your house for you. (Okay, we made that last one up.) Premarin climbed to become the best-selling drug in the United States for several years running.

Of course all of these claims were unsubstantiated, and despite decades of growing claims for HT, growing approval at FDA never followed suit, and the drug remained officially used only to treat hot flashes and vaginal dryness.

The history of how the WHI came to be what it was is most definitely a David and Goliath story. Goliath, in this case, is Wyeth-Ayerst, the giant drugmaker responsible for Premarin. It rankled the high-ups at Wyeth to know that until the drug was officially approved by the FDA to treat heart disease, all they had to help market that blockbuster drug for the heart was a growing collection of observational studies, small clinical trials, and some very good word of mouth. Wyeth wanted federal approval to use Premarin for heart disease prevention and didn't think it would take too much effort to get it.

What Wyeth didn't count on was a David in the form of a feisty, brilliant women's-health activist named Cindy Pearson. Coming to the hearings in her professional capacity as director of the National Women's Health Network, Pearson urged the FDA to withhold approval until the right kind of research could be done. In this case, the stone that David hurled at the giant was aspirin: Pearson pointed out that no drug had ever been approved for cardio protection in men— not even aspirin—unless it was verified by clinical trials using placebos as a control. The FDA staffers at the meeting, who luckily included the longtime women's-health movement friend and activist Phillip Corfman, were convinced, and the stage was set for the WHI.

Wyeth must have believed in its product: it must have been sure of the results, because not only did it let the trial go forward, assuming it would justify its heart claims once and for all, but it donated enough Prempro and Premarin for thousands of women to take the pills over a decade and a half.

How big was the WHI? It involved 161,808 women, cost millions of dollars, and lasted fifteen years, from 1991 to 2006. The trial had two major parts: the randomized clinical trial and the observational study. In many cases, women who were rejected or dropped from the clinical trial were encouraged to join the observational one. Between 1993 and 1998, 27,347 women between the ages of fifty and seventy-nine were enlisted to participate in either the estrogen-plus-progestin group or the estrogen-only section. The women involved in the trial seemed to get what drugmakers struggled to understand: that women wanted real knowledge not just to protect their own health but to pass down to later generations. At a 2006 conference honoring participants, woman after woman said that she was motivated to join the WHI out of a sense of obligation to daughters and granddaughters, to the larger community of women.

Because the WHI is so massive, it can be hard to fully understand all the findings. As some experts are quick to point out, "there's still debate today about how to interpret the results."[10] Some writers and scientists have kept very busy recently in trashing the study.

We think it is important to understand both the praise and the criticism, both the breadth of this massive piece of science and its very real limitations.

What Was the WHI Intended to Do?

The WHI was designed to test several aspects of older women's health: the potential benefits of low-fat diets, calcium and vitamin D consumption, and, of course, hormone use. WHI investigators wanted to know what benefits or risks long-term HT and ET use might have for women's health. In particular, they were interested in the potential cardioprotectivity of hormone use (that is, would women taking HT and ET have fewer heart attacks and strokes than women on a placebo). Additionally, they wanted answers about HT's ability to maintain bone density and its relationship to breast cancer.

One of the major criticisms to emerge since the end of the trial is that the participants were already postmenopausal and, on the whole, significantly older than most women who would want to use hormones. They started taking HT and ET years or even decades after they had finished the disruptions of hot flashing and night sweating.

Although it might seem counterintuitive, the investigators had a few really good reasons for choosing this group of women. First, they already knew that HT and ET would quell internal heat waves; the study wasn't testing for that. Having women who were flashing in the trial would only serve to "unblind" the group, making it very clear which women were receiving the drug and which were taking sugar pills.

A second major reason that doctors decided to test older women was that the primary goal of the trial was to look at the ability of the drugs to prevent heart attacks. Quite simply, most women won't see their risk of heart attack rise at all until after age fifty-five, and the danger won't go up significantly for most until their seventies. The WHI was meant to be a long-term trial, but not *that* long, and investigators needed a test group that could provide answers in under two decades.

Despite the good reasons for choosing an older population, this decision placed some pretty serious limitations on the trial. First of all, most women will start taking HT when they are premenopausal. By starting women on the drugs later, it was harder to tell if the problems these women had as a result of taking HT were applicable to younger women, and it prompted many scientists and commentators to argue that the timing of HT was a key issue. It made room for the argument that not all of the negative health findings of the WHI were applicable to younger women taking the drug. Both claims are intriguing but unproven.

Other criticisms of the WHI were logistical. Some study subjects didn't take their pills or keep to regimens tightly enough. If too many women dropped out or stopped taking the treatment, it would change the statistical validity of the data that emerged.[11]

Another criticism is that many of the results of the WHI weren't statistically significant; that means, at least mathematically speaking, they could have been the result of chance instead of hormones. In most of those cases, though, the numbers were close enough to this meaningful line to warrant caution, and study subjects were advised of the results.

What Did the Study Find Out about HT and ET?

In a population of ten thousand women, those who took estrogen and progestin pills had an average of eight more strokes, seven more heart attacks, eight additional cases of breast cancer, eighteen extra blood clots in the legs or lungs, and twenty-three more cases of dementia (women over sixty-five). On the plus side, there were five fewer hip fractures and six fewer cases of colon cancer in HT users than the placebo group. This means, for example, that in any given year, thirty-seven women taking HT would have heart attacks when compared with thirty in the placebo group; ten women taking HT would get colon cancer and sixteen in the placebo group.

For women who took estrogen only, there were seven additional blood clots, twelve more cases of dementia (women over sixty-five), and twelve extra strokes. Those who took estrogen only also had seven fewer cases of breast cancer and six fewer hip fractures.

The only people in the estrogen-only wing of the trial were hysterectomized women. This is because taking estrogen alone increases the chance of developing cancer of the uterus; by pairing estrogen use with progesterone, this risk could be reduced. Unfortunately, it turned out that adding progesterone raised the risk of breast cancer.

As might be expected, women who took estrogen alone had notably less breast cancer than their estrogen-plus-progestin counterparts, and had fewer heart attacks. They also had more strokes and blood clots. You might say it's a choice between health above the waist (less breast cancer without progesterone) or below (less endometrial cancer with estrogen plus progestin).

These numbers should help you understand a few things. First of all, while you would have an increased risk of developing heart attacks, breast cancer, and blood clots if you took hormones, this certainly doesn't mean you *will* have these problems. Even with the increased risk, the numbers of people with each problem are very small, but the risk is very serious and should be weighed and understood accordingly. We would add that recent opinion on the WHI has suggested that while estrogen was "bad" for older women, it might be healthier for younger women. This seems to us like it might be looking at things backwards. We would point out that just because HT is less unhealthy for young women doesn't mean it is good for them.

Now let's look specifically at what we know and don't know about what hormones do in different parts of our bodies.

The Bottom Line

Heart

The WHI confirmed that HT and ET should not be used to treat or prevent heart disease. It just doesn't work. Whether hormone drugs actually hurt the heart (as seems likely) or simply fail to offer the protection we hoped for is debatable.

One of the most controversial theories in response to the WHI is the idea that timing of hormone use is what makes the difference between HT helping or hurting the heart. Proponents of this view argue that the problem with the WHI wasn't the estrogen, it was the age of the study subjects. If HT and ET were administered when a woman was young and first menopausal, this argument reasons that she would be in a position to receive the benefits.

This idea is primarily based on specific subpopulations within the general WHI group. For example, women who started the hormones within ten years of menopause had an 11 percent lower risk of heart disease. Compare that with women who started at least ten years after, who had a 22 percent higher risk. For women taking estrogen only, between ages fifty and fifty-nine, the risk of heart disease was 37 percent lower than the placebo, and likewise, their older counterparts had a risk 11 percent higher. Data from the Nurses

Health Study seems to agree with this analysis. The problem with this theory is not just that it is based on information that is largely statistically insignificant, but it is also completely untested. It is all very well to suggest that taking HT at the right age might help your heart. But now that we know HT at older ages can hurt you, it seems like quite a gamble to suggest women should play a dangerous guessing game, trying to pick a point that is early enough to see benefits while avoiding risks. Until there is much more information about this highly contested theory, it seems like a better idea to protect the heart by exercising, maintaining a sensible weight, and decreasing stress levels.

A *New England Journal of Medicine* study made waves in the summer of 2007 by looking at younger WHI women and heart problems.[12] The study suggested that while HT and ET use hurt older hearts, it might have provided some benefit for younger participants. What wasn't made clear in the media when the study was reported was that the data being analyzed was from the estrogen-only arm of the trial and therefore was looking at hysterectomized women, the majority of whom had gone through menopause surgically. A further important point about this study: it actually looked at "coronary artery calcification," not heart attacks, and was therefore analyzing a risk factor for heart problems rather than actual cardiac events.

Stroke

When the blood flow to the brain is seriously disrupted, either by blood clots and artery blockers or by hemorrhaging, the result is a stroke.

For many years, HT and ET advocates tried to argue that the drugs would decrease stroke risk. This never made any sense to us, since, among other reasons, other estrogen and progestin drugs like birth control pills had been documented to cause strokes in otherwise low-risk populations (especially women who were too young to worry about such things.)

The WHI found that, indeed, taking HT and ET raises your risk of stroke: 151 patients in the estrogen-plus-progestin group had strokes, compared with only 107 in the placebo group (1.8 percent of the total population compared with 1.3 percent). That's a 41 percent increase over 5.2 years.[13] For women taking estrogen only, the risk was even higher.

Keep in mind that strokes aren't common until after age sixty-five, and you should consider that this risk will go up as you age.

Cancer

One of the most talked-about news stories of 2006 came out of the Twenty-ninth Annual Breast Cancer Symposium, where doctors reported an unheard-of 7 percent drop in breast cancer rates in 2003. Although admitting that the connection to hormones wasn't certain, Dr. Peter Ravdin of the Anderson Cancer Center in Houston explained this trend, saying, "It seems that it was the decrease in the use of hormone therapy."[14] Other researchers confirmed Ravdin's findings in the *Journal of Clinical Oncology*, where a team of researchers led by Christina A. Clarke found that as HT use dropped 68 percent between 2001 and 2003, breast cancer rates fell between 10 and 11 percent.[15] Clarke added, "This drop was sustained in 2004, which tells us that the decline wasn't just a fluke."

The truth is that the increased breast cancer rates were the least unexpected thing about the WHI findings; as we discussed earlier, scientists have suspected a possible breast cancer link for nearly as long as HT drugs have been around.

Among other things, HT and ET can make the breast tissue dense. This means that it is harder to spot tumors and potential cancers. In the first two years of the WHI, women taking hormones actually had less breast cancer diagnosed than their placebo-popping counterparts. By year three this had equalized, and after the fourth year, breast cancer among hormone users surged. It seems likely, in retrospect, that in the early years hormone takers had as much breast cancer as their counterparts but the cancers simply weren't being detected because their breasts were too dense. When you consider how important early diagnosis and treatment are, the effect of hormones on breasts becomes even more concerning.

It may be that HT makes a difference in the *type* of breast cancer a woman develops. While the majority of breast cancers begin in the milk ducts, hormone users are more likely to get lobular cancers. This is bad, because while ductal cancers form lumps that are more easily detected, lobular cancers are hard to spot.

Because women in the estrogen-only wing of the trial weren't at the same high increased risk of breast cancer as their combined estrogen-plus-progestin counterparts, some scientists have theorized that progestin—and particularly the kind of progestin found in Premarin, medroxyprogesterone acetate—is responsible for this terrible side effect of taking HT.

If you are a woman with a family history of breast cancer, or if you have suffered from the disease in the past, you shouldn't take hormones.

In terms of other types of cancer, the results are mixed. Hormone treatment seems to lower the risk of colon cancer somewhat, although because (as with the breast) cancers in HT users are diagnosed later, the death rates in users and nonusers is about the same. There seems to be a slightly higher risk of ovarian cancer with hormone use. While breast and colon cancer are common, ovarian and uterine cancer are less likely to occur.

Bones

While the ability of HT to maintain bone mass has been demonstrated, and the WHI findings support a modest reduction in fracture rates among women taking estrogen and combined drugs, we still don't recommend hormones for this purpose.

Although women on hormones have denser bones and fewer breaks, these benefits are lost as soon as hormone use stops. This means that to keep seeing gains for your skeleton, you would need to keep popping pills. Since we now know that long-term hormone use is a bad idea, it seems best to suggest finding other ways to keep bones healthy and whole (note that we aren't advocating a switch to bisphosphonates!—read chapter 19 for more on this). In a 2003 study, doctors from the University of California, San Diego, compared fracture rates in current and former hormone users. Tara Parker-Pope explains, "Women who were using hormones at the time of the study had the highest bone density at every age. Current users were 25 percent less likely to suffer a fracture during the year-long study than non–hormone users—but only as long as she was still taking the drugs."[16] It turned out that women who had stopped using the drugs more than five years before the trial had bone densities analogous with women who had never tried HT.[17]

Brain Effects and Dementia

Before the WHI many women took HT for one reason: they thought it would prevent Alzheimer's disease. Part of this perception was a deliberate conflation of Alzheimer's with the mild, transient "fuzzy brain" many women experience during the change. Of course this largely undocumented but frequently experienced problem has *nothing* to do with the progressive, fatal disease that slowly wipes away memories and eventually cognition.

As with so many presumed but unproven benefits of HT, there were several small trials that suggested a benefit for Alzheimer's prevention. There were also observational studies, including the Manhattan Study of Aging and the Baltimore Longitudinal Study of Aging. Both trials found the risk of developing Alzheimer's to be 50 percent lower in hormone users.

However, just as long-held assumptions about the heart were toppled by the WHI, so were many ideas about the supposed benefits of estrogen for Alzheimer's. The WHI Memory Study (WHIMS) found a stunning difference in Alzheimer's rates between hormone users and the placebo users: those receiving hormones had a 76 percent *higher* risk of developing dementia.[18] Given this contradictory data, we would discourage anyone from going on or staying on estrogen to prevent Alzheimer's or other memory disorders.

Other Health Considerations with HT

There are so many different health effects associated with taking hormones, both positive and negative, that it would take an entire book to go through them all completely. Let's just talk about a few of the WHI findings that got a little less attention than the heart and breast cancer results.

In 1974 a Boston study published in the *New England Journal of Medicine*[19] showed the negative effects of estrogen therapy on the gallbladder. Although lower-dose hormone preparations have contributed to fewer incidences of this problem, it is still a real concern for women contemplating HT. The HERS trial found that users had a small risk increase: study authors estimated that estrogen users would have one additional gallbladder surgery for every 185 users, an increased relative risk of 38 percent over the placebo group.[20] These findings were confirmed by the WHI, where investigators estimated the increased risk to be higher than previously suspected. The WHI found that for every group of ten thousand women, there will be an average of seventy-eight women on hormones who develop gallbladder problems compared with forty-seven women who are hormone free.[21]

For years, some hormone advocates insisted that HT would help alleviate urinary incontinence. This was, as it turned out, another myth. Far from helping with incontinence, it exacerbated the problem. This increase was seen in all types of urinary incontinence, and it happened quickly—after one year.[22] You definitely shouldn't take HT or ET to prevent this problem, and if you have a history or a family history of it, you might want to think twice before taking hormones for other reasons.

In general, HT use was associated with a higher rate of gynecological surgeries, breast tenderness, and bleeding. It is estimated that while only 5 percent of the placebo group experienced bleeding and spotting, 51 percent of the women on hormones struggled with this problem. More women on the drug had hysterectomies and dilation and curettages (D and Cs).[23] This is ironic, because women who have hysterectomies experience more brutal menopause symptoms and often have to rely on estrogen: in this way, hormones become both the cause of, and later the solution to, women's health problems. In other words, they are only able to solve the problems they have first created.

This goes to a larger issue: while ET and HT are well known to be good at alleviating hot flashes, night sweats, and vaginal dryness, the drugs haven't been shown to actually improve quality of life. This is sort of a "little picture/big picture" comparison. While specifically

HT is able to address certain problems such as hot flashes, it isn't capable of fixing the bigger issues, and women who take it aren't happier overall than those who don't. The WHI investigators wrote that "[HT] resulted in no significant effects on general health, vitality, mental health, depressive symptoms, or sexual satisfaction."[24] If the proof is in the pudding, then when it comes to HT, you should probably skip dessert.

Speaking of sweets, and to finish discussing the WHI on a positive note, it is possible that women who take hormones are at a slightly reduced risk of developing diabetes.[25] This benefit may be specific to the estrogen-only arm of the trial and should be understood as modest. There are better ways to prevent diabetes, and this benefit shouldn't be seen as a reason to initiate HT.

Estrogen Basics

Estrogen isn't one hormone but the name of a group of hormones. Like members of a close family, these compounds can be very similar in certain ways and completely different in others. There are three principal forms of estrogen found in the human body: *estrone, estradiol*, and *estriol*. Estradiol is the primary estrogen produced by the ovaries. Estrone is formed from estradiol; it is a weak estrogen and is the most abundant found in the body after menopause. Estriol is produced in large amounts during pregnancy and is a product of the breakdown of estradiol. Before menopause, estradiol is the predominant estrogen. After menopause, estradiol levels drop more, so that estrone becomes the predominant estrogen.

Estradiol is produced by the ovaries each month and is the estrogen most constant in our bodies throughout life. Estrone is the estrogen associated with the menopausal woman; it is made in the adrenal glands and the ovaries and is derived from body fat.

Receptive Listening: Understanding
Estrogen Receptors

Like all good hormones, estrogens are messengers: they travel through the body carrying important information between the brain and various parts of your body. When the postman delivers letters, he matches the address on the envelope to the address on the house or mailbox. As estrogen moves through the body, it carries a sort of biological "address." It knows it has found the right house when this "address" matches up with the cells in a certain organ or tissue.

This happens because those cells have a tiny protein molecule called an *estrogen receptor* that helps the hormone bind to target tissues. Just as no other house in New York has Barbara's exact apartment, building, and zip code number, so target tissues are the only ones in the body that have estrogen receptor proteins. (Although the breast and uterus are the main "destinations" of estrogen, they are not the only ones. Estrogen molecules also act on the brain, bone, liver, and heart and a number of other really significant places.) Only estrogen (and closely related molecules) can bind to these tiny sites.

Before an estrogen molecule enters a cell, the estrogen receptor lies dormant and doesn't change the cell at all. When the two meet, all of this changes. It's sort of like a couple falling in love. You may always have a part of you that is capable of love, but until that right person enters your life, it just lies in wait and doesn't alter the way you act or the person you are. Then one day you meet, and you start to be reshaped. Well, estrogen receptors are sort of the same. When estrogen molecules enter their cells, they completely change. Literally they transform their shape in the binding process, and this allows them to alter the cell and the way it behaves, starting on the genetic level. Just like a new love starts to change the way you like or dislike certain things, so the estrogen/tissue binding begins to turn on and off different switches in the DNA.

Also like love, some estrogen-cell matches are good ones, and some can be dangerous or disastrous. In the liver, for example, the entrance of estrogen causes an increase in the amount of HDL cholesterol (the "good" cholesterol) and decreases the amount of LDL cholesterol (thought to be "bad.") Here, estrogen and target tissue are a match made in heaven. (Remember, now, that we are talking about natural estrogen that your body makes, not the kind you take by pill or patch or apply as a cream. This makes a big difference.)

Sometimes, though, just like love, estrogen-tissue binding can go badly. In certain types of breast cancer, for example, estrogen can actually increase the growth of dangerous cells. In this case, the readiness of breast tissue to merge with estrogen and cause the rapid growth of cells is a really bad thing. The worst part is that this happens through the same process—the proliferation of certain types of cells—that is responsible for many positive functions in the breast and uterus, including the ability to lactate or menstruate, and for maintaining bone mass.

How does this necessary process go bad? During each monthly cycle, just as the uterus produces lots of cells that would cushion and nourish a potential fetus (cells that are then cleaned out when you have your period), so the breast grows cells that line the milk glands, in preparation for a potential pregnancy. When that pregnancy doesn't happen, the cells wither and die. So for the entire reproductive period, women are experiencing monthly the rapid growth and rapid death of breast cells.

Sometimes this process goes wrong. This has to do with DNA replication, which occurs every time a new cell is made. As the cell prepares to grow, DNA copies itself, like a paper running through a photocopy machine. When this happens, there are sometimes small errors or problems with the copy.

When mistakes like this transpire on a cellular level, it is called a *mutation*, and in the breast and uterus it can lead to uncontrolled cell growth. This DNA change can happen through heredity (getting the predisposition for mutation passed down to you from Mom and Dad), through outside forces such as radiation or chemicals, or simply through bad luck—sudden errors in DNA duplication. However it happens, the result can be the existence of dangerous cells.

Estrogen doesn't cause cell mutation. What it does do, though, is cause the replication and proliferation of dangerous cells once they exist. And this makes the likelihood of developing and spreading cancer much greater.

For a long time, scientists figured that all estrogen receptors were the same. Of course, this never made much sense to begin with; there is almost nothing in life that is "one size fits all." But for decades scientists hoped that, as Natalie Angier puts it, "there was only one type of estrogen receptor, one peerless, versatile molecular docking site with which estrogen must unite if the tissue of the uterus, breast or elsewhere are to respond."[26]

With this theory, it would make sense that taking hormone pills would work in your body in much the way natural hormones do. This would have been wonderful: like a great beach book where you know every twist of the plot before it happens and everything comes to a comfortable conclusion. Unfortunately, it turns out that this story is a lot more complicated. The narrative took a drastic turn when scientists discovered a second type of estrogen receptor. They started calling the original kind alpha and the new one beta.

This discovery was significant. First, it demonstrated that estrogens affected and changed the body in ways that went far beyond the breasts and the uterus—sites of alpha receptors—to organs not thought of as particularly influenced by sex hormones—like kidneys, lungs, and bladder—that have beta receptors. It meant that almost every organ in the body was in some way acted on by estrogens. When asked if there was any part of the body that estrogen did not work on, Professor Benita S. Katzenellenbogen of the University of Illinois, Urbana, responded, "I used to think so. Now I have my doubts."[27]

Second, it shows how little we understand about the mechanisms through which various estrogens and tissues bond. We are still not sure how differently beta receptors work in terms of encouraging diverse genes or binding in unique ways with a range of estrogens. It turns out, for example, that beta receptors can be up to ten times faster than alpha at binding with certain types of plant estrogens, such as the ones found in soy and kidney beans.

Perhaps the most salient point is that all this new estrogen research underscores how crude our understanding is of how hormones—and by extension hormone drugs—work. If we could create a compound that acted on one type of tissue but not on others or was able to accomplish the good estrogen effects while avoiding the bad, the story might be different. Unfortunately, right now, we are as able to do that as we are to put fat on only in the breasts while avoiding it on the stomach or bottom.

Hormone Preparations

Many pills, patches, and injectibles are based on only one human estrogen rather than a mix of the three estrogen compounds. While some of these hormones may be natural in the sense that they are similar to the hormones found in our bodies, limiting your hormone replacement to one type of estrogen could create an overall imbalance, since the principal blueprint for estrogen in the human female body is based on three compounds, not one.

So far, there is no substantial evidence to suggest that one estrogen drug carries different risks from any other. Although the WHI was performed using Prempro and Premarin, the FDA warns women to assume that the health hazards observed with those specific drugs would apply generally. The Million Woman Study in the United Kingdom backed up this conclusion, finding that different preparations and different methods of administering them made little to no difference in risks and benefits of the drugs.[28] More trials comparing one estrogen product to another are necessary to fully clarify this issue.

As with birth control pills, different women feel better or worse on different pills. It is nearly impossible to predict how individuals will fare on various preparations, so it is up to patients to decide if they feel like experimenting until they find the right drug.

Conjugated Estrogen

"Conjugated" means chemically combining two or more estrogen compounds. When you are talking about *conjugated estrogen*, you are usually talking about Premarin. You are also talking about the specific product tested in the WHI and many of the major studies we have. (Premarin is made by collecting urine from pregnant horses, then processing it in a lab.)

The conjugated estrogens in the brands Cenestin and Enjuvia are made by combining a variety of plant esters. While the makers of these drugs claim that they are chemically similar to Premarin, Wyeth (which makes Premarin) insists the horse esters in its product provide unique benefits that can't be duplicated.

When you take conjugated estrogens, your body converts them into active estrogens and uses them as it would the estrogen your ovaries produce. Premarin is a mixture of more than ten different estrogens, including estrone (which we make in our own bodies) and equilin and equilenin (horse estrogen, which, of course, we don't make in our own bodies). Because it comes from an animal, Wyeth

Estrogen-Only Products*

PRODUCT	WHAT IS IT?	WHAT DOES IT DO?	WHAT FORM DOES IT COME IN?	OTHER INFORMATION
Conjugated estrogens (Premarin)	A combination of several estrogens, including some derived from pregnant mares' urine.	Helps reduce hot flashing, night sweating. Aids with vaginal dryness and atrophy.	Available as a regular and low-dose pill, a combined pill, and a vaginal cream.	Should be used for the shortest possible duration and in the smallest amount due to risk of blood clotting, heart attack, breast cancer, stroke, etc. It is possible that equilin, one of the horse esters, may tax your liver more than non-equine esters.

*All prescription medications.

(continued)

PRODUCT	WHAT IS IT?	WHAT DOES IT DO?	WHAT FORM DOES IT COME IN?	OTHER INFORMATION
Plant-based conjugated estrogen (brand names include Cenestin and Enjuvia)	Made from combining multiple estrogens from plants.	Same as Premarin.	Available in pill form.	Not approved for long-term use. May or may not be similar to Premarin.
Estradiol-based estrogens (brand names include Estrace, Activella, and Gynodiol (oral), and Estraderm, Climara, Vivelle, FemPatch, Vivelle-Dot (patches), and Estring (vaginal ring)	This is "bioidentical" meaning it is chemically the same as the estrogen your body produces. It is derived from plants. Taken orally, it is metabolized by the liver and converted to estrone, the most abundant postmenopausal estrogen.	Used to treat flashing, sweating, and vaginal dryness and atrophy.	Usually prescribed as oral tablets or patches. Also available as a ring and a vaginal cream. For specific dosing, ask doctor or see patient package insert. Available in generic form.	Same precautions as conjugated estrogens, except perhaps slightly less risk to the liver. Also watch out for interaction with several other drugs—ask your doctor for a list of these, or check package inserts.

| Estropipate-based estrogens (brand names include Ogen and Ortho-Est) | Another plant-derived estrogen, this one is made from purified crystalline estrone. In effect, when you take estropipate, you're getting the final by-product of estradiol and conjugated estrogens, since the liver converts other estrogens into estrone. | Often prescribed for women who have bad side effects from the other estrogens, such as breast tenderness and bloating. These drugs are used to treat flashing, sweating, and vaginal dryness. | Standard dosage for Ogen tablets ranges from one 0.625 mg tablet to two 2.5 mg tablets per day. Tablets should be taken in cycles of 3 weeks on and 1 week off. Standard dosage of Ortho-Est ranges from half a tablet to 4 tablets per day at 1.25 mg or 1 to 8 tablets at 0.625 mg (again, three weeks on, one week off). Available in generic form. | Same side effects as with other estrogen products. |

(continued)

PRODUCT	WHAT IS IT?	WHAT DOES IT DO?	WHAT FORM DOES IT COME IN?	OTHER INFORMATION
Esterified estrogens (brand names include Estratab, Estratest, Menest)	A mixture of synthetic estrogens.	Used to curb flashing, sweating, and vaginal dryness.	Tablets: standard doses: 0.3 mg, 0.625 mg, and 2.5 mg. Available in generic form.	Same concerns as other estrogen products; check for specific possible drug interactions.
Ethinyl estradiol	Synthetic estrogen used mostly in birth control but occasionally as HT.	Used to curb flashing, sweating, and vaginal dryness.	Tablets. Available in generic form.	Same concerns as other estrogen products; check for specific possible drug interactions.

considers it "natural." We would remind you that estrogen made or processed in a lab is never "natural," whether it is chemically identical to your body's or not.

Estrogen Plus Progestin (Combined Therapy)

In the early days of hormone replacement therapy, women received estrogen only. As reports grew of increased rates of endometrial cancer among women on "unopposed" estrogen, doctors and pharmaceutical companies came up with the idea of adding progestins for a few days in each cycle. This way, once the progestin was stopped, the uterus would shed its lining, thus decreasing the risk for cancer.

Estrogen and progesterone can be combined in various ways. In cyclical therapy, you take estrogen daily, add progestin for a few days of the month, and then stop the progestin. You'll get a period as soon as the progestin is stopped. Many women continue to bleed monthly on combined therapy even though ovulation has stopped (although the bleeding should eventually cease). Continuous therapy came about because many women complained about the bleeding. In this option, you take estrogen and progestin continuously, but use a lower dose of progestin. The thought is that the continuous level of progestin will be too low to cause bleeding but high enough to block the potentially cancer-causing effects of estrogen. While the continuous approach may cause less bleeding than the cyclical approach, it doesn't wholly eliminate the bleeding.

Combined Therapy

PRODUCT	WHAT IS IT?	WHAT DOES IT DO?	WHAT FORM DOES IT COME IN?	OTHER INFORMATION
Combined estradiol and norgestinate (brand names include Ortho-Prefest)	This pill combines a natural estrogen with a synthetic progestin.	Used to treat hot flashes, night sweats, and vaginal dryness.	Ortho-Prefest has a pulsatile delivery system: two different pills, one with just estrogen, and one with estrogen and progestin.	Same side effects as other estrogen and progestin products. Check for specific drug interactions.

(continued)

PRODUCT	WHAT IS IT?	WHAT DOES IT DO?	WHAT FORM DOES IT COME IN?	OTHER INFORMATION
Combined estradiol and norethin-drone acetate (brand names include Activella, Combi-Patch, FemHRT)	Both estrogen and progestin are plant-based, but only the estrogen is bioidentical.	Used to treat hot flashes, night sweats, and vaginal dryness.	Available in pill and patch form. Check specific product for dosing. This is continuous HRT, so you get both estrogen and progestin daily. Typically after a few months, you stop having your period completely. In some women it takes a little longer, and often in the first few months you may experience break-through bleeding.	Same side effects as other estrogen and progestin products.

| Conjugated estrogen and medroxy-progesterone (MPA) (brand names include Prempro and Premphase) | This combines Premarin and Provera. It was the drug used and tested in the Women's Health Initiative Estrogen Plus Progestin Trial. | Used to treat hot flashes, night sweats, and vaginal dryness. | Standard dose for Prempro is 0.625 mg conjugated estrogen/ 2.5 mg MPA daily. Premphase contains 0.625 mg of Premarin and 2.5 mg of MPA. Prempro is continuous therapy, and estrogen and progestin are taken every day. With Premphase, estrogen is taken every day and the progestin is added to the estrogen pill for the last two weeks of the menstrual cycle. | Same side effects as other estrogen and progestin products. |

(continued)

PRODUCT	WHAT IS IT?	WHAT DOES IT DO?	WHAT FORM DOES IT COME IN?	OTHER INFORMATION
Esterified estrogens and methyl-testosterone (brand names include Estratest, Estratest HS, Menogen, Menogen HS)	Combines estrogen and testosterone.	Some research has suggested that testosterone is especially important for a woman who has undergone surgical menopause. When you have your ovaries removed, you aren't producing the tiny amount of testosterone that a woman with ovaries does, even after menopause. The result can be terrible hot flashing and sexual problems.	These non-Premarin-based estrogen/testosterone combinations have significantly less testosterone than their equine alternatives.	Studies have found that testosterone may raise blood pressure. Same concerns as with other estrogen drugs.

| Conjugated estrogen with methyl-testosterone | This is Premarin and testosterone. | Some research has suggested that testosterone is especially important for a woman who has undergone surgical menopause. When you have your ovaries removed, you aren't producing the tiny amount of testosterone that a woman with ovaries does, even after menopause. The result can be terrible hot flashing and sexual problems. | Tablet form. | Studies have found that testosterone may raise blood pressure. Same concerns as with other estrogen drugs. |

Progestin

While estrogen gets all the attention, progesterone is just as essential to our bodies. Progesterone is the name of the naturally occurring hormone. When it is synthesized in a lab, we call it progestin. Progesterone is made from cholesterol and is influential in the second half of the menstrual cycle. It is a *precursor* to other hormones, which means it can create estrogen and testosterone; it can also help to balance them.

Since the results of the WHI, progestin has been a hormone with a bad reputation, accused of causing the unanticipated heart attacks in the combination estrogen-plus-progestin group.

This new distrust was added to the many other reasons why women and their doctors were already unhappy with progestin, including the fact that it causes irregular bleeding, breast tenderness, and constipation. The bleeding is one of the main reasons women go off hormone regimens; although most women will adjust to the drug and stop bleeding excessively after the first several months, this side effect is enough to drive many women to rip up their prescription slips.

Because of these problems, many doctors wish they could just do away with progestin supplementation all together. The risk of uterine cancer makes this impossible, but some doctors recently have been experimenting with giving patients very small, occasional doses of progestin to counteract estrogen instead of the regular dosing most patients have become accustomed to. Dr. Steven R. Goldstein of New York University is among those advocating "long-cycle therapy,"[29] in which women are given just one or two doses of progestin a year and monitored with transvaginal ultrasound. Not only is this new methodology untested—who knows if the small amount of progestin is enough in the long run to prevent cancer?—it is also expensive and not always covered by insurance. In general, until we have a lot more information about how both hormones work, we advise against this kind of experimentation on your body. In fact, in September 2007 Jacques Rossouw, one of the central scientists in the WHI, told Barbara he would not give ET alone to women with uteruses in any circumstances.

Most women take progestin in either continuous or cyclic doses. Some HT treatments combine estrogen and progestin in one pill, like oral contraceptives. Other regimens require taking two pills, one estrogen and one progestin.

There are two types of progestin: natural progestin (either the kind made in your body or its manufactured chemical twin), also called progesterone; and synthetic progestins. Most people assume that a synthetic hormone is made in a lab, whereas the natural hormone originates in nature. This is not the case. Both are made in the lab, and even synthetics can be concocted from natural products. The difference between the two is not their source, whether they come from soy or yam or are developed in a test tube. The distinction lies in their basic molecular arrangement. If the chemical structure of the product identically matches that of a woman's natural occurring hormone, it is considered to be natural. But pharmaceutical companies have little incentive to spend millions of dollars to research and manufacture a product they can't exclusively patent, as is the case with natural hormones. However, the device that delivers a hormone, such as a patch or an applicator tube for a cream, can be patented, which is why some pharmaceutical companies market so-called bioidentical-hormones with patented delivery methods. Synthetic hormones, on the other hand, are made by altering the molecular structure of a hormone enough so that it can be patented. But natural estrogen and progesterone are available and FDA-approved, just like the synthetics, and can be prescribed by your doctor.

Do not take progestin without first talking to your doctor if you have a bleeding or blood-clotting disorder, breast cancer, cancer of a genital organ, liver disease, or undiagnosed vaginal bleeding.

Possible serious side effects of progestin therapy include an allergic reaction (difficulty breathing; closing of your throat; swelling of your lips, tongue, or face; or hives); shortness of breath or pain in your chest; a sudden severe headache; visual changes; a painful red, swollen leg; numbness or tingling in an arm or a leg; prolonged heavy vaginal bleeding; stomach or side pain; or yellowing of your skin or eyes.

Other side effects may be more likely to occur, such as dizziness, drowsiness, headache, breast pain or tenderness, abdominal pain or distension, diarrhea, vaginal discharge, or mood changes, anxiety, and irritability.

Some doctors believe that the type of progestin you take can make a big difference in how dangerous it might be. Medroxyprogesterone acetate (MPA) has been singled out as potentially dangerous. Despite this, the Million Woman Study in Great Britain looked at HT use in British women between the ages of fifty-four and sixty-four and found that none of the synthetic progestins—MPA, norethisterone, or norgestrel—were better or worse in terms of breast cancer risk.

This has led some to theorize that the safety difference lies between synthetic progestin and micronized progesterone. The Postmenopausal Estrogen/Progestin Intervention Trial (PEPI), one of the few to look at both progestin and progesterone, suggested that there might be differences in how they act in the body but much more research would be needed to substantiate this theory.

Testosterone

Certain pills combine estrogen and testosterone, and some doctors have begun prescribing testosterone off label for the treatment of sexual problems. Although we think of testosterone as a "male" hormone, women actually make it in our ovaries. Women produce a fraction of the testosterone that men make and, like other sex hormones, we create much less of it following menopause.

Since Viagra proved that sex drugs could be big business, several drug companies have pursued creating testosterone drugs to serve as a pink equivalent to the "little blue pill." In 2004, the FDA rejected an application from Procter & Gamble (P & G) to approve the testosterone patch Intrinsia. The reason was that despite some limited clinical evidence that the patch increased desire in women who were using it, long-term safety data weren't available. In the wake of the WHI revelations, the FDA was wary of approving any new, potentially dangerous hormone preparations. P & G is currently retooling and retesting the drug, and a *New York Times* article noted that other companies were working to make their own "T" products, including gels and nasal sprays.[30] The testosterone patch was approved in Europe.

You should know that if you are taking testosterone alone for sexual problems, you are using a drug for off-label reasons with no long-term safety data. Another major problem with testosterone therapy, as the eminent New York University sexologist Leonore Tiefer points out, is that taking a quick-fix approach to sexual problems ignores social and relational factors that are more important for most women than any chemical imbalance in determining how they feel about sex.

In terms of menopause symptoms, there are no solid data to sug-

Examples of Available Progesterones

PRODUCT	WHAT IS IT?	WHAT DOES IT DO?	WHAT FORM DOES IT COME IN?	OTHER INFORMATION
Prometrium	A natural form of finely ground (micronized) progesterone made from wild yams.	Causes the shedding of the uterine lining as in menstruation and possibly helps prevent overgrowth of the lining that can lead to heavy bleeding.	It can be taken orally or as a vaginal suppository. The common dose is 200 mg capsules taken once a day for 12 days per cycle and 100 to 200 mg a day for continuous therapy.	This treatment is only for women who haven't had hysterectomies. If you are allergic to peanuts, you shouldn't use this product as it contains peanut oil.

(continued)

PRODUCT	WHAT IS IT?	WHAT DOES IT DO?	WHAT FORM DOES IT COME IN?	OTHER INFORMATION
Crinone	Progesterone vaginal gel.	Causes the shedding of the uterine lining as in menstruation.	Applied to the vagina, the gel adheres to the walls of the vagina so that the progesterone can be absorbed locally with minimal absorption into the bloodstream. In theory this means fewer side effects.	Do not use at the same time as other vaginal products. If you are using another vaginal product, use it at least six hours before or after a dose of topical progesterone.

gest that testosterone helps calm them.[31] You should also know that testosterone may lower your "good" cholesterol and put you at a greater risk for high blood pressure. It can also cause weight gain, facial hair and acne, and lowering of the voice.

SERMs

Often referred to as "designer" hormones, selective estrogen-receptor modulators (SERMs) burst onto the scene in the 1990s. The first SERM, tamoxifen, was used to treat breast cancer patients

Examples of Available Progestins

PRODUCT	WHAT IS IT?	WHAT DOES IT DO?	WHAT FORM DOES IT COME IN?	OTHER INFORMATION
Medroxy-progesterone (brand names include Amen, Curretab, Cycrin, and Provera)	The most commonly prescribed progestin, this synthetic is made by adding a chemical group to proges-terone.	Treats irregular uterine bleeding.	Dosages vary according to brand of prescription.	Drugs that contain pro-gestins like Provera may cause a greater risk of devel-oping breast cancer. If you are taking one of these drugs, you should avoid smoking, which can increase risks of blood clot-ting. Avoid salt, which can cause fluid retention and excess sun. Weight gain and swelling are common side effects. There are sev-eral drugs that can adversely interact with these prescrip-tions, so check a full list before taking them.

(continued)

PRODUCT	WHAT IS IT?	WHAT DOES IT DO?	WHAT FORM DOES IT COME IN?	OTHER INFORMATION
Noreth-indrone acetate (brand names include Aygestin and Norlutate)	This synthetic proges-terone is made from testosterone.	It is often prescribed to women who have had problems dealing with side effects from Provera or Cycrin and is said to help reduce the breast tenderness and bloat-ing that are often caused by MPA.	Common dosage for Aygestin is 2.5 to 10 mg for 5 to 10 days. Common dosage for Norlutate is 2.5 to 10 mg from the 5th through the 25th day of your cycle.	Same as other progestin drugs—don't take if you have a history of blood clotting, liver problems, or breast cancer.
Micronor	A progestin-only birth control pill that is similar to Aygestin.	Used to stop break-through bleeding.	It's a very low-dose progestin—only 0.35 mg daily. Because it's so low, it is often pres-cribed in continuous HT.	Same risks as other progestin drugs, although anything that can be used as a contraceptive generally has higher levels of hormones.

Levengestrel IUD (brand name: Mirena)	Birth control device thought to curtail bad menopausal bleeding.	Device continuously delivers progestin for up to five years.	Hormone-releasing device.	Device must be implanted and removed. Carries additional risks associated with all IUDs, including unpredictable bleeding and ovarian cysts.

because it would act like an estrogen on some tissues while blocking estrogen on others; in other words, it can positively influence bone as other HT does but without breast-cancer-promoting tendencies. A 1998 study found that invasive breast cancer rates were reduced by 49 percent when women took tamoxifen. Women taking the drug were also notably more likely to develop endometrial cancer, pulmonary embolism, strokes, and deep vein thrombosis.[32] As the National Women's Health Network points out, "In most older women with no risk factors other than age . . . the negative effects of taking the drug outweighed the benefits."[33] In other words, if you haven't had breast cancer and aren't at high risk for it, this probably isn't the best option for you.

Another popular brand-name SERM is called Evista (raloxifene). It is marketed to menopausal women for the improvement and maintenance of bone density. It isn't prescribed for other menopausal symptoms and may actually *increase* your risk for hot flashes. The initial results from the STAR trial—a large study of Evista with 16,000 women—found that the drug was on par with tamoxifin as a breast cancer reducer and seemed to cause fewer endometrial cancers and blood clots when compared with its sister drug.

"Natural" Hormones

No one would argue that Suzanne Somers isn't an excellent sales-woman. After making the ThighMaster a popular household item, the former sitcom star and breast cancer survivor turned her pen toward singing the praises of so-called bioidentical hormones.

Since the results of the WHI, "natural" hormones have gotten a big boost because women perceive them to be more gentle or somehow safer than their pharmaceutical sisters. Unfortunately, this perception isn't borne out by evidence or chemistry.

When you hear the terms *natural* or *bioidentical* attached to a hormone, chances are that this means the chemical you are using is chemically the same as one that you produce in your body. It could also mean that the product is derived from a "natural" source—a plant estrogen, for example. This latter definition is immediately dubious because, of course, the mare's urine used in Premarin is a "natural" product, but certainly not lacking in chemical processing and refinement.

There is no solid evidence showing that "natural" hormones are safer than or significantly different from synthetic ones. As Dr. Isaac Schiff, the chief of obstetrics and gynecology at Massachusetts General Hospital, explains, "We just don't have the information. . . . No one has proven that the bioidentical is any safer or any more harmful than Premarin."[34]

What is so upsetting about Suzanne Somers's claims is that they are grounded in the old idea that hormones will keep you young. Somers herself is quoted in the *New York Times* calling bioidenticals the "juice of youth." Somers's plan is based on regimens created by a former actress named T. S. Wiley. Although Wiley sometimes calls herself a molecular biologist, in reality she holds a regular undergraduate degree from a school in Missouri.[35] While we don't believe that doctors are the only ones who can offer solid health advice, we are suspicious of people who misrepresent themselves in order to sell products or services. Without being mean, we feel it is fair to suggest that Somers's history of special diet, exercise, and admitted plastic surgery are evidence that hormones alone haven't kept her young.

Many natural hormones, prescription and otherwise, come from compounding pharmacies. A compounding pharmacy is a place that blends or customizes different combinations of drugs, including hormones. They are licensed and monitored in all fifty states by pharmacy boards.[36] Among other things, a compounding pharmacy can create a discontinued medication, blend a chemical with different bulks and binders (for example, micronized progesterone is usually suspended in peanut oil; a compounding pharmacist could create an alternative for women with nut allergies), tailor dosages to meet individual patient needs, and prepare the medication in different or more easily useable forms.

Particularly for menopausal women, compounding pharmacies have gained a reputation as a safe haven in the estrogen sea where a caring practitioner gives you individual attention and makes a product tailored to your needs. But like many "alternative" or "natural" medicines, the products created in compounding pharmacies are often undertested. And while a particular estrogen or progestin may be FDA approved, the combination generated by your pharmacist is not—there are no trials on that dosage.

If you decide to use a compounding pharmacy, make sure it meets the highest standards required legally by your state. Ask if the pharmacy has ever had to recall products or had liability claims filed against it. Find out how long it has been in business.

Another charismatic seller of natural products over the years was the now-deceased Dr. John Lee. Dr. Lee wrote a best-selling book called *What Your Doctor May Not Tell You about Menopause*, in which he championed progestins for menopause symptoms, particularly advocating "natural" progesterone. Lee's theory was that women's menopausal woes stem from an excess of estrogen and a dearth of progestin. He also, more controversially, argued that natural progestins don't carry the health hazards of synthetics.

In truth, there is no evidence that natural progestins are safer, and although they may provide some hot-flash relief, there is no proof that they benefit bones and some evidence that they can cause postmenopausal bleeding. Natural progesterone cream ranges from the blatantly synthetic (those that are chemically identical to progestins used in oral HT) to those made from soybeans and yams. The National Women's Health Network writes that "it is unclear if any active components of wild yam can be absorbed through the skin, but whether or not they are, eating or applying wild yam extract or diosgenin will not result in increased progesterone levels in humans because we cannot convert diosgenin into progesterone.... It's as much of a stretch to consider natural progesterone an herbal product as it would be to consider the birth control pill (whose genesis is the same plant) an herbal product."[37]

Some other "natural" hormones include dehydroepiandrosterone (DHEA), estriol, melatonin, and ipraflavone. DHEA is made by the adrenal glands and has become a popular dietary supplement in the past couple decades. Like so many hormone supplements, it is touted as a "youth" pill. Although both men and women take the drug, it produces very different effects in different genders, including raising testosterone levels and lowering "good" cholesterol levels in women's bodies. In general, it seems to have a lot of the same questions surrounding it that we see with testosterone.

Estriol (most frequently taken as the main ingredient in the preparation tri-est,) is a "weak" estrogen thought to provide some of the benefits of HT without the breast and endometrial cancer risk. Tri-est is a combination of 80 percent estriol, 10 percent estrone, and 10 percent estradiol. There is no evidence that estroil has any anti-cancer effects, and more research would be needed to prove that it doesn't bear cancer risks.

Melatonin is an herb used by many Americans to regulate sleep. Most people don't realize that it is actually a hormone. Natural melatonin levels rise when we sleep, and so the idea is that taking supplements can help balance hormones and cure insomnia. Although taking the herb for limited amounts of time is probably safe, there are no long-term data to support using it over time.

Ipriflavone is a synthetic chemical sold over the counter as a dietary supplement. It is used for strengthening bones, but there is evidence that it isn't effective in increasing skeletal density when used alone.

The bottom line, we believe, is that a natural hormone is made in your body, not in a lab, warehouse, or pharmacy. Once you take into account the risks inherent in less-tested products, we don't see a problem with using natural hormones. Just realize they probably carry the same risks as prescription HT and ET.

Of Pills, Patches, and Creams

Does how you take a hormone make a difference in how safe it is or what it does in your body? The answer isn't entirely clear, but new evidence suggests the answer is a definite maybe.

There are two major ways that your body processes hormones. When you take estrogen as a pill or through a patch or an injection, the hormones circulate through the bloodstream to all parts of the body. This is called *systemic therapy*. When you use a vaginal cream, suppository, or ring, you are using *local therapy* that doesn't enter the blood. It has been theorized that local therapy is safer because the drug is metabolized differently in the body and avoids acting on certain tissues. There are two important things to keep in mind. First, it can be difficult to be sure that a chemical is acting locally and not systemically. The vaginal ring, for example, which seems like a local device, delivers hormones strong enough to be absorbed and enter the blood. Second, different women react in different ways to the same dosages. It can be tough to tell with some creams if they are being absorbed into the body in high enough quantities to provide their desired health effects.

If you are using a progestin cream, it is important not to assume that it will counterbalance an oral estrogen. Studies suggest that many progestin creams are absorbed weakly and won't provide the endometrial protection offered by oral progestin. This is true of both prescription and over-the-counter creams. If you have a uterus and are taking estrogen, make sure you are taking a progestin that will provide endometrial protection.

Some recent evidence has provided more support for the idea that gels and patches are a safer way to get your hormones. A French trial called the Estrogen and Thromboembolism Risk study (ES-THER) found that women who used patches and gels reduced their risk of blood clots. When compared with oral estrogen users, the women using alternative delivery systems had blood-clotting rates closer to non–hormone users.[38] Since blood clotting is one of the most serious health risks associated with HT use, this is a big deal. We would caution simply that more information is needed. Scientists made similar safety arguments about oral contraceptive patches, saying they would be safer because they didn't pass through the digestive system but entered the bloodstream directly. Unfortunately, it turned out that with the birth control patch, clotting rates were higher. More time will tell if HT patches are indeed safer.

What about Birth Control Pills?

Birth control pills are often used as hormone replacement when a woman is perimenopausal. The hormone levels in the pill are higher than those in menopausal estrogens. Since, as the WHI showed, estrogen and progestin supplementation becomes more damaging to the body and more dangerous as we age, you should assume the same thing is true with oral contraceptives. Because oral contraceptives are stronger than HT and ET, this should perhaps weigh more heavily in a decision to use or not use hormonal birth control as you age. Once you are menopausal—once birth control is no longer necessary, there is no reason to stick with the pill.

What If You Want to Get Off HT or ET?

HT proponent Tara Parker-Pope calls it the "dirty secret" of estrogen drugs: when women started getting off HT in massive numbers, doctors began observing that these women experienced something akin to drug withdrawal. Hot flashes that had been absent for years or were never a problem returned with a vengeance. Urogenital problems and mood swings started showing up.

Does going off HT or ET cause withdrawal symptoms? And if so, why do some doctors insist that it doesn't?

In the winter of 2006, Laura and Barbara were attending a meeting on sexuality after sixty-five on Manhattan's Upper East Side. When Laura asked about the difficulties of getting off HT, two thirty-something gynecologists looked her straight in the face and insisted that there were no adverse effects of dumping such a strong drug even after decades of use. Unfortunately, this simply isn't true. WHI investigators reported in the *Journal of the American Medical Association (JAMA)* that more than 50 percent of the women who had hot flashes before taking HT experienced them again when they went off the drug. In addition, 6.4 percent of women who never had hot flashes started having them after estrogen use stopped. In addition, vasomotor problems, joint stiffness, depression, and vaginal dryness also occurred after discontinuing hormones.[39]

If you are thinking of going off HT or ET, don't get discouraged. As Deborah Grady and George F. Sawaya note, most women are able to adjust to symptoms and 75 percent don't have serious problems giving up estrogen.[40] Perhaps, though, if you went on HT to fight severe menopause symptoms, you shouldn't try and go off "cold turkey." Instead try slowly tapering down on your dose. If you find your symptoms become unbearable, go back on and try again in a few months or a year, this time more slowly.

So Who Should Take HT and ET?

In all of the excitement about hormones in the past decade, one of the most important things to keep in mind is that historically women took ET and HT for two very different reasons. The first—the one the drugs were approved for—was treating menopausal symptoms, specifically hot flashes and night sweats, and delaying bone loss. The second major use of estrogens was as preventative medicine to avoid chronic disease and fight the more general problems of aging.

Today we know that long-term use of HT for preventative purposes isn't a good idea. Perhaps it will never be a good idea, but at the very least we need a lot more information before healthy women will begin throwing potentially dangerous chemicals into their bodies.

For the short-term treatment of menopause symptoms, however, estrogen drugs are still useful, although—and this is key—not safe.

We do not believe that every woman who has a hot flash should run out and request a prescription. There is a big difference between the hot flashing and night sweating that many women experience and the severe, debilitating problems suffered by a small group.

If your flashing is making your life hell and letting your work get out of hand, if you are in so much discomfort physically that it is starting to affect you emotionally, a little bit of HT or ET might provide much-needed relief.

That said, in all the recent news about the possible benefits of HT for younger women, the head scientists at the WHI are clear: HT isn't good for young women; it is simply less dangerous for younger women than for those "more distant from the menopause."[41]

Make a list: in one column write all the reasons why you want to get symptom relief, and in the other honestly list the risks, one by one. Remember, not every woman who takes hormones will develop these sometimes fatal health problems, but some will. Imagine that the two sides of your page are different ends of a scale and be honest with yourself about which way it is tipping.

If you decide to take hormones, be smart about it. Take the smallest amount you can and think of it as a temporary solution. After a short time, begin to taper off your dose. If you find that the unbearable symptoms return, go back on the drug. Try again after another period of time, a couple of months or even a year. Always remember that like an antibiotic, HT is extremely useful to some people for short amounts of time but isn't intended for long-term use.

Keep in mind that just because menopause symptoms don't feel good doesn't mean they are dangerous. As Barbara has been saying for decades, no woman ever died of a hot flash. At the same time, if you are really suffering, the risks aren't high enough that you should be terrified to try HT for your symptoms.

We don't recommend using hormone treatments for bone maintenance. Because most studies suggest that increased bone density is reliant on continued hormone use, and because we know that long-term treatment is dangerous, this isn't the best solution for keeping your bones well.

If you have had a hysterectomy, and in particular if you have had an oophorectomy, you may find that taking estrogen is more necessary. Women who are thrown into menopause by surgery often experience particularly intense and persistent menopause symptoms and are also at risk for a number of different serious health problems. The jury is still out, but it may turn out that women who've undergone total hysterectomies aren't simply palliated by ET; they may actually receive health benefits that women who go through natural menopause do not. Dr. Jacques Rossouw of the WHI reaffirms that estrogen therapy is standard treatment for women who've had surgery.[42]

Reasons Not to Take HT and ET

1. History of or significant risk factors for breast cancer.
2. History of blood clots or family history of heart disease and stroke.
3. Known heart disease.
4. Liver disease.
5. If you are or if you hope to become pregnant.
6. If you have a history of unexplained vaginal bleeding.
7. Any history of or significant family history of reproductive cancers.

So many women in recent generations found natural menopause to be uncharted territory. Their mothers and grandmothers had all undergone hysterectomies, and there was no one they could reliably turn to for information about the natural twists and turns of the change. Likewise, women now must chart the path of a predominantly hormone-free menopause. It won't look like their mom's or even their friend's.

Barbara, too, finds herself in uncharted territory. T. S. Eliot once wrote that "the end of all our exploring will be to arrive where we started, and know the place for the first time."[43] At a recent party with friends, a longtime acquaintance in her mid-forties started bending Barbara's ear about her hot flashes. What should she do, the talented editor wondered, to curb her crippling night sweats? Perhaps antidepressants or untested but available natural supplements?

Barbara thought for a few minutes: Although her friend was really suffering, she couldn't forget about the new hazards awaiting women from the untested fleets of HT alternatives now being pushed on a populace overeager for remedies. Suddenly Barbara found herself offering advice that even five years ago would have been unlikely to come from her mouth: "Perhaps," Barbara said, "you should try a little HT."

11

menopause, naturally? what we know about the wild west of natural, alternative, and bioidentical menopause medicine

The obstacles to discovery — the illusions
of knowledge — are also part of our story.
—DANIEL BOORSTIN, PREFACE TO *The Discoverers*

W hen conventional medicine fails you," a friend of Laura's told her confidently in a recent conversation, "you have no choice but to take matters into your own hands." She was explaining her reasons for switching from a pharmaceutical to an herbal regimen to treat chronic insomnia exacerbated by hot flashes and night sweats.

Laura's friend's attitude is typical of many people's feelings about herbal and alternative medicine. Taking supplements can give us a sense of freedom and confidence in our ability to help ourselves.

For centuries, women have turned to herbal and natural medicines as a way of taking control and creating hope for our health during years when our well-being was ignored. Many women persecuted as witches in medieval and Renaissance Europe were actually providers of alternative care to a populace that couldn't afford doctors.

As Barbara Ehrenreich and Deirdre English note in their classic 1973 pamphlet *Witches, Midwives and Nurses: A History of Women Healers,* "Many herbal remedies developed by witches still have their place in modern pharmacology."[1] The violence with which many alternative-care providers were suppressed had two implications for the future of medicine. First, it showed the fierce resolve of the medical establishment in consolidating authority and relegating the mostly female lay healers to the periphery of modern medicine. Importantly, this was done in part by locating medical professionalism in the universities and removing it from the home. Second, in doing so, it created a sense that these alternative practitioners possessed a shadowy, potentially powerful sphere of knowledge. Alternative practitioners have taken many forms and roles over the years: "Healers and herbalists, bonesetters and barbers, shamans and spiritualists have offered the public a multiplicity of ways to address the confusion and suffering that accompany disease."[2]

These days, it's not just the people without access to mainstream health care who are exploring herbal options. In fact, studies suggest that the majority of complementary and alternative medicine users are affluent and have high levels of education.[3] So how many women use herbal medicines? According to an October 2003 article in the *Archives of Internal Medicine,* the use of botanicals and dietary supplements increased by an estimated 380 percent between 1990 and 1997, with sales of over $600 million in 1998 for herbal products alone.[4] Nearly one in six American women took at least one herb by the year 2000,[5] and the numbers keep going up. Among peri- and postmenopausal women, usage of botanical dietary supplements may be as high as 79 percent.[6]

We are among the millions of Americans who have come to trust and treasure herbal treatments. Barbara likes chamomile tea for insomnia, peppermint for indigestion, and for respiratory infection echinacea is (or was) her choice.[7] Today she hesitates to take her once-beloved remedies as the shameful facts on lack of quality control are coming to light. How can the very real need for nonpharmaceutical approaches to medicine be balanced against evidence that supplement makers are becoming like unregulated versions of their drug company counterparts? How can we guard ourselves against an unsafe supply and a serious dearth of clinical knowledge on natural, alternative, and bioidentical menopause medicines?

A Drug by Any Other Name, or Welcome to the Wild, Wild West

The first thing to realize about an alternative drug is that it is exactly that—a drug. Just because something says it is "natural" doesn't mean that it isn't having a profound effect on your body, both good and bad. The chemicals in these botanicals work a lot like their synthetic counterparts and can interact with other herb and prescription medications in potentially dangerous ways. People taking herbs often forget this because they can buy them over the counter or because they equate the word *natural* with "gentle" or "safe." The truth is that you can end up taking way too much of certain chemicals such as estrogens in herbal form. Many prescription pharmaceuticals have primary botanical ingredients, and many more are simple chemical variations on naturally occurring compounds.

The accessibility of alternative medicines adds to patients feeling that they are in charge of their health decisions. The flip side of this freedom is a certain amount of danger. Herbs, supplements, and natural remedies are not regulated by the government, which means you can never be sure, chemically speaking, what you are getting. Just because the bottle in your medicine chest with the pretty label says it is red clover doesn't mean it *is* red clover.

Take a walk down the aisle of your local health-food store or vitamin store, and you are truly in the Wild West, a space where anything goes. At some point botanical and supplemental medicine came to be the least regulated part of the world of medicine. Although there are many honest natural medicine makers out there, there are also lots of folks who, like their pharmaceutical counterparts, are out to make a buck at any cost.

Complementary and Alternative Medicine

The role of complementary and alternative medicine (CAM) in America is only expanding, and menopausal women are a big part of this change. The National Institutes of Health (NIH) defines CAM as diverse products and medical practices that aren't part of conventional medicine. This is a scaled-down, more politically correct version of an older, broadly used definition that insisted CAM was any medical practice not taught in U.S. medical schools.[8] Both of these classifications rely on the old relationship between doctors and alternative practitioners, an adversarial dynamic in which mainstream medical doctors and natural healers were at odds, two opposing teams competing for the bodies and minds of the general populace.

Although these tensions still exist between science and belief, the lab and the living room, doctors are increasingly accepting of and are learning about alternative medicine. Health insurance has begun to cover certain types of alternative treatments. Americans agree with this approach: while 50 percent of us use CAM as part of our health regimens, only 4 percent use it exclusively. CAM products and procedures have become an "adjunct" to our more conventional practices.[9]

New terms reflect this change in thinking: in addition to "alternative," CAM is now called "complementary" medicine, suggesting its relationship with the mainstream and "integrative," which bespeaks an even closer, less hierarchical dynamic with the doctor's office. In a larger way, the embracing of alternative medicine by the general public suggests a big shift in the way we relate to our doctors and our bodies.

What still separates herbs and pharmaceuticals is a base of real scientific evidence. Very few CAM products have any sort of clinical trials, and the trials that do happen are flimsy by the standards of FDA requirements for prescription drugs. This has led some doctors to dismiss supplements as modern-day snake oil. As one doctor explains, "There is no alternative medicine. There is only scientifically proven, evidence-based medicine supported by solid data or unproven medicine, for which scientific evidence is lacking."[10] We don't buy such a viewpoint; it's like insisting there is only one language worth speaking. But we do worry about the safety and health of those embracing alternatives.

Why Aren't Natural Medicines Regulated?

After a period of decline, natural medicines were making a big come-back in 1980s America. All of this came to a screeching halt when a supplement called L-tryptophan was pulled from the market after a series of patients became disabled and even died after taking it. Then President George H. W. Bush, the Congress, and a young FDA director named David Kessler began moving to give the government more control of supplement regulation and more ways to insure product safety.

In response, a conglomerate of natural product makers mounted an epic campaign to oppose new laws and regulations. Using television and print ads, the group convinced average Americans that the government was trying to take away their natural medicines. The result of this battle was the passage of the Dietary Supplements Health and Education Act (DSHEA), a deceptively named bill that has made insuring product quality and safety of supplements and vitamins basically impossible. Rather than providing more consumer protection, this new law set back the clock, removing most of the natural-medicine regulation of the twentieth century.[11]

How Bad Is the Botanical Supplement Supply in the United States?

Before taking any drug, including natural medicines, the two most basic questions to ask are "Is it safe?" and "Does it work?"

The answer to the first question may eliminate the need to ask the second. Indeed, if most studies of product quality in the botanical and dietary supplemen industry are to be believed, then most herbals lack basic label a curacy, purity, and product-to-product consistency.

There are several way that botanical medicine labels can mislead.[12] The first is blatant the contents may not be what they say they are. This could be because many botanicals degrade quickly over time, so if a product sits too long on shelves it may end up being chemically useless.

Some products are contaminated with impurities, including occasional traces of prescription products. Many consumers take potentially unsafe herbs without even knowing it. Herbs are often grown in countries with lax agricultural policies, and dangerous chemicals such as DDT have been found in things as benign as green tea. Supplement capsules may not contain the amount of a given herb that their packages claim. A June 2000 *New York Times* expose found that one-quarter of thirty brands of ginkgo biloba, an herbal extract used to enhance memory, did not have adequate levels of the active ingredients listed on the label.[13]

Because there are no official government recommendations regarding doses on herbs (this isn't true with vitamins), supplement manufacturers are left to provide their own suggestions regarding how much of their product you should take. When you look on the "Supplement Facts" box on the back of your herbal medicines, you will usually find a list of the active herbs, and where you would see a number or percentage indicating the daily value (DV) each pill holds, there is often a star or an asterisk. The reason is that for the vast majority of botanicals, there is no established or uniform DV. So when the supplement makers give their individual dosing advice, the numbers have been shown to be vastly different from company to company and bottle to bottle.

In addressing the problem of standardization, Judith Garrard[14] makes two salient points: first, many herbal products that bear the same name aren't the same thing: there are three different species of echinacea, for example, which can work differently and at different strengths in the body.[15] Labels may not let you know what kind of echinacea you are getting in a given jar. A 1995 *Consumer Reports* review of the popular herb ginseng found that of the ten brands it reviewed, two different types of ginseng were represented.[16]

Different parts of a plant may be used to create very different products. Again, these variations may not be apparent from product packaging. If studies have tested the usefulness of a plant's root, and capsules contain dried leaves, we don't really know anything about that product. Indeed, even the way a plant is grown and picked can have remarkable effects on the potency of products produced from it.

This is further complicated by the fact that we don't have a thorough chemical understanding of many popular herbs, let alone their less ubiquitous counterparts. Red clover is one of the most popular menopause herbs and one for which there are some of the most standardized studies. Despite this fact, in a report published in 2006 in the *Journal of Alternative and Complementary Medicine*, researchers identified twenty-two compounds in red clover and measured twenty: they write, "This represents a significant improvement in the characterization of red clover supplements because currently only four of the isoflavone components (daidzein, genistein, formononetin, and biochanin A) are measured and reported in clinical studies."[17]

Judith Garrard's second point is that how you make and take a product make a difference. If you are drinking St. John's wort tea, your body is getting something different from the capsules you might opt to take instead. If you are using soy cream on your body, this isn't comparable to munching down on a plate of tofu or edamame.

This is also true for the way a product is manufactured. Herbal medicines get a lot of mileage out of claiming ancestry from "traditional" processes. Unfortunately, the ways many botanicals are extracted and processed bear little or no resemblance to methods used by ancient peoples. Supplement makers, obviously, use very different methods of extraction; the use of strong chemicals to extract the active ingredients can make a traditionally helpful or benign herb dangerous.[18]

As one thorough analysis concludes, "In some cases, description on product labels were so vague about plant parts, or even the plant species, that experienced pharmacists on the study team were not able to discern ingredient information. If pharmacists trained to interpret pharmaceutical product descriptions are unable to understand the labels for some of these products, how can a layperson make sense of them, much less compare products with a benchmark or with one another or convey this information to their physician?"[19]

A Soybean a Day? Menopause Supplements' Safety and Efficacy

So do natural remedies work? Let's look at the evidence for a few of the most popular natural products for menopause.

Black Cohosh

At a recent cocktail party, a beautiful, stylishly dressed friend talked at length about her hot flashes and bothersome night sweats. When Laura asked her what she doing now to aid her discomforts, she didn't hesitate: "My dear," she enthused, flipping her blond curls, "*everyone* is taking black cohosh!"

Although certainly not everyone is taking it, black cohosh, or *Cimicifuga racemosa*, is probably the best-known herb specifically associated with menopause. A plant that grows wild throughout the East Coast of the United States and Canada, and a relative of the buttercup, black cohosh has long been used to relieve vaginal dryness and quell hot flashes.[20]

Like many alternative drugs, black cohosh has a long history; it was used by the Native Americans and has been employed as a folk remedy for hundreds of years.[21] It was the main ingredient in U.S. patent medicines such as Lydia Pinkham's vegetable compound, and its root extract has been used for decades in Germany and other European nations.

Scientists are still trying to understand how black cohosh works and are actively engaged in isolating and identifying its different elements.[22] The central mystery is whether black cohosh functions by acting like estrogen in the body or through other means. While the plant has some known estrogen-like activity, it is also possible that it contains nonhormonal agents as well. This ambiguity has been used by some to suggest that black cohosh is safe for women who have had breast cancer, but such a recommendation is at this point irresponsible.

So why might it work? Triterpene glycosides, which are extracted from the root rhizome of the plant, likely act like an estrogen and are a progesterone precursor. The drug suppresses female luteinizing hormone, a chemical associated with triggering hot flashes.

In terms of good clinical evidence on black cohosh, the results continue to be mixed and confusing. In 2002, Dr. Adriane Fugh-Berman, a women's-health activist and professor at Georgetown Medical School, and Dr. Fredi Kronenberg, a professor of physiology at Columbia, surveyed scientific studies on complementary and alternative treatments for menopausal symptoms.[23] Their review, published in the *Annals of Internal Medicine,* found that in ten clinical trials using herbs to treat hot flashes, only black cohosh demonstrated a beneficial result. These positive findings were couched in the news that improvements with black cohosh were not markedly different from hormone treatment or placebos. In other words, you'd receive the same symptom relief from simply thinking that you were taking black cohosh as you'd get from actually using it. There is no solid evidence that black cohosh builds bone.

Most trials use a product called Remifemin as their form of black cohosh. This kind of standardization testing one product is lacking many herbal trials, but it should be noted that the formula for Remifemin has changed over the years—the dose has risen from 2 mg per tablet to 20 mg—probably making old and new data incomparable.

Adverse effects of taking black cohosh can include nausea, vomiting, dizziness, visual disturbances, trouble with the nervous system, and reduced heart rate. As the American Pharmaceutical Association pointed out at its 2000 annual meeting: "Because it contains salicylic acid [an active ingredient in aspirin and anti-acne drugs] and an anticoagulant, black cohosh may interact with salicylates or salicylic acid containing herbs and any anticoagulant containing substance. This could cause increased bleeding or affect platelet aggregation."

Many different black cohosh preparations, including Remifemin, are available in health-food stores and some drugstores. No more than 40 mg per day is recommended. Because long-term toxicity has not been studied, many nutritionists recommend discontinuing black cohosh for a few months after six months of continuous use. There has also been some recent concern about liver damage in cohosh users,[24] another good reason not to overdo your dosages and to take the herb for the shortest amount of time possible.

Soy

Soy goods, ranging from vegetarian food to supplements to bath scrubs and lotions, have touted this little bean as the great hope of menopausal health. By some estimates, Americans will spend between $3 billion and $4 billion this year on soy food alone. This figure excludes the money that will go to soy supplements. But does soy serve as a safe and efficient menopause aid? The evidence, as with most natural remedies, has been mixed.

Why are soybeans so healthful? One reason is that they are unique among plant foods in supplying all the essential amino acids that the human body needs. Soy protein is similar to meat protein but contains less saturated fat. In 1999, the American Heart Association and the FDA recommended it to aid in lowering cholesterol. Soy contains compounds called *flavonoids*, chemicals found in fruits, vegetables, legumes, whole grains, nuts, seeds, herbs, and spices that are thought to be useful for certain health concerns. Like so many "natural" menopause aids, it works phytoestrogenically.

Soy came to be one of the natural remedies of choice for menopausal women for a number of reasons. A big one was the discrepancy in hot flashes and breast cancer rates between American and Japanese women. Doctors wondered what lifestyle difference could account for the relative ease with which women in Japan navigated the menopause transition. One difference they could find was the large amount of soy consumed traditionally as part of a Japanese diet.

Today, the scientific community is still split on soy: some believe fervently that it will not only ease hot flashing but actually work to prevent breast cancer. Others counter that as a phytoestrogen, soy might feed breast cancer just as HT and other hormone preparations do.

The argument for soy begins with its status as a "weak" estrogen. The isoflavones genistein and daidzein are plant hormones that can mimic or block the effects of biological estrogen. Because of this, soy seemed to hold promise that it might act as a natural cancer fighter.

If it did help, it would be because breast cancer basically feeds off estrogen. It's possible that because plant estrogens aren't as strong, they are able to block more powerful human hormones from getting to estrogen receptors, depriving the cancer of its way of growing.[25] Such claims, however, aren't substantiated, and because the relationship between cancer and estrogen is so potentially deadly, it seems unwise to knowingly introduce any estrogen, even a weak one, if you have had, have, or are at high risk for breast cancer.

But what about hot flashes? When soy has been given to women in controlled studies, the benefits in preventing hot flashes have been negligible. In a trial of postmenopausal women in Italy, those taking soy reported 45 percent fewer moderate or severe hot flashes after twelve weeks of treatment, but women in the placebo group reported a 30 percent improvement.[26] Again, most studies aren't big enough or nearly long enough to give us truly useful information.

Those who do take soy should consider possible side effects. First, soy is highly allergenic. Additionally, some physicians have reported cases of patients developing symptoms of hypothyroidism on high doses. This is probably because genistein interferes with a key enzyme in the thyroid gland, thyroxine peroxidase. Like a decision to take HT, a decision to use large amounts of a phytoestrogen must be weighed carefully against potential risks.

There is evidence that soy supplements—which we don't recommend taking—have the same quality-control problems seen in other natural products. One study looked at thirteen different soy products available over the counter at drug and grocery stores. Each soy preparation was tested four times. Researchers found that "in all products tested, only 4 of the 13 products have 90%–100% of the labeled amounts and 6 of the 13 products had greater than 85% of the labeled amounts."[27] In addition, at least one of the products was self-inconsistent, having content that "has changed over time," and five of the products had more than 5 percent unknown impurities, with two being more than 40 percent impure. The study authors conclude, "A lack of clear standard allows for the marketing of more expensive products that are not superior, a poor predicament for the industry and consumers."

Does this mean we should all cut soy from our diets? Of course not. There are too many proven health benefits from this powerful little bean. What it does mean is that we should avoid megadosing. The best way to enjoy soy's benefits and avoid its risks, at least until science can give us more information, it to get our soy through food consumption as a natural by-product of a healthy diet. As little as a cup and a half of soy milk, half a cup of tofu, or two tablespoons of roasted soy nuts a day can provide the recommended 50 mg per day, and if you are prone to thyroid or breast problems, you may actually want to limit your consumption.

Red Clover

After black cohosh, red clover is one of the most frequently used menopause herbs. Promensil, a popular menopause treatment, counts red clover as its main ingredient. A medicinal herb used by American Indians to treat a variety of ailments from cancer to whooping cough, it is taken in many parts of the world and is found in creams to counteract skin irritation.[28] Red clover is rich in isoflavones, containing high concentrations of four major ones: formononetin, biochanin A, daidzein, and genistein. You may recognize a few of these as the active chemicals in soy, and you may have already guessed that red clover works phytoestrogenically.

In 2001, a group of researchers from George Washington University and Columbia University reviewed the scientific evidence for red clover's effectiveness in the September issue of *Menopause: The Journal of the North American Menopause Society.* They felt there were two good clinical trials in which women were randomly given either red clover extracts or a placebo for three months. Neither trial found red clover to be better than the placebo for hot flashes or vaginal dryness. Like other phytoestrogens, we're still unsure what effect it has on breast tissue.

Although red clover is on the FDA's "generally recognized as safe" list, anyone taking it should be mindful of some important facts. First, some types of clover contain coumarins. These are chemical compounds that reduce blood clotting. Because of this, women taking blood-thinning drugs such as warfarin, heparin, clopidogrel, or even over-the-counter thinners such as aspirin should consult a doctor before using red clover.

Evening Primrose Oil and Other Fatty Acids

Evening primrose is a biennial herb common to North America. Usually taken in capsule form or sold as an oil, it is derived from the seeds of the evening primrose plant. It is often recommended because it contains potentially heart-healthy fatty acids, including linoleic acid and gamma linoleic acid. It has long been postulated that a shortage in fatty acids may be associated with PMS and other menstrual problems, and it has recently been suggested that perhaps primrose could help treat menopause problems as well.

While evening primrose does contain fatty acids, it is also highly estrogenic. Because of this, it has all the risks that any estrogen substance does, including a possible link between evening primrose use and increased risk of breast cancer. In addition to such risks, clinical data haven't demonstrated strong success in treating any ailments with evening primrose except for mastalgia (sore breasts), and the herb may cause gastrointestinal problems. A British study published in 1994 randomized and blinded (meaning even the scientists conducting the experiment didn't know which women were receiving clover and which placebo) fifty-six women who were experiencing lots of hot flashes. The study found, ironically, that flashing in the placebo group went down while women actually receiving the oil had the same number of hot flashes as they did at the start of the trial.[29]

Another source of fatty acids is flax seeds. A rich source of lignans, they may be helpful in relieving hot flashes and mood swings and alleviating vaginal dryness. Like evening primrose oil, what effect they have is probably based on their phytoestrogenicity. Two tablespoons a day can be ground in a coffee grinder and sprinkled on cereal, soups, salads, or casseroles. Flax can also be taken in capsule form, with 500 mg per day being the recommended dosage. An added benefit: they are a good source of omega-3 fatty acids.

Dong Quai, Chasteberry, and the Importance of the Placebo Effect

Dong quai, or *Angelica sinensis,* is a plant that grows on cold, damp mountain slopes in China, Japan, and Korea. It has been widely used in Asia for nearly two thousand years and has recently found popularity in the United States for treating gynecological problems.

Because it is relatively new to the American herb market, there has been very little research conducted on the safety and effectiveness of dong quai. One 1997 study[30] attempted to determine whether dong quai can be useful for women suffering from hot flashes and other major menopausal symptoms. Seventy-one women were divided into two groups. One group received 4.5 grams of dong quai root daily for six months, while the other group got a placebo. Researchers determined that for hot flashes, the herb was no better than a sugar pill. Although a traditional Chinese healer would probably recommend dong quai in combination with some other herbs, and the study's failure to replicate this might have impacted results, the information from this trial is relevant, as dong quai is often sold alone in the United States.

Side effects from taking dong quai include excessive blood thinning, a laxative effect, internal bleeding, skin irritation, severe rash, sensitivity to sunlight, and potential carcinogenicity. Dong quai can also make it hard for the body to retain vitamin B12, which can aggravate anemia and cause weakness. All told, there isn't good evidence for this herb, and there are a lot of reasons not to take it.

A similar case can be made about chasteberry, or *Vitex agnus-castus*, which some women take to prevent hot flashes.

Chasteberry, like dong quai, was originally used to treat menstrual irregularities, painful menstruation, and breast pain. While it may function phytoestrogenically, the fruit itself has a dopamine-like activity that inhibits prolactin release, increasing progesterone in the luteal phase of the menstrual cycle.

There is little clinical evidence that chasteberry has any positive effect beyond a placebo; however, adverse effects include stomach problems, itching, rash, alopecia (hair loss), headaches, and fatigue. It can also interact negatively with drugs that work on dopamine receptors (e.g., metoclopramide) and birth control pills. On the balance, the dangers of chasteberry seem to far outweigh any suspected benefits. (As a side note, two of the herb's names—chasteberry and monk's pepper—suggest another, possibly undesirable effect: a decrease in interest in sex.)

Ginseng

In the excellent guide *The Truth about Hormone Replacement Therapy*, the National Women's Health Network reminds us that "Siberian ginseng" is a completely different plant from ginseng, despite similar uses.[31]

A Swedish trial published in 1999 tested American ginseng for its usefulness in treating hot flashes and menopause symptoms. The study found no significant results, and hot flashes weren't decreased.[32]

Natural Progesterone Creams

Perhaps no preparation illustrates the psychological distance and chemical closeness of herbals and pharmaceuticals like the burgeoning popularity of so-called natural progesterone creams.

In March 2004, a paper based on a two-year study conducted at the Clinical Research Foundation at Bassett Health Care in Cooperstown, New York, found that over-the-counter progesterone cream was absorbed into the blood in the same amounts as FDA-approved capsules. In other words "natural" progesterone cream was found to be just as strong as prescription hormones. This means that the millions of women who are using these creams every year are potentially at risk for heart disease and other HT risk factors. Women should understand that when it comes to estrogen and progesterone, "natural" doesn't mean "mild" or "low dose."

For more information on these popular remedies, read chapter 10.

Alternative Practitioners

A number of alternative nonchemical practices are increasingly being used for various medical problems. These usually involve seeking the help of an alternative practitioner. Like a doctor, an alternative practitioner, such as an acupuncturist, a chiropractor, or a naturopath, must be chosen with care, and you should put in the time to make sure the person you are working with is properly licensed and certified.

When searching for a practitioner, start by asking your doctor for a referral. You should also go online to search for professional organizations for the type of service you are seeking. Contact them and ask about licensed, credentialed people in your area.

Do a little research about what sorts of training and certification are required by your state for various kinds of care. Make sure that the practitioners you decide to use have those qualifications. The National Center for Complementary and Alternative Medicine (NCCAM) suggests checking out the Directory Information Resources Online (DIRLINE), a database at the National Library of Medicine that keeps locations and descriptions of a variety of health organizations (dirline.nlm.nih.gov).[33]

The only alternative therapy that has been extensively tested for treating menopause symptoms is acupuncture. A Chinese medical system that's been in use for more than two thousand years, acupuncture has gained broad acceptance even among mainstream medical doctors in the past two decades. NCCAM estimates that somewhere around 10 million adults have used acupuncture at one time in the United States, and that each year around 2 million Americans participate in the practice.[34]

An acupuncturist inserts small needles into different points of the body. It is generally painless, although improper needle placement or patient movement can lead to soreness. As long as you seek out a qualified practitioner, the process is considered generally safe. Make sure that your acupuncturist uses a new set of disposable needles each time you go in for treatment.

There have been several studies testing acupuncture's ability to treat menopause symptoms. One problem with any study involving acupuncture is the difficulty of creating a control. Some scientists have done it, though, and it is interesting to note that while acupuncture is found to be significantly helpful for menopause problems in uncontrolled studies, studies that compared acupuncture to placebo treatments don't show the same benefits. Janet S. Carpenter explains that in controlled trials, "acupuncture did not consistently improve hot flashes, sleep disturbances or mood."[35]

Reflexology uses foot massage to rebalance bodily energies and by extension promote healing. There is one randomized controlled clinical trial of the process for menopause symptoms. Thirty-five women were given nine sessions of foot reflexology and thirty-one women received a foot massage with no reflexology. The study found no difference between the treatment and placebo groups.[36]

Magnet therapy seeks to use magnetic fields to treat a variety of ailments. In a placebo-controlled clinical trial, the procedure was less effective than placebos for decreasing hot flashes and improving quality of life.

Although it's certainly not yet widespread, some insurance companies have started to cover CAM therapies and medicines.

Getting Information for Yourself

You may encounter other herbs and natural supplements that aren't specifically covered here. First, be aware that this probably means, at least where menopausal complaints are concerned, that the product doesn't have much clinical information to support it. You should be able to do your own research, though, and we think that is a good idea with any product you are regularly putting in your body.

The National Center for Complementary and Alternative Medicine (NCCAM) is a government agency devoted to funding and encouraging new scientific research on herbal medicines. As Dan Hurley and others have documented,[37] the center was founded by members of Congress who were particularly sympathetic to the supplement industry, and although NCCAM continues to be overly optimistic and easily convinced about the potential of different herbs and practices, it is still a good place to start in getting "the basics" about different products. Use the NCCAM Web site as a starting point and take what it says with a grain of salt.

ConsumerLab.com is a wonderful resource for getting specific information about hundreds of products. Located in White Plains, New York, and headed by Dr. Tod Cooperman, ConsumerLab publishes extensive reports about individual product purity as well as giving helpful overviews of herbs and supplements. Report summaries are free, and full reports are available to members for $27 a year. (Dr. Cooperman obviously can't test *all* brands on the market, so if yours doesn't make his list, don't assume it is necessarily of inferior quality.)

We also recommend using the National Library of Medicine's Medline Plus (nlm.nih.gov/medlineplus/) and the Mayo Clinic (mayoclinic.com) Web sites as good general resources.

In general, we feel that a big problem with herb use in the United

States is that people take a "Why not?" approach to using many kinds of supplemental products. We think people would benefit from taking the approach we recommend with prescription drugs—that is, a "Why should I?" attitude. Start by assuming you don't want to take something, and see if the evidence can change your mind.

Far too many menopausal women end up consuming chemical soups involving combinations of vitamins, herbs, and pharmaceuticals. This is a bad idea for so many reasons, but the most obvious is that you run the risk of getting way too much estrogen. In general, if you are going to take herbs and nutrients, we suggest doing so in food form rather than in supplements. This eliminates inconsistencies in extraction methods and lessens the risk of megadosing. This isn't always possible but should be considered when it is.

Likewise, we advise avoiding combination supplements with vague names like "menopause therapy." Be wary—especially if these preparations don't tell you exactly which herbs are in them. Even if the ingredients are listed, we recommend avoiding combination supplements because they complicate safety decisions.

We agree with many doctors that complementary and alternative medicine will benefit from a better relationship with science and a more open dynamic with "mainstream" medicine. Far from feeling that herbal medicine should be co-opted by doctors, we would argue that there are too many patient-health issues at stake to accept the sometimes antagonistic relationship between these two schools of wellness. Most of us—including doctors—struggle with the complexities of scientific testing. But anyone can understand the story of a friend who says an herb has helped her. Most of us aren't fluent in the thick statistics used to generate claims of "efficacy" in medical journal articles, but we understand a caring alternative practitioner telling us about how Native American wisdom might work for us.

This issue of language gets to the heart of a subject where many doctors fail: communicating in simple, clear ways that make patients feel they are a part of their health care decisions. This is one place where doctors have much to learn from their counterparts in natural medicine.

There are many reasons why doctor-patient (and doctor-herbalist) communication is important. The first is that patients often fail to tell their doctors about the botanical drugs they are taking, and doctors aren't always trained to ask. This means that patients miss out on the benefits of their doctors' knowledge about their supplements and may not get crucial information about drug interactions.[38] One of the most dangerous results of not thinking of herbal medicines as drugs is that they can interact with pharmaceuticals and prescription medications, and the results can be disastrous.[39] Indeed, a fifth of those who take prescription drugs—as many as 15 million adults—also take herbs or supplements and may be at risk.[40]

Of Pearls and Swine

There is a lot of wisdom to be found in alternative and complementary medicine. It can feel good to participate in wellness traditions that stretch back far before Western medicine, and it can make us feel connected to the human community and in control of our medical destinies.

There is also a lot of danger. Until regulation and supply are better, until real long-term, double-blinded, placebo-controlled trials of herbs are available, botanical medicines remain riddled with questions, concerns, and caveats.

In an excellent editorial in the *Journal of the American Medical Association*, Dr. Wayne B. Jonas summarizes this world with brilliant brevity: "Alternative medicine is here to stay. It is no longer an option to ignore it or treat it as something outside the normal processes of science and medicine. The challenge is to move forward carefully, using both reason and wisdom, as we attempt to separate the pearls from the mud."[41]

12

the skinny on menopausal weight

is gain really just part of the change?

A diet slightly richer in humble pie might
do nutrition experts some good.

—STEVEN SHAPIN

We are about to introduce you to the best diet guru around. This expert can help you figure out the only diet plan that will work for you and is the only one who can help you lose and maintain weight.

No, we're not talking about the author of some new, hot weight-loss book. We're talking about you.

We're not the only ones who think so. A number of recent studies have concluded that nutritional knowledge and self-awareness outstrip food limitations and rules in their ability to help you find and keep a weight that is healthy and attractive.

While this may come as a surprise to you, it will come as no surprise that Americans are obsessed with weight—mostly how to lose it. Harvard professor Steven Shapin notes that "a fifth of American men and more than a third of American women say they would like to lose at least twenty pounds."

Many women find that they put on some weight at midlife that they just can't seem to take off. That weight tends to be in places they didn't put on weight before: the belly instead of the hips, for example. For years, there has been an assumption both in popular culture and in medical literature that menopause is the reason for this gain.

But do extra midlife pounds really happen as part of the menopause transition or are they just part of the more general aging process? If men start to get bigger as they get older, why do so many cultural messages emphasize midlife weight gain as a female problem?

What to Expect When You're Expanding

For decades, the notion that menopause and extra pounds come hand in hand has gone relatively unchallenged. Menopause philosopher Susun Weed writes eloquently about her own weight issues, noting, "I had some killer hot flashes, but the most difficult part of menopause for me was gaining weight. I knew it was going to happen; I knew it was supposed to happen. But I never thought it would happen."[1] At first Weed felt bad about her new full figure: "My modern prejudices surged to the fore—'Yuck. You look disgusting. You're overweight . . . ' I knew it wasn't true. But despite years of feminism and consciousness raising on every ism, from ageism to weightism, there was my culture yelling at me in my own mind every time I looked in the mirror." After a lot of work on self-acceptance (not to mention encouragement from her partner), Weed finally concluded that "the best ally you can have on your menopausal journey is an 'extra' ten pounds."

While Weed is right about a lot of things—confused cultural messages about weight gain, and the potential health benefits of a small amount of extra weight (we'll talk about that below)—she never stops to examine her beliefs about the source of her surplus pounds.

Although we're not sure why, we know that women seem to start putting on weight at an accelerated rate between the ages of thirty-five and fifty-five.[2] Although certainly not all women will fight an intensified battle of the bulge, the number of obese women in the general population rises with each decade of life until the sixties and seventies, when it slows down a little.[3]

The amount of this gain seems to be about an average of a pound a year during the menopause transition. The Healthy Women's Study, a long-term trial out of Pittsburgh, found that after three years, pre- and perimenopausal women gained an average of five pounds; 20 percent of the women gained ten pounds during the first three years of the study.[4]

The nutrition expert Artemis Simopoulos notes that midlife weight gain used to be just that—before the 1960s and '70s, women in the United States and Canada would gradually, naturally increase body weight in their thirties, forties, and fifties, at which point the extra pounds would stop coming. Now she says, the gain is greater and the plateau is virtually nonexistent. Why the recent trend toward continuing to gain weight in later decades? Simopoulos cites familiar culprits—dietary changes that include diets high in trans fats, soft drinks with large amounts of fructose, and too many omega-6 fatty acids. She notes that women also drink more alcohol than in previous generations, no longer smoke at the same rates (unfortunately one way to keep off pounds), and live more sedentary lives. Simopoulos is firm in asserting that mid- and late-life weight gain has "nothing to do with menopause."[5]

Although some studies have observed weight gain to be more pronounced around the change, a link is still unproven, and information from various trials is conflicting.

Something that people trying to sell "menopause" products won't remind you of is that men put on weight at midlife too. Women and men gain weight differently, but by the time they hit their forties, fifties, and above, they are both trying to avoid expanding. Rose Frisch of the Harvard School of Public Health explains that while women have higher body fat at younger ages—26 to 28 percent for women versus 12 to 14 percent for men—men soon catch up, with both sexes having around 30 to 40 percent body fat. A 1996 study from Grant Medical College in Bombay found that while only 10 percent of young men (seventeen to twenty) in the trial were obese, a whopping 90 percent were obese by the time they reached their late thirties and early forties.[6] Women start out bigger but stay on average smaller than their male counterparts. In fact, recent research finds that 65 percent of men are carrying too much fat, compared with only 55 percent of women.[7] This is a gap that is widening, not narrowing, and some estimates suggest that in five years, as many as 75 percent of men will have unhealthy body mass indexes. The number of overweight women is growing steadily, too, just not as quickly as the number of men.

Why We Gain Weight: Reasons and Rationales

Conventional wisdom has long imagined roller-coaster hormones to be the cause of unwanted weight. There certainly seems to be a relationship between hormones and body size.

This is clear in the years before girls get their first periods. A friend of Barbara's wisely observed that her young daughter's friends "all seemed to be putting on extra weight. . . . It must be because they are getting ready for their first period." Girls tend to put on weight just before menarche and lose it several years later as hormones even out.

It is possible that a similar phenomenon occurs around menopause. Rather than hormones "causing" weight gain, it seems feasible that the shock of fluctuating chemicals surging throughout the body sets off warning signals. Our bodies, partly because of an evolutionary development that is no longer useful for people not living hunter-gather lifestyles, react to situations of external and internal stress by storing extra fat, giving us a little extra protection and energy for whatever tough times or challenges lie ahead. As in puberty, weight gain during perimenopause can be temporary for most women. Once hormone levels stabilize, extra pounds should come off. So why, unlike previous generations, is it that so many women have the opposite experience?

Metabolic Slowdown and Muscle Change

Although hormone levels seem to have a relationship to weight gain, they don't seem to be the main cause; they are really more of a supporting character in a larger story. Doctors at the Mayo Clinic explain, "As you get older, the amount of muscle tends to decrease and fat accounts for more of your weight. Metabolism also slows naturally with age. Together, these change your calorie needs."[8]

Although it certainly isn't established, some doctors believe that muscle loss speeds up around the time of menopause; Dr. Ian Maclean Smith of the Department of Internal Medicine at the University of Iowa notes that "loss of muscle increases sixfold at the time of menopause, so it may have a connection with estrogen."[9] This doesn't mean, though, that menopause *causes* either muscle loss or weight gain, just as menopause doesn't *cause* heart disease. Rather, if there is a relationship at all, it seems likely that hormones lost at menopause play a protective role for a number of problems.

The National Library of Medicine notes that while both men and women lose lean body mass and muscle tissue, "muscle changes often begin in the 20's in men and the 40's in women."[10] Just as men gain body fat later in life than their female counterparts, so it seems possible that women, either because of estrogen decline or for some other, not yet understood reason, lose muscle later on. In an article on midlife weight gain in the *Journal of Postgraduate Menopause*, Laurey Simkin-Silverman and Rena Wing note that weight changes are "more strongly associated with aging than with menopause."[11]

We've all heard that as we age, our metabolism (the mechanism through which your body makes food into energy) slows down. Again, this is something that happens to both men and women. Laura's younger brother, still in his early twenties, while gleefully consuming an entire pizza justifies his gluttonous ways by saying, "Well, I have to enjoy this while I can—I won't be able to eat this way forever." Indeed, we can all look back nostalgically to the days when we didn't give a second thought to ordering dessert or finishing our French fries. Metabolism may not be the culprit, however.

The Mayo Clinic reminds us that while "common belief holds that a slim person's metabolism is high and an overweight person's metabolism is low . . . this isn't usually the case; the real culprit in weight gain is usually inactivity. When you put on weight, it is probably because you are taking in too many calories and not expending enough of them, not because your body is processing them too slowly."

Since muscle requires more calories to maintain than fat, a good way to keep eating and not gain weight is to exercise. While starting—and sticking with—a good exercise program is important for your overall health and well-being, it can be particularly helpful with weight control. Specifically, starting a good strength-training regimen, that is, lifting and bearing weights, can help prevent muscle loss as well as rebuild and maintain lost muscle. Aerobic exercise raises metabolic rates as well. Although it may be harder to get the results you want from your workout as you get older, putting in even small amounts of effort on fitness can make a big difference.

As Adam Greenberg and his colleagues at Tufts University have discovered, muscle loss at midlife may not be a completely inevitable process: ". . . while some of that [muscle loss] may be attributed to the aging process, most of the blame rests on lowered activity levels."[12] This is both really good and really frustrating news. It means that we can do something about keeping ourselves healthy as we age, but it also means we have to take responsibility for some of the ways our bodies change.

The Thyroid

The thyroid gland, a receiver and creator of powerful hormones that regulate how much energy your body needs and uses, plays an important part in controlling metabolism.

One thing that can cause weight gain (or loss) is a thyroid that isn't functioning properly.[13] The thyroid gland sits at the base of your neck; its appearance is often compared to that of a butterfly. The hypothalamus, the part of the brain responsible for triggering reproductive hormones, is also the gland that makes your thyroid work. The hypothalamus sends messenger chemicals to the pituitary, a small oval gland at the base of the brain. The pituitary, in turn, releases thyroid-stimulating hormone, or TSH. This chemical moves on to the thyroid, signaling it to perform its jobs.

When something goes wrong with the thyroid, it is sort of like the game telephone—the complicated messages between the brain and the body get scrambled. The result is that the body either uses too much energy, resulting in weight loss, or it doesn't use enough, resulting in weight gain.

Artemis Simopoulos says that as we age, our thyroids naturally slow down a little, along with our metabolisms. This means that even if you don't have a thyroid problem per se, you may still put on weight if your thyroid function starts to decrease.

Diabetes

You know the saying "you are what you eat"? Well, you may not actually become that pecan pie or bag of chips, but if you are eating too many high-sugar, refined carbohydrate foods, you may find that your blood is getting a little too sugary as well. The anthropologist Ethne Barnes notes that "the most prevalent disease in the United States related to diet and obesity is diabetes type II."[14] The growing number of diabetes and prediabetes cases in America is indeed disturbing. The *New York Times* notes that "one in three children born in the United States five years ago are expected to become diabetic in their lifetimes. . . . The forecast is even bleaker for Latinos: one in every two."[15] The *Times* calls the growth an "epidemic," comparing it with AIDS and cancer, and the American Diabetes Association predicts that the disease could actually be responsible for "lowering the average life expectancy of Americans for the first time in more than a century."

Sugar, or glucose, is a very important nutrient. It feeds your brain and does other useful things in the body. Like so many good things, if you have too much of it, it can turn from friend to foe, from nutrient to poison. You get glucose from consuming food, but your muscles and your liver are also sources of natural glucose.

Insulin is another chemical that helps your body consume and use nutrients. Its job is to help sugar get out of the blood and into the cells of your body, where it can be used.

Some people don't make enough insulin, and others become *insulin-resistant*, meaning that their bodies don't respond to insulin. Think about your cells as a very exclusive club and the sugar as people waiting patiently behind the velvet ropes. Insulin is the important friend who can help get them inside. If insulin either doesn't show up or shows up and isn't recognized by the bouncer, sugar has to keep waiting in line, while more sugar builds up behind it, waiting to get in. If the line gets too long, that is, if too much sugar amasses in the blood, you can develop diabetes. Also, as tissues become insulin-resistant, the body begins to store fat that it once would have burnt off.

Prediabetes is just what it sounds like: the sugar in your blood is too high but not yet at disease levels. Far from being an exclusive club, your body becomes a bad neighborhood. It's not certain that it will become crime-ridden, but all the conditions and warning signs are there that problems are on the way. According to the National Diabetes Information Clearinghouse, people with prediabetes are at a greater risk than those without risk factors for the disease, for stroke, heart disease, and vision loss.[16]

There are two types of diabetes. Type 1 (sometimes called juvenile diabetes) occurs when the body can't make insulin. It is usually diagnosed when people are children or young adults. Type 2, the form of the disease that particularly concerns midlife and aging people, can develop at any time in the life span. You develop Type 2 when your body tries to compensate for high levels of sugar in the blood by making more insulin. At first this works, and blood sugar goes down. But at some point, the body stops reacting to the insulin. Even though the body keeps making more and more of the stuff, the cells aren't responding, and the blood sugar level remains dangerously high. Eventually the body slows down and stops making so much insulin. Around 90 percent of diabetes cases are Type 2.[17]

Unlike Type 1, Type 2 diabetes is related to certain lifestyle factors. Weighing too much and not getting enough exercise are both major risk factors for developing the disease. We are not suggesting that people cause their own diabetes. Rather, we know that overeating and underexercising can be major contributors to an illness that probably also has a genetic component. As one doctor wisely put it, "Genetics may load the gun, but human behavior pulls the trigger."[18]

What is a normal glucose level? Well, it depends on your body. The National Institute of Diabetes and Digestive and Kidney Diseases stresses that target glucose levels are an individual matter and should be adjusted as such. Generally, though, a "normal" range is considered to be between 70 and 120 milligrams of glucose per deciliter of blood.

Women who have gestational diabetes—that is, who develop temporary diabetes during pregnancy—need to be especially careful. They are at a much higher risk for developing Type 2 diabetes later in life.[19]

If you have insulin resistance, or prediabetes, you have a compelling reason to lose weight. You may have unique nutritional needs, though. While it is difficult for everyone to lose weight, people with blood sugar problems have particular nutritional concerns. Some recent studies confirm what certain diet gurus have long believed: the glycemic content of foods must be monitored more closely by individuals with blood sugar problems. The glycemic index—a scale invented in 1981 that rates each food with a number based on sugar content—is one way to do that.[20] It assigns a numerical value to foods that corresponds to the amount of glucose in that item. By adding up numbers of things eaten over the course of a day, a person can estimate how much glucose they've taken in.[21] To see the index go to www.glycemicindex.com.

Fat Genes: Understanding the Role of Genetics and Willpower in Weight Loss

The role of genetics in weight control is still being studied. We all know that genes play a significant role in what shape and size you are; common sense as well as science tell us this. But to what extent is being overweight something we are born with and to what extent is it something within our control?

Several genes and the chemicals they produce are being studied right now in the hopes of understanding the relationship between genes and nutritional free will. Although so far these studies are leading to more questions than answers, they provide a hint of the complicated relationship between the eating habits you acquire and the body you are born with.

Leptin

When the hormone leptin was first discovered at New York's Rockefeller University in 1994, hopes were very high that it would represent a major breakthrough in the science of weight-loss drugs. Dr. Jeffery Friedman discovered that when leptin was injected into mice who were bred to be obese, the mice lost weight. Leptin worked in part by letting the brain know that the body was full. If you didn't have enough of it, your brain wasn't able to tell the body to stop eating, even when you had taken in more than enough calories. If leptin was injected into humans, it stood to reason, researchers thought, that it would help the stomach, brain, and body reconnect.

As with so many hypotheses, the reality turned out to be much more complicated than the scientists originally anticipated. Mice don't make leptin naturally, whereas humans do. In fact, overweight people have higher leptin levels than thin people.[22] It seems possible that as with insulin, the body can become resistant to leptin. For a small segment of the population who, like the mice, don't naturally make leptin or don't make enough of it, it seems that injecting it has the same weight-loss benefits. For most people, though, it has no effect. Scientists still have a long way to go in understanding the function of leptin before it can be used to develop antiobesity drugs.

One thing we do know: crash dieting lowers the levels of leptin in your body and signals your brain that it needs to eat. The brain tries to compensate, and slowed metabolism is one of the ways the body tries to prevent itself from getting into dangerous nutritional situations. This is probably one reason why extreme nutritional restrictions don't seem to work for weight loss.

Friedman notes, however, that exercise doesn't seem to lower leptin levels (as opposed to dieting, which does).[23] This may be one reason exercise is such a fantastic weight-loss tool: it helps increase how many calories you need without triggering your body's hunger and starvation protection mechanisms.

The leptin studies begin to raise some very important questions about weight control, willpower, and genetics. Do we get fat because of some underlying biological cause? Or is the sudden rise in American obesity really just evidence of a national lack of self-control? Friedman's answer is interesting. He believes that willpower and simply choosing to eat or not eat are important within a ten- to fifteen-pound weight-loss range. Want to lose that holiday weight or slim down for your son's wedding? Then muster up your self-control, create a plan of attack, and stick to it. This situation changes when you need to lose twenty-five pounds or more. Friedman explains, "By the time you're in a situation where you have to lose substantial amounts of weight, willpower really doesn't appear by itself to be terribly effective."[24] The bigger you are, Friedman feels, the more biology plays a role in making weight loss difficult.

Ghrelin

Not getting enough sleep lately? It might be contributing to your extra pounds. It seems possible that skimping on z's can be a factor in weight gain. Americans in general get a lot less sleep than they used to. It is estimated that the average person sleeps for about two fewer hours than they did fifty years ago. Women who don't get enough rest—that is, more than seven hours a night—are much more likely to carry some extra pounds. When you are sleepy, your appetite increases.[25] The reason is that as levels of leptin decrease, levels of ghrelin, a chemical that has been associated in studies with obesity[26] and is an appetite stimulant, increase. Your body becomes confused and can't tell the difference between fatigue and hunger. At least two studies (one at Columbia University and another at Bristol University, United Kingdom, and the University of Chicago) suggest that when you don't get proper sleep, you are much more likely to become obese.[27]

Perilipin

A new discovery that has a lot of people excited is a gene called perilipin (alternately plin). Perilipin creates a protein that may settle around fat droplets and prevent them from being broken down. To find out more, researchers tested 150 obese patients over the course of a year.[28] These patients were put on a low-calorie diet, and their weight was measured over the course of the trial. People who had perilipin mutations showed little to no success with low-calorie diets. Those who didn't tended to lose "significant" weight.

Sometimes genetic mutations are part of an evolutionary process; our bodies change to try to protect us. Jose Ordovas, one of the scientists who worked on the trial, explains, "That may sound funny these days, but in old times, fat was difficult to hold on to, so this protein protected it."[29]

Perilipin has scientists excited because more study might help them identify in advance individuals who would be resistant to traditional weight-loss methods and address their needs differently. It might also, in time, lead to the development of genetically specific weight-loss drugs (although that day is still far off).

SHBG

Another theory involves sex hormone binding globulin (SHBG), a molecule that attaches itself to testosterone. The levels of this chemical drop noticeably in the body around the time of menopause, which allows more testosterone to flow throughout the body. Women with more testosterone tend, like men, to put on more fat in the upper body. This may be one reason why midsection weight gain could be so prominent at menopause. Since we know that estrogen decline around menopause means that the ratio of estrogen to testosterone shifts, with testosterone levels declining at a slower rate than estrogen, this seems like an intriguing theory as to why midlife women put on weight, but there still isn't any good science to substantiate it.

Weight-Loss Drugs

If scientists could identify and understand the genetic components of weight loss a little better, they could potentially develop better drugs to help people get and stay thin. Until that great day, however, when we are able to really understand the relationships among metabolism, nutrition, and weight, consumers would be wise to be wary of weight-loss drugs. Some of the biggest pharmaceutical disgraces of the second half of the twentieth century involved prescription weight-loss preparations.

Early advertising campaigns aimed at getting women to start smoking centered on the ability of the chemicals in cigarettes to quell hunger. In 1917, the makers of Lucky Strikes ran an ad showing ladies' jowls and proclaiming, "Avoid that future shadow!"[30] A 1936 ad would urge, "Reach for a Lucky instead of a sweet!"

In 1944 Abbott Laboratories, an Illinois pill maker, decided to try to have an existing compound approved to treat obesity. The drug, called Desoxyn (desoxyephedrine), was an amphetamine; it had originally been approved in November 1943 to treat depression, alcoholism, hay fever, postencephalitic Parkinson syndrome, and narcolepsy.[31] While Desoxyn was eventually approved for weight loss, immediate controversy began to swarm around the emerging drug class.

In 1946, the new acting medical director of the FDA, Walton Van Winkle, worried that Desoxyn exposed patients "unnecessarily to a potent drug."[32] At issue were both concerns about the drug's safety as a powerful amphetamine and its potential for addiction. Having gone on record with its misgivings, the FDA turned away from the issue for several years. After stricter regulations came into place in the 1960s and '70s, weight-loss drugs lost popularity because of their reputation for being addictive.

In the 1990s prescriptions of amphetamine weight-loss drugs began to explode. There were many reasons for the sudden and dramatic revival—drugs had been reconfigured to make them less addictive, for one—but the major actor behind the change was the impact of one study that got a lot of attention from the press. It wasn't a good study; in fact, more than two-thirds of the original study participants dropped out over the course of it, and of the ones who remained nearly all regained the weight they lost.

What the study suggested was that two chemicals, fenfluramine and phentermine, when taken together as the cocktail fen-phen would help people drop pounds. Before the long-term safety implications of this off-label combo could be tested, American Home Products rushed the approval of a combined product, Redux, that quickly became a blockbuster. The problem with this new wonder drug was that people taking it started experiencing some serious side effects. These included mood swings, memory trouble, and, most alarming, heart problems. In 1997, seven doctors published a study revealing that twenty-four female patients on fen-phen had abnormal echocardiograms and valve abnormalities. The drug was pulled, but eventually more than fifty thousand cases of heart valve damage and primary pulmonary hypertension would be documented.

The two biggest weight-loss drugs currently on the market are Meridia (sibutramine) and Xenical (orlistat). Both have had significant safety questions posed about them.

Meridia in particular has raised alarms. It was approved by the FDA just months after the withdrawal of Redux, despite evidence that it also caused (different) heart problems. In 2002, the drug was withdrawn from the market in Italy after two young women died. The rest of Europe and the United States, however, did not follow suit.

Meridia works by blocking signals from the brain about hunger.[33] In a review of twenty-nine trials on the drug, it was found to be associated with minimal weight loss and modest increases in heart rate and blood pressure, which counterbalanced improvements in triglycerides.[34] Dr. Michael Andersen observes, "If a patient loses 10 or 15 pounds with diet and Meridia, it's not uncommon to see them gain a lot of it back."[35]

The watchdog group Public Citizen has filed several petitions with the FDA calling for the drug's withdrawal, with no success. However, a new trial, the Sibutramine in Cardiovascular Outcomes (SCOUT) Trial, will look at nine thousand patients over five years. As Eric Coleman explains, "This will be the first trial to verify or refute the long-held assumption that drug-induced weight loss—in this case, with sibutramine—reduces the risk for fatal and nonfatal cardiovascular disease."[36] We feel it should be mentioned, however, that five years is too brief a time to establish any sort of long-term safety data.

Xenical (orlistat), the other available drug on the market, works in the gut by blocking fat absorption in the intestines.[37] It was approved by the FDA in 1999 and is sold by Roche Labs. A 2002 *Journal of Hypertension* study found that Xenical helped patients lose about 2 to 3 percent of their body weight.[38] The drug can cause digestive problems; one trial found that up to 50 percent of patients taking the drug had gastrointestinal distress.[39] As with Meridia, patients who lose weight with the drug often gain it back.

In the spring of 2007, an over-the-counter version of Xenical, branded Alli, started popping up in drug and grocery stores around the nation. Quite apart from the safety concerns surrounding abuse with an over-the-counter diet aid that has such far-reaching effects on the body, Alli has some . . . well . . . less-than-pleasant side effects. For users who don't adhere to the low-fat diet suggested by the drugmaker GlaxoSmithKline, the result can be soiled pants. Indeed, drugmakers suggest that because of the accident potential, people trying the drug should do so on a day off work and wear dark pants, or carry a change of clothes if this isn't an option.[40]

Another new pharmaceutical in the works had some doctors very excited when trials of it were announced in 2004 and 2005. It is called Acomplia (rimonabant), and it was discovered first as a way to help curb the appetite cravings associated with marijuana smoking.[41]

Unfortunately, despite initial excitement about the pill, results so far have been less than encouraging. In his long-awaited report in the February 15, 2006, issue of the *Journal of the American Medical Association (JAMA)*, the lead study author Dr. F. Xavier Pi-Sunyer noted, "it must be acknowledged that the trial was limited by a high drop-out rate [50 percent] and that long-term effects of the drug require further study." In an accompanying editorial, Denise Simons-Morton pointed out that the study had some of the serious but classic problems of other weight-loss drug trials. These included a massive drop-out group.[42] As Jeanne Whalen explains, Acomplia "still hasn't hit the market in the U.S.," and the FDA is asking for more data before it will consider approving it.[43] The hesitation by the FDA to "rush to judgment" seems to us like a step in the right direction of putting patient safety first. While growing obesity rates indeed constitute a national health crisis, allowing undertested drugs to flood the market, carrying untold health hazards, is not the solution.

Herbal weight-loss supplements have proliferated in recent years in health-food stores. Particularly those containing extracts of a plant called hoodia have gotten a lot of visibility through high-profile advertising campaigns. We will make this very simple for you: there are no miracle weight-loss supplements that are both effective and safe. Most over-the-counter weight-loss pills use some kind of stimulant to curb hunger. They vary from the ineffective to the dangerous, and we suspect you already have some sense that taking them isn't the best way to lose weight.

You Are What You Eat: The Perils of Plan Diets

It seems like every couple years a new fad takes over, and suddenly there are five or six best-selling books or expensive programs espousing their method as the only one that will possibly help you reach your goals. We've gone through high-carb, low-fat, vegetarian, low-carb, and back again. We've Weight-Watchered, Slim-Fasted, Jenny-Craiged, Atkinsed, and South-Beached. Why, then, do we still struggle with obesity on such a massive scale?

The *Journal of the American Medical Association* estimates that there are a thousand available diet books on the market,[44] and *U.S. News & World Report* says that Americans spend "more than $33 billion a year on diet books, foods, programs, gadgets and DVD's in the hopes of losing weight."[45]

We all know that most plan diets aren't long-term solutions. Dr. Stephen Hawks of Brigham Young University says, "You would be hard pressed to review the dietary literature and conclude that you can give people a set of dietary guidelines or restrictions that they will be able to follow in the long term and manage their weight successfully."[46]

A recent trial published in *JAMA* set out to compare four major types of diets: the Atkins, a low-carbohydrate, high-protein option; the Ornish, a low-fat vegetarian diet; the Weight Watchers, a portion and calorie control plan; and the Zone, a diet that aims at creating certain ratios of carbohydrates to proteins and fats.[47] Unlike people in the real world who sign up for these diets, the people in the trial received extensive specific counseling and monitoring to ensure they were sticking with the program they were assigned to.

Scientists conducting the trial found that while people lost "modest" amounts of weight on each program, there was "no statistical significance"[48] between the quantity of weight lost on one plan when compared with another. In other words, the programs were all equally limited in their ability to promote weight loss and all about the same in terms of the amount of weight people shed when they adhered to them.

The study authors concluded that success on a given diet is at least somewhat dependent on whether the diet is right for you. Even though the weight-loss results were the same for all four plans, the actual effects the diet plans had on the body were different. People are different, and so should their diets be. You may need to try several before you find one that works for you. Also, a diet isn't a lifelong eating plan; the best way to lose weight is to find a way to make healthful meals that work for your lifestyle and goals. The truth is that eating healthfully and getting plenty of exercise continue to play the biggest role in weight maintenance. For more information on these, check out chapters 13 and 14.

You have to be patient with yourself during menopause. It's a time of massive, far-reaching change. If you put on a couple pounds during menopause, give yourself a break. Understand that this may be part of your body's way of dealing with the stress of big biological change. Once you are postmenopausal, commit to taking off weight in a healthy way through eating nutritiously and exercising. Don't waste your time and money on diet crazes or take risks with your health by swallowing marginally useful, potentially harmful pills.

13

minding your peas and caveats

menopause nutrition and eating healthfully in the second half of life

What would happen, for example, if we were to start thinking about food as less of a thing and more of a relationship?

—Michael Pollan

In a January 2007 *New York Times* article, the food anthropologist Michael Pollan wrote some deceptively simple advice: "Eat food. Not too much. Mostly plants. That, more or less, is the short answer to the supposedly incredibly complicated and confusing question of what we humans should eat in order to be maximally healthy."[1]

After decades of national debate about what foods will help us live healthier, longer lives, such a basic premise is really, of course, the preface to an intricate conversation about the nature of food. What exactly is it? Why do we eat? What will our relationships with food be?

Perhaps most important, what does it mean to "eat right"? And why are there so many conflicting cultural messages about it? Different books on menopause will give you completely different nutritional regimens, let alone more general advice manuals on eating and health. How can you make good choices, to make sensible, lasting changes without just falling for the latest trend?

Without getting too philosophical, lets ask ourselves exactly what food means in our society. Is it vegetables, fruits, and raw products of nature that come together bound by taste and culture? Or is it something conveniently packaged on a store shelf, waiting to fill certain calorie quotients without taking up time or making a dent in our increasingly busy lives? Our relationship with food has everything to do with our ability to make nutritional choices that will help us age healthfully.

Many women find around midlife that they have gotten into some pretty bad habits. While they were busy being the dynamic, busy, accomplished people they are, they grew rather sedentary. There were lots of reasons not to start a formal exercise program, lots of things to do besides worry about the fat and calorie content of dinner each night, and more important things to worry about than a cookie (or three) with a cup of coffee after dinner.

Really listen to your body; it will tell you what it needs. Don't assume that because you have eaten the same thing each day for twenty years, you still need as much food. Wait until you actually feel hungry to eat. Think long and hard before you reach for that chip. Are you doing it out of habit? If you are actually hungry, don't fight it. Rather, try to satisfy your hunger in a healthful way. Eat a meal with lots of vegetables instead of four carrot sticks followed by half a container of cottage cheese followed by a chocolate bar followed by chips. You get the idea.

Many people prefer to have guidelines in terms of what they eat. The U.S. Department of Agriculture (USDA) recommends that a sedentary woman between the ages of thirty-one and fifty take in around 1,800 calories a day, 2,000 if she is moderately active, and 2,200 if she is active. Over the age of fifty-one, this recommendation becomes 1,600 calories a day for sedentary women, 1,800 for the moderately active, and 2,000 to 2,200 for the active.[2] If you find you are putting on weight and want to stop, try to eat slightly smaller portions. This can be as simple as making an effort to leave something on your plate when you go to a restaurant, or just being aware of serving sizes and limiting yourself to one or two. Instead of filling that bowl with ice cream, try enjoying one healthy scoop.

Have water instead of that bottle of juice or cut out one dessert or snack item a day. Have a plain hamburger instead of a cheeseburger or broiled chicken breast instead of fried. Making little changes one at a time is the best way to discover how many excess calories you have been eating.

Make sure you are eating healthfully: it is possible to be both overeating and malnourished. In her book *Diseases and Human Evolution*, anthropologist Ethne Barnes makes the point that sometimes we overeat to compensate for nutritional deficiencies in our food. Barnes writes, "There may be plenty to eat, but not everything people eat has nutritive value. People subsisting primarily on highly processed foods often eat more than they need because they are starved for nutrients."[3]

Portion Control

It seems these days that the phenomenon of "portion distortion" is becoming an omnipresent reality of twenty-first-century life. An appetizer at a popular chain restaurant can provide many of an average woman's calories for an entire day, let alone an entree and a dessert. As we watch news report after news report bemoaning how overweight Americans are, and we wring our hands and ask why, one major reason doctors and nutritionists keep coming back to is how much we are eating.

Unfortunately, restaurant food doesn't (except in specifically requested, rare instances) come with a nutrition facts box. The consumer is left to guess how many calories they are consuming. This is changing as cities like New York pilot programs to force restaurants to provide such information.

Two researchers at the University of Arkansas, Scot Burton and Betsy Creyer, believe that if restaurants were forced to put such information in menus and on ordering boards, many people would opt to eat less and more healthfully. In their research, the two found that "the majority of people consistently underestimate"[4] how many calories are in their food when they eat out. Burton explains, "Our findings illustrate how poorly consumers understand the nutritional content of many of the meals they eat outside the home. Reasonable consumers know that a large number of these items aren't healthy, but they still do not realize how unhealthy the meals can be and the possible effects of frequent, long-term consumption."

Restaurant meals have been shown to be significantly higher in calories than home-prepared ones—around 600 additional calories and 44 more grams of fat.[5] That's pretty serious business if you are someone who eats out with any frequency. Simply preparing meals at home more often might be one good way to lose weight without even trying.

There is no doubt that portions in restaurants and in other commercially prepared foods have gotten bigger. According to the National Heart, Lung, and Blood Institute (NHLBI), twenty years ago a breakfast bagel had around 140 calories.[6] Today the same item has around 350 calories or more. A cheeseburger used to have around 330 calories, while today it packs a whopping 600 to 700 calories. Soda and juice used to come in single-serving containers of around 6.5 to 8.0 ounces; today, they are more likely to be in 16- to 20-ounce bottles.

Forty years ago, no one had heard the term *supersized*, and most people ate the majority of their meals at home. Today, many people eat out as often as they eat in. According to researchers at the University of Arkansas, Americans eat 54 billion meals a year at restaurants.[7] When we eat out, we want to feel we are getting as much bang for our buck as possible. Large portions may represent greater economic value, but if you get used to eating the oversized portions offered by restaurants and start to expect the same mounds of fries or rice or even buttered vegetables every day, you will be consuming calories far in excess of your daily requirements. Other lifestyle changes have made it less likely than ever that we will burn off these extra calories: cars take us nearly everywhere, and work hours have gotten longer, making it harder to carve out time for recreation or exercise.

A little information can go a long way in terms of reeducating yourself about food. Much of this information is available on the Internet. The NHLBI, the American Diabetes Association, and the

American Dietetic Association are all excellent sources. Of course the Food and Drug Administration (FDA) also has not only its famous food pyramid, which is under near-constant revision, but detailed information about nutritional choices. The FDA is also trying to incorporate physical activity into the pyramid, as well as encourage people to personalize it based on height, weight, and daily calorie goals. The institution's Web site provides more information on this, but perhaps the most economic diet plan around might be simple adherence to FDA recommendations on portion size.

The NHLBI's Web site makes this information easy to, um, digest by comparing an amount of food with another item. For example, a portion the size of a fist is about the size of a serving of breakfast cereal. A pancake should be about the size of a compact disc, and a cup of salad around the size of a baseball. A portion of meat is about the size of an average palm and an ounce of cheese is about the size of two dice. Thinking about food this way can be simpler than trying to think in grams and ounces.

Vitamin Pills: Do They Work?

Vitamins are the original micronutrient and the bedrock of the supplement industry. Macronutrients such as carbohydrates and fat are taking turns as cultural whipping boys, but micronutrients have gone relatively unchallenged in Western life for decades.

Is a vitamin pill a food? The government of the United States thinks so. With the passage of the Dietary Supplement Health and Education Act of 1994 (DSHEA), all so-called natural supplements were legally classified as foods. What this means, among other things, is that vitamin makers don't have to prove the safety and efficacy of their products to the FDA before they start selling them.

Despite the fact that we spend a ton of time wondering if we are getting the right vitamins and minerals, we don't spend much time learning or wondering what they actually are, and we certainly don't question whether they do what they say they will do. Most basically, a vitamin is an organic substance needed by the body in small amounts to maintain health and proper functioning. These molecules help important chemical reactions in the body to happen.

Although the scientific understanding of vitamins is a recent phenomenon, humans have observed for centuries that certain foods could help cure illness or prevent serious health problems. Ancient Egyptians would eat liver to prevent night blindness thousands of years before we would figure out that liver contains high levels of vitamin A, and in the eighteenth century, an English physician, James Lind, noticed that sailors who drank lime juice, rich in what we now know as vitamin C, didn't succumb to scurvy, a sometimes fatal illness common among sailors on long trips without access to fresh fruit and vegetables.

After discovering that unpolished rice would prevent the ravages of a disease called beriberi, the nineteenth-century Dutch doctor and Nobel Prize winner Christiaan Eijkman suggested that perhaps certain foods had certain qualities that made them indispensable to healthy humans. Science was on the way to making a distinction between those qualities and the foods that contained them.

The term *vitamin* was born when Casimir Funk coined it around 1912 to describe a nutrient he had recently isolated that was responsible for beriberi. The word caught on and soon came to mean nutrients in general. The race to isolate and identify these health-giving compounds was now moving full speed ahead. Chronicler of the supplement industry Dan Hurley writes, "In the four short years between 1912 and 1916, vitamins A, B, B1, and C were all discovered; the necessity of dietary minerals, such as calcium and iron, was also quickly established."[8]

Originally, scientists took a "more is better" approach with vitamins, urging doses far beyond what would now meet the FDA's recommended daily intake (RDI). This practice came to be known as "megadosing," and it has been exposed as a potentially dangerous practice. Vitamins, like foods, are best in moderation. This is because "malnutrition" doesn't just mean not getting enough vitamins or foods; it can mean getting too many—an unbalanced intake.

Something we don't spend enough time talking about is the biological difference between vitamins naturally occurring in food and the kind many of us take every day in capsule form. Vitamins in supplement form fall into the same category as many natural and herbal supplements as far as government regulation is concerned. That means, unfortunately, that the FDA doesn't have much regulatory responsibility or control over vitamins.[9] Herbs and vitamins have an interesting relationship; they're almost always sold in stores together, and one bolsters sales of the other. It's estimated that vitamin pills account for somewhere around $7 billion in sales, a huge percentage of the total supplement industry.[10]

Do vitamins work? Obviously in many cases they do, but the evidence for multivitamins isn't stunning. If you take one every day and feel good, by all means keep doing so. Actually we would recommend it unless one makes you feel bad. Just make sure you're not taking one with doses that far exceed the FDA recommendations. Be aware that some vitamin makers hold a more-is-better philosophy despite evidence that too much of a nutrient can hurt you. For a brief time, the amount of a given vitamin that could go into a supplement was regulated, but since the passage of the DSHEA, this is no longer the case. It seems important to note that since the passage of this law, adverse events related to taking vitamins have jumped by 62 percent.[11] Although people do overdose on vitamins, very few end up getting seriously ill and even fewer die (but most deaths, sadly, are among young children).

Building Stronger Foods

The idea of adding nutrients to food is an old one. In the 1830s, long before most vitamins were synthesized, a French chemist proposed that adding iodine to salt could prevent goiter or swelling of the thyroid.

In America in the twentieth century, vitamin D was added to milk in the 1930s, and vitamins, minerals, and proteins were used to "fortify" breads, breakfast cereals, and other grain products. More recently, fluoride was added to the water to promote oral health, and in the 1990s, the FDA began requiring the addition of folate to various grain products to prevent birth defects.

Some of these changes have led to unparalleled improvements in public health. Others are less well proven, and given the dangers of overconsuming certain nutrients, it is worth asking if having food manufacturers slip these compounds quietly into food really helps consumers become active participants in their own well-being. Still, on the balance, most government-mandated add-ins have helped public health far more than they have hurt it.

In recent years, food companies have begun adding all sorts of chemicals, nutrients, and herbs to food. Again we find ourselves at a moment where the best thing for most Americans would be to eat less, yet food makers using new technologies are creating nutrient-loaded foods and suggesting that eating more of them will be better for you—this water has vitamins, that candy bar has added protein, that sugary iced tea contains St. John's wort or guarana.

Reedeming Fat: Dr. Artemis Simopoulos and Essential Fatty Acids

Fat has gotten really bad press in the past three decades, so let's list some good things about fats: They help to make cell membranes. Your brain is made up mostly of fat and needs it to function efficiently. Finally, fat can help you absorb nutrients: the antioxidant lycopene, found in tomatoes and other red vegetables, is taken in by the body at a much higher rate when it is accompanied by a little fat.[12]

Fats can be divided into three major categories: saturated, monounsaturated, and polyunsaturated. The names come from the specific chemical bonds that hold them together. You can figure out how much of any kind of fat is in a certain food by either checking the nutrition information box on the back of labeled food or looking up the information online or in food information books for unmarked products.

Saturated fats come mostly from animal products; they are usually solid or waxy at room temperature. (There are exceptions—palm oil and coconut oil, to name two.) Common sources of saturated fat include whole milk, red meat, butter, poultry, and coconut and palm oil. Saturated fat should make up less than 10 percent of your total calories each day.[13]

Unsaturated fat comes in three varieties: monounsaturated, polyunsaturated, and trans fats. These are usually deemed the "healthy fats" by most information sources, but remember that too much of *any* fat isn't healthy, and there is much evidence that trans fats are actually dangerous. Although there is no specific limit set on how much unsaturated fat you can eat, it is suggested that people get no more than 35 percent of their total calories from fat.

Monounsaturated fat is typically liquid at room temperature and cloudy when refrigerated. It is the main type of fat in olive oil, many nuts, and oily vegetables like avocados. Polyunsaturated fats, which are always liquid, are found in many vegetable oils, certain nuts, and fish. Omega-3 fatty acids are found in bigger quantities in polyunsaturated fats. Dr. Artemis Simopoulos, who has been on the front line of research and education about this particular type of fat for many years, argues that creating a balance between omega-3s and their more common counterparts omega-6s is essential to reshaping our increasingly problematic modern diets.

Omega-3s are common in green plants, vegetables, and in the products of animals who consume large quantities of greens, as well as in fish like salmon and mackerel. We have come to think of them as "fish oil" products, and indeed, the fats of many fish are rich in them. The sources of omega-3s are much broader, though, and Dr. Simopoulos suggests eating a diet rich in vegetables and greens.

Trans fats, which include hydrogenated oils, are mostly the product of twentieth-century food science. Since World War II, the United States has become a packaged-food nation. Foods increasingly needed to stay fresh for longer periods of time as they were transported across the country and eventually across the world and sat for months on supermarket shelves. Trans fats helped make this possible because they stay solid at higher temperatures. The 1970s margarines that contained trans fats were touted as healthier alternatives to saturated-fat butter. A generation of mothers was convinced that feeding margarine to their children would be good for them. It turned out that hydrogenates were much less healthy—particularly for the heart—than plain old saturated fats. While the older, natural fat was indeed responsible for raising levels of LDL ("bad") cholesterol, the new techno-fat, it turned out, did this as well, *and* made rates of HDL ("good") cholesterol plummet.

People are beginning to pay serious attention to the dangers of trans fats. In December 2006, New York City announced that it would ban all trans fats from its restaurants by 2008. Some health experts cautioned the city not to rush food purveyors lest they simply substitute other unhealthy fats.[14] Other major American cities are likely to follow New York's example, with Chicago already developing a less restrictive version of the plan.

Food labels now list the amount of trans fats in prepared foods. We strongly suggest cutting down or eliminating them from your diet, especially now that they are increasingly easy to identify and avoid.

Fat of the Land: Traditional Diets and Essential Fatty Acids

Dr. Artemis Simopoulos was on vacation in her native country of Greece and was spending time on her family's farm in the northwest Peloponnese. The homestead was idyllic; lined with olive and fruit trees and populated by free-roaming chickens. Watching the birds one day, Simopolous noticed they were munching on grasses. She had always assumed that chickens preferred corn and feed. When she queried her father, he told her that the birds naturally ate grasses, insects, and worms.

Dr. Simopoulos began wondering if chickens that ate a "traditional" diet had a different nutritional content from chickens fed on grain or corn. Collecting some eggs, she brought them back to the United States for lab comparison with the regular supermarket eggs. What she found was dramatic: the grass-fed chickens produced eggs with a ratio of 1:1 of omega-3s to omega-6s. The supermarket eggs had a ratio of 1:20 of omega-3s to omega-6s.

For a long time, Dr. Simopoulos had been doing research on essential fatty acids, trying to figure out what sort of a difference they made in diet. In the 1960s, a fifteen-year study found that men on the island of Crete were healthier than their counterparts around the globe. Intrigued with this good news about her homeland, she set out to understand the parts of the Greek diet that made it so healthful.

Among other things, the men of Crete were eating a lot of wild plants instead of the grains more common in Western society. Those plants, it turned out, were richer in omega-3s, and the overall diet provided a better balance between omega-3s and 6s. The men also ate meat and eggs from animals that fed on grasses.

Although omega-3s seem to confer some health benefits, among them decreasing inflammation and helping to prevent coronary heart disease, the different balance of fatty acids echoed a seismic alteration in lifestyle—in the basic ways that people got, ate, and understood food.

What Michael Pollan calls "our national eating disorder" may be caused in part by the fact that while historical diets developed very slowly—the product of evolution, environment, and time—our modern diet is the product of massive and rapid change. Simopolous argues that bodies "expect" to be fed the same types and rations of fat that nourished our cave-dwelling ancestors: When we eat French fries cooked in partially hydrogenated vegetable oil instead of wild plants, or wolf down a fat-laden hamburger heaped with mayonnaise instead of meat from a lean, free-ranging game animal, our bodies register the insult.[15]

This brings us back to Pollan's simple plan: if you want to be healthy, eat less meat and dairy and lots of plants—more than you are eating now.

A final thought for menopausal women: be careful about interactions between estrogen and alcohol. Whether you are taking hormone therapy or just grappling with the ups and downs of perimenopause, you should know that those glasses of wine are interacting with your hormones. Among other things, it can accentuate the effects, meaning it will take fewer drinks to see alcohol-related changes in the body. We're not just talking about getting drunk more easily. We mean that all the bad things that can happen when you drink too much will happen more easily if you mix alcohol and high estrogen levels.

14

change of pace
menopause and exercise

Take exercise: for while inaction weakens the body, work strengthens it; the former brings on premature old age, the latter prolongs youth.
— A. Cornelius Celsus, first-century Roman medical writer

there are always so many reasons why people either don't exercise or don't do it enough. They're busy, lazy, confused about what exercises to do, think joining a gym is too expensive, they're too old . . . this list goes on.

You really are never too old to start: the National Institutes of Health (NIH) reports that exercise and physical activity can "improve the health of people who are 90 or older, who are frail or who have the diseases that seem to accompany aging."[1] So you healthy meno-babes out there have no excuse. Forty? C'mon. Fifty? No problem. Sixty? Why not?

First, let's be clear about what we mean when we say "exercise." We mean any sort of movement that gets you using your body in a healthy and active way, from walking down the stairs of your apartment building to running a marathon, from carrying your own groceries home to becoming an expert yoga practitioner, from taking ten-minute walks to becoming a regular gym rat. You don't have to spend hours a week at a fancy gym. You might start by doing a couple of hours of yoga and tai chi each week. Perhaps you simply commit to engaging regularly in an activity like gardening or house-work that gets you moving. The point is to do *something* on a daily basis.

Exercise is like religion in American culture: it is spoken of in mystic terms, and we are assured daily by countless media sources that if we do enough of it or the right sort of it, we will avoid a host of terrible things, including chronic disease, obesity, and cancer. The Mayo Clinic estimates that "you can reduce your risk of dying prematurely by almost half if you exercise every day or nearly every day."[2] Still, even the most optimistic proponents must admit limitations.

The truth is that nothing will prevent us from dying and that data on exercise suggest simply that it can *delay* the onset of chronic disease. Still, there are so many benefits that we find it hard to over-state how good exercise is for you. Exercise is particularly important for midlife women because of its preventive powers but also for its ability to alleviate certain menopause symptoms.

Menopause is also a great time to make changes that will help your health for the rest of your life. The National Institute on Aging explains, "When older people lose their ability to do things on their own, it doesn't happen just because they have aged. More likely it is because they have become inactive. Older inactive adults lose ground in four areas that are important for staying healthy and independent: endurance, strength, balance and flexibility."[3]

Knowing When to Say When: How Much Exercise Is Enough?

One of the most confusing things about starting a workout regimen is accepting that no one knows how much you should be exercising to reap the many health benefits. The magic number, quoted by every fitness expert, governmental and otherwise, is thirty minutes of exer-cise daily.[4] The truth, however, is that because exercise and activity are so difficult to measure and because people's individual metabo-lisms and bodies are so different, no one really knows how much is enough. Still, thirty minutes a day is a good and realistic goal for many women.

Very few people exercise every day, and many don't exercise for thirty minutes at a time if they do. We believe that's okay—whatever your engagement with fitness, you can find benefits. In fact, we worry about increasingly strict guidelines. It seems to us that while they may be challenging for some people, they can be discouraging for others. As Madelyn Fernstrom, director of the Weight Management Center at the University of Pittsburgh, says, the bar is sometimes set "so high that most people will say, 'Forget it, I'll do nothing.'"[5]

Although as someone wise once observed, people tend to "overestimate the time they spend being active just as they tend to underestimate how many calories they consume," we want to encourage you not to get discouraged by the numbers game. It is a good idea to keep a journal of your physical activity to give you a more realistic idea of how much work you are doing. This will help you to push yourself and improve in realistic, gradual ways. But don't let anyone, even a doctor, tell you that your efforts aren't good enough.

There have been some shocking oversights in the creation of exercise guidelines over the years.

A study published in the August 4, 2005, issue of the *New England Journal of Medicine* reminded readers that, as Dr. Martha Gulati, a cardiologist at Rush University Medical Center in Chicago, says, "The current American College of Cardiology and American Heart Association exercise guidelines and standards are based on exclusively male data."[6] And not even a large sample of men—only 224 of them.[7]

To compensate for this, Gulati and her colleagues developed a chart to help adjust and predict exercise capacity for women based on their age. Their study is particularly valuable for menopausal and midlife women because it looked at a population of 5,721 women with no heart disease or mobility problems and who were age thirty-five and older. They found that women who weren't able to exercise enough were twice as likely to die as those who worked out more.

The Basics

There are four basic areas of fitness where we begin to fall behind as we age if we aren't careful: endurance, flexibility, strength, and balance (we think of it like this: Exercise For Stronger Bodies). Each of these areas has to do with a set of things we do in the world and has a group of exercises that promote maintaining it.

Most medical guidelines wisely suggest that we try to get a little exercise for each of these things. Some activities accomplish more than one of these goals: yoga, for example, can provide both flexibility and balance training.

If you have never exercised before, it is always a good idea to discuss your plans with your doctor. If you suffer from any sort of chronic or serious illness or if you are elderly, this is particularly important. Your health care professional can advise you about exercises that should be avoided or could be particularly dangerous for you. Likewise, she can tell you if there is something you might really benefit from. Another good idea is to discuss specific health considerations with instructors at your gym or community center who are teaching exercise classes.

In It for the Long Haul: Endurance and Cardiovascular Exercise

When we talk about endurance, we mean our ability to keep going, stay energetic, and get things done. An endurance runner isn't someone who runs fast but someone who runs far. A person who has good endurance is someone who can get through a workday without feeling tired or finish cleaning the house without getting out of breath. As we age, it is very easy to begin to slow down a little in this department. Endurance exercise, sometimes called aerobic exercise, is designed to help keep our energy up by increasing our heart rate and breathing for longer periods of time, increasing the amount of oxygen coming into our bodies.[8] Oxygen, in combination with fat and sugar (glucose) is used by the body to make adenosine triphosphate (ATP), a substance in our cells that is essential in storing and releasing energy.

This type of exercise is great for weight loss; it burns lots of calories and can help boost your metabolism. More important, it strengthens the heart and lungs as well as lowering blood pressure and improving circulation. Regularly performing aerobic activities can help prevent a heart attack.

If you haven't been exercising, it will take time to build up your stamina. Start by doing as little as five minutes of exercise at a time. Again, because fitness levels are so different, walking may be an endurance activity for you, while your friend may require something more vigorous. In general, any cardiovascular exercise performed at low to medium intensity will do. Some basic cardiovascular activities include running, working on a stair machine or an elliptical trainer, playing tennis, swimming, walking up and down stairs, jumping rope, practicing martial arts, and bike riding.

One simple way to gauge how hard you are working is to try speaking. If you are working moderately hard, you should be able to converse without too much trouble. If you are performing vigorous activities, you may find it more difficult. However, you shouldn't be gasping or breathing so hard that you can't talk.[9]

Always start a workout by warming up. A warm-up should take between five and ten minutes; it should slowly increase your breathing and let more blood flow to your heart and lungs. As you warm up, your body temperature rises and your muscles warm.[10] Conversely, when you cool down, you allow your breathing to return to normal gradually, which puts less of a strain on your heart than if you stop exercising abruptly and prevents a certain amount of muscle soreness. You want to be sure that the warm-up and cool-down don't take longer than the main part of your workout.

You can gauge your progress by keeping track of your activity level. Before you begin your new regimen, try measuring how far you can walk in five minutes. You can do this by counting blocks, miles, or just the number of times you walk up and down the hallway or around the house. Write down your results. Note when and how far you can increase the distance you go.

As you begin exercising, challenge yourself but don't push yourself too hard. You shouldn't experience dizziness or chest pain. The Mayo Clinic recommends seeking a doctor's immediate advice if you start feeling "tightness in your chest or severe shortness of breath, chest pain or pain in your arms or jaw or you experience heart palpitation, dizziness or faintness."[11]

Remember to drink lots of water. Not only is it important to stay hydrated, but it will actually help you feel more energetic. Also, don't

exercise in temperatures that are too hot or too cold. Not only is trying to exercise in high heat or cold dangerous, it just doesn't make
sense: when you feel uncomfortable, it is very unlikely you will get
the best or longest workout of which you are capable.

Although your goal may be thirty minutes of aerobic exercise a
day, you may want to break that up into ten-minute segments, which
are easier to fit into a busy schedule. Go for a ten-minute walk or run
before work, take a ten-minute walk break in the middle of the day,
and then do a final one when you get home. However you choose to
integrate exercise into your life, it should be in a form that makes the
most sense for you and that creates the situation in which you are
most likely to stick to your fitness plans.

How can you gauge how hard you are working? One common
measure is to take your pulse, or times per minute that the heart
beats; each age level has a different target heart rate. According to
the NIH, those numbers are:

AGE	PULSE IN BEATS PER MINUTE
40	126–153
50	119–145
60	112–136
70	105–128
80	98–119
90	91–111
100	84–102

It is important to realize that many medications can alter or affect heart rate. This includes a class of drugs called beta-blockers,
which are prescribed for high blood pressure and heart problems
(some eyedrops used for glaucoma also contain beta-blockers). These
drugs can slow your heart rate so that no matter how hard you exercise, you may not be able to achieve target heart rates. It *doesn't* mean
that the exercises aren't working or that you shouldn't do them, just
that pulse isn't a good way for you to measure your progress.

You are urged not to measure activity in target heart rate if "you take medication that changes your heart rate, you have a pacemaker, if you have an irregular heart rhythm called atrial fibrillation, or you have any other condition that affects your pulse rate." [12]

If you do decide to use this measure, remember that you aren't trying to raise your nonexercising heart rate; quite the opposite. Your heart rate should go up when you are exercising and actually drop a little bit when you aren't.

Another way of measuring your exercise is to use the Borg scale. No, we're not talking about *Star Trek* villains. The scale is named after a Swedish psychology professor, Gunnar Borg, who developed the scale to help people measure subjective experiences like physical effort or pain. The scale below is particularly recommended for midlife and older adults; you can measure your exercise by rating how much effort you think you are expending on a given activity on a scale from 6 (very, very light effort) to 20 (maximum effort).

The Borg Scale

NUMBER	EFFORT
6	Least effort
7–8	Very, very light
9–10	Very light
11–12	Fairly light
13–14	Somewhat hard
15–16	Hard
17–18	Very hard
19–20	Very, very hard
Above 20	Maximum effort

With endurance exercise, you want to work your way up from light effort to your main goal, something in the zone between fairly light and somewhat hard.

Setting the Right Tone: The Benefits of Strength Training

Most people can do their bodies a lot of good when they spend a little time each week performing weight-bearing activities (weight or strength training). Weight-bearing exercise is one of the best and safest things you can do to maintain bone mass, build muscle (which we know burns more calories than fat), and help in balancing blood sugar.

If you are just getting started, go slowly. If you belong to a gym or are joining one, try taking a basic strength-training class and let the instructor know it is your first time. If you are working at home, consider getting a book or a video. If you are looking for a really economical way to do these exercises, send for the excellent and free brochure put out by the National Institute on Aging, available on its Web site (http://www.nia.nih.gov). It provides detailed instructions on the sort of exercises you should be performing and the proper way to do them. Regardless, you should get some sort of outside advice to be sure you are exercising the muscles you should be and not lifting in a way that could be dangerous.

Start by testing some light weights of different sizes. Try to find one that you can comfortably lift between ten and fifteen times. You may find, if you are just starting out, that you want to perform the exercises without weights; your own arms will provide some good basic resistance. Depending on the sort of exercise you are performing, you may find that you need a heavier or a lighter weight. Certain muscles will be stronger than others, either because of biology or lifestyle; be ready to adjust for this. Most strength-training classes will recommend having a "lighter" set and a "heavier" set of weights for this reason. You may want to do the same thing at home.

A good goal is to perform strength exercises two to three times each week. Don't worry if you only do it once a week at first; get used to the feel of the exercises and then try to do them a little more often. Try not to move the weights too quickly—take three to five seconds to lift and lower. If you find you are thrusting or wrenching, it is likely you are using a weight that is too heavy. Not only are you in danger of overworking muscles, but you can hurt your joints if you are lifting improperly. Remember to breathe out as you lift the weight and in as you lower. If you don't, you might be letting your blood pressure get dangerously high. More practically, it will also be less painful if you are diligent about getting air into your body.

As with endurance exercise, we aren't suggesting you should never challenge yourself, but don't work the same group of muscles two days in a row; your body needs a day to recover. Edward Lasowski, a doctor who specializes in sports medicine and rehabilitation, recommends performing ten basic weight-training exercises to work each major muscle group: "Divided into exercises for your arms and shoulders, abdomen and chest, back and legs, you can complete these exercises in 20 to 30 minutes."[13]

If you have a little pain the next day, don't worry—it's normal. One way that muscles form is by repairing small tears generated through use. If you are so sore or exhausted that you have trouble performing daily tasks, however, you have overdone it. If you have overworked parts of your body, just take several days to rest and let yourself heal.

Aging Gracefully: The Importance of Balance and Flexibility Training

Balance training is an often overlooked but extremely important type of fitness that is particularly good for preventing fractures and injuries. It helps us to be confident as we walk or run, convinced that we needn't worry about dangerous falls. It also helps prevent smaller injuries like sprains and muscle tears. Many people are afraid to start exercising later in life because they are concerned about hurting themselves, but the majority of sports and fitness injuries are actually the result of bad balance, not poor endurance or strength.

Almost every kind of sport requires good balance, but so do most of our everyday actions. As one expert explains, balance "is the foundation of movement, whether you want to run faster or walk without pain."[14] Whenever you experience a slight change in terrain (and this could be from pavement to dirt path on a hike or simply from carpet to tile in your house) you need to adjust your center of gravity. Another term for this shift is *agility*, which just means the ability to change your balance and use the full necessary range of motion. As we move, we are constantly losing and regaining our balance.[15] If we are agile, we are able to make those adjustments with greater ease.

Unfortunately, as we age, we are not only more likely to fall but more apt to incur serious injury when we do. So it is all the more important to get in a good program of balance exercise at a younger age that will prevent the potential problems of bad balance at an older one. The *American Journal of Preventative Medicine* reported in 2003 that a combination of strength and balance training can reduce falls by 40 percent.[16]

When you are getting started, try this test. Stand on one foot and measure how long you are able to stay that way. Stand near a counter or something that you can grab when you feel yourself losing your balance. Write down how long you were able to keep the posture. Each month, try the test again and check your progress.

Tai chi is a great form of balance training that is safe for even the oldest and least mobile individuals. There are well over a hundred forms of the exercise, and you can probably find classes that are more or less rigorous based on your fitness and skill level. Not only is the exercise good for balance, but it enhances the cardiovascular system as well. A ten-year study that combined research from Yale, Harvard, and Emory universities found that tai chi could reduce falls by up to 47 percent.[17]

You certainly don't need expensive equipment or a gym membership to reap the benefits of balance training. Try doing the dishes or performing another stationary household chore while standing on one foot. The fitness trainer Cheryl Bradshaw recommends twisting from side to side while playing with children or, while watching television, "sit on the floor with your legs out in front of you. Keep your back straight and pretend there's a lemon between your shoulder blades that you're trying to squeeze."[18] Even simply pulling the stomach into the spine can help to strengthen the core muscles.

Yoga, another excellent exercise practice for developing balance, focuses on exercising both the body and mind and works on building a greater connection between the two. Although there are many different varieties of yoga, most work on achieving and holding poses or postures that have names ranging from the frightening (Baby Cobra), to the humorous (Downward Facing Dog), to the mysterious (Inverted Warrior). If you are practicing the series of postures called Sun Salutes, for example, you are getting some amount of cardiovascular engagement and strength training using the best and potentially heaviest weight out there—your own body.

Yoga also helps with flexibility. Flexibility training, like balance, is an essential, important part of exercising that often goes ignored. Flexibility allows joints to move fully and smoothly. When you exercise, your muscles tighten up and shorten; stretching provides a helpful counterbalance.

While it is a good idea to do a little bit of stretching as part of your warm-up and cool-down, it is also a good idea to do more extensive stretching several times (perhaps two or three times) a week for between twenty and sixty minutes.[19]

With flexibility training, you should aim to work at about the same range on the Borg scale as you do with endurance exercise; it should be somewhat hard. If you are taking a class, the instructor will make sure you hold stretches for the right amount of time. If you are working at home, the American College of Sports Medicine recommends holding each stretch for about thirty seconds.

The No-Nonsense Guide to Exercise Excuses

As we said at the beginning of the chapter, people can come up with a lot of reasons not to get in shape. Because we understand this (we use many of these excuses from time to time ourselves) we have compiled a list of some of the most popular excuses with our suggestions for overcoming them.

Not Enough Time

When it comes to working out, we need to be creative. Think about ways you can multitask. Rake leaves, mow the lawn, or weed the garden. Start walking to the store or to work, if that is possible for you, or park farther away in the parking lot. Use the stairs at work instead of elevators.

Playing baseball in the backyard, going biking in the neighborhood, or doing other kid-centered activities can be a great source of exercise that accomplishes the other goal of spending time with your family. Organizing walks or runs with friends can also combine exercise with spending time with loved ones.

Self-Consciousness

We've all been there: we're trying to take an exercise class, or going hiking with a group of friends, or even just enjoying a soccer game at a family picnic, when someone younger or more agile than us comes along and makes us feel old, out of shape, and generally self-conscious or embarrassed about our bodies and our ability to move them. Rather than letting this discourage you, find a space where you *do* feel comfortable. This can be a friend's basement, a gym with more of your peers, or even your own backyard.

Too Many Disruptions

One of the hardest but most important parts of exercising is probably sticking to it and making sure you work out regularly. To keep your routine, plan ahead. Write down your exercise plan in your datebook at the beginning of the week just as you might jot down an appointment, and hold yourself to it.

I've Tried to Exercise Before — Unsuccessfully

So you've tried to exercise before. You've done the whole New Year's resolution thing—join a gym, start eating right, change your life—before, only to return to your old habits.

Why do so many well-laid fitness plans fail? Many times it's because of the three Bs: burnout, boredom, and big bills. When you first start exercising, instead of just doing that step class you had planned on, you find yourself staying for the weight training and yoga as well. This works at first but a few weeks or months later, you find the idea of going to the gym daunting.

If this sounds like you, don't worry. You simply need to start being realistic about what kind of daily and weekly commitment you are able to make and sustain. Overexercising can feel so good at first but can quickly burn you out and tempt you to stop working out altogether, and you may also be putting yourself at risk by damaging muscles and tissues. This can provide an even less negotiable reason to stop working out—injury. Doctors classify working out compulsively with eating disorders as dangerous behavior.

If you're bored try some variety. Perhaps you can try a step aerobics class on Mondays and a yoga class on Wednesdays. Maybe you can play tennis once a week with friends and go on hikes other days. Whatever sort of exercises you perform, try to mix them up.

Another way to keep things interesting is to include friends. Start a walking group or try hitting the gym with a couple of pals. It gives you someone to motivate you (you will be less likely to skip the gym if you are meeting someone there) and you can support each other through the challenges of getting in shape.

Tightening the Belt: Exercise on a Budget

Another reason many people don't stick with workout goals is that gyms and other health-fitness tools can be really expensive. A gym membership is typically between $40 and $100 a month, although certainly there are more and less expensive options out there. And of course, personal training, massage, and other gym features cost additional money, not to mention the price of proper sneakers and workout attire. But if you are working on a tight budget, you can still find a workout program that can be healthy for you.

First, check with your employer: many companies will pay for all or part of a gym membership. Second, explore classes at a local community center. YMCAs and other community organizations often offer classes and equipment at a fraction of the cost of a gym. Many low-income housing communities and senior centers offer similar opportunities.

Another way to do group exercise on a budget is to buy a couple of fitness videos and have friends over to work out with you. Of course, starting a walking or jogging group is completely free.

While some exercise equipment can be extremely costly, there are less expensive alternatives such as jump ropes, hand weights, exercise balls, and resistance tubing and bands. Strength training on a budget can be a little tricky. If you aren't taking classes, a good way to get started is to buy small hand weights (three- or five-pound weights) plus a video. A subscription to a health magazine such as *Shape* or *Prevention* will provide advice on all four major types of exercise as well as nutrition and healthy eating. If you can't afford a subscription, library membership is free. If you walk to the library to read about exercise, you'll have doubled your benefit!

If you can't afford or simply don't want to spend money on hand weights, you can make your own for next to nothing. Fill empty laundry detergent bottles or milk containers with water, and you have a free effective hand weight; you can make it lighter or heavier simply by emptying or filling the container.[20] Cans of food can make great hand weights. Wrap packaging tape around the cans to make handles; a sixteen-ounce can is one pound.

If you have a little more cash at your disposal, you can look into used exercise equipment at the Salvation Army and similar thrift stores; you can also save money by shopping online.

Flexibility and balance training are fairly easy to do on a budget. Go to the library and pick up a copy of *Yoga for Dummies, The Complete Idiot's Guide to Exercise,* or Bob Greene's *Get with the Program.* Laura highly recommends the Living Arts Yoga video series, particularly the *Total Yoga* program with Tracey Rich and Ganga White.

If you live in a community that you think would benefit from greater fitness education, consider getting involved and spearheading the activity yourself. You could really make a difference in not only your own health but that of those around you as well.

section three
the pause

15

mindful menopause
memory, cognition, and alzheimer's disease

Women and elephants never forget.

—DOROTHY PARKER

I never forget a face, but in your case, I'll make an exception.

—GROUCHO MARX

O f all the classic signs of aging, few are more expected or more feared than memory problems. This is one area where we all behave like aging starlets at the plastic surgeon; we are willing to spend tons of money, take big risks, and basically try anything if it will help our brains stay healthy.

Some age-related decline in memory is to be expected, but as the years go by we start to take sudden blanks, blocks, and slipups more seriously. We no longer laugh when we find our remote control in the refrigerator or our glasses on top of our head after a lengthy search. What if this really is the first sign of something truly serious?

"Truly serious" is, of course, the specter of Alzheimer's disease. Every year millions of Americans suffer and die from this terrible, long-lasting illness that slowly robs individuals of their independence, their memories, their ability to interact with loved ones, and eventually their powers of speech. Directors of horror films couldn't come up with a scarier way to die. As baby boomers approach the passage between middle age and senior status, there is overwhelming interest around what can be done to reduce the odds of developing Alzheimer's, and the race to find drugs that can slow or even prevent the illness has become a major public-health priority.

What does this have to do with menopause? Many menopausal women have insisted for a long time that something big is going on in the brain at midlife; they feel their ability to manage multiple tasks, remember names and faces, and retain information slipping. Whatever this phenomenon might be, one thing it most certainly is not is the first sign of Alzheimer's.

Doctors did insist for years, however, that hormone therapy (HT) and estrogen therapy (ET) could prevent and slow Alzheimer's. The "estrogen for Alzheimer's" craze started in 1994 with the publication of a paper in the *American Journal of Epidemiology*.[1] As with treating heart disease, however, using ET to prevent Alzheimer's was always an off-label prescription. Also as with heart disease, the Women's Health Initiative (WHI) showed that HT and ET actually *increase* a woman's likelihood of developing the dread disease.

So what is the truth about menopause and memory? And how can we do our best to help our brains age healthfully?

Is Midlife Memory Loss Inevitable?

Although there is almost no scientific documentation of a connection between memory problems and menopause, many women going through the transition take it for granted that they forgot that appointment or flubbed that friend's name at a party because of raging hormones.

Of all the so-called menopausal symptoms, none is more mysterious or less scientifically explored than "brain fog" or memory problems. Does this phenomenon really exist?

Too many women describe this struggle for it to be untrue. That said, we think the problems have been exaggerated and their significance and causality distorted. Natalie F. Woods and her colleagues reported data from the Seattle Midlife Women's Study noting that while women felt they had more memory problems than they did ten or twenty years earlier, in reality, most women demonstrated little decline or abnormality.[2] The study showed two significant things. First, it found that perimenopause seemed to cause some memory problems that ended when the women entered menopause. Like hot flashes, some cognitive trouble may be a temporary side effect of the hormonal roller coaster your body is on. When things quiet down, the brain returns to normal.

Second, it seems that whatever effect hormonal status has on the brain, stress, depression, and illness all have a greater impact, and menopause can be a very stressful time.[3] You may never have so many things going on in your life that need your management and attention as you do in the years between thirty-five and sixty-five. Stress can have a negative effect on many aspects of our health, but it is particularly hard on our brain. We have such powerful reactions to stress because for many of our hunter-gatherer ancestors, their lives may have depended on the ability to react quickly to dangerous forces in their environments. Unfortunately, when we live with a high level of intense anxiety day in and day out, we can actually damage our brains.

Our body works very hard to maintain homeostasis, that is, to keep temperature and levels of chemicals in the body as constant as possible. When we come in contact with something very stressful, our bodies secrete two hormones designed to help us respond with energy and alertness to whatever potential danger looms near: adrenaline (or epinephrine) and cortisol. These messengers cause dramatic changes in the body. In situations of danger—in the short term—these are good changes. In the long term, however, these chemicals can damage existing neurons, disrupt memory formation, and limit the growth of new brain cells.[4] The more frequently this biochemical chain of events is triggered, the more likely it will happen again with less cause.

Depression makes this situation worse. Robert Sapolsky writes in *Scientific American* that "stress brings about cell death in the hippocampus," a sea horse–shaped part of the brain involved in memory processes, "and studies have found that this brain region is 10 to 20 percent smaller in depressed individuals."[5] There may be a connection between psychological distress and Alzheimer's. Researchers at the Rush Alzheimer's Disease Center studied eight hundred Catholic clergy members and found that those who dealt poorly with stressful situations were more likely to develop the disease and also to decline more quickly when suffering from it.[6]

Another thing that can potentially make the menopausal mind falter is sleep problems. Although no one is exactly sure why we sleep, scientists are increasingly confident that it has something to do with how we learn and retain knowledge. It may be that we are trying to sort through the information taken in during the course of a day, getting rid of useless stuff and encoding the things we need to keep. Another possibility is that we are giving the brain—ever-watchful and hardworking during the day—a chance to relax, detox, and get strong. A third possibility is that snoozing allows us to cement procedural knowledge such as how to dance salsa or speak French.[7] When roller-coasting hormones—or whatever causes menopausal sleep trouble—are keeping us up at nights, it can take a serious toll on our memories. Exactly how much damage is done is debatable. *Time* magazine writes that, "After about 18 hours without sleep, your reaction time begins to slow from a quarter of a second to half a second and then longer. . . . After 20 hours, your reaction time, studies show, is roughly the same as someone who has a blood alcohol level of .08—high enough to get you arrested for driving under the influence in 49 states."[8] This sounds very dramatic and other studies have found less or nearly no effect on memory from sleep deprivation.

In general, when you are tired, it is easier to feel overwhelmed and unable to cope if you forget that important name at the wrong moment or accidentally miss your dentist appointment.

Estrogen and Memory

What role does estrogen play in the brain? The truth is, we don't know. Many studies have failed to find conclusive "cause and effect" links between midlife hormone changes and memory. British researchers at the University of Sheffield found "an absence of evidence linking perceived memory problems to the menopause," adding that anxiety and depression were "the main significant predictors of perceived memory difficulties."

Cathryn Jakobson Ramin, whose book *Carved in Sand: When*

Attention Fails and Memory Fades at Midlife describes her experiences with midlife memory problems, makes the case for estrogen as a factor, writing, "Sufficient levels of the hormone are essential for neurons to properly utilize the neurotransmitter acetylcoline, critical for optimal function of the hippocampus and frontal lobes. Estrogen also increases the rate of neurogenesis and helps neurons build new synaptic and dendritic connections, limiting the damage wrought by an overabundance of midlife cortisol." In other words, it may help neurotransmitters function, neurons grow, and damaged brain cells repair.

The problem is that while your body's natural estrogen may indeed do these things, there is good clinical evidence that taking HT and ET does not. Doctors theorize that whatever benefit estrogen might give the brain can only be had during a certain "window," as with heart disease. Perhaps, they argue, the Women's Health Initiative Memory Study (WHIMS) results were tainted because they studied older women taking the drug; if you were to take estrogen during perimenopause and immediately postmenopause, the results might be different.

This seems like a big "if" to us, and we would want a lot more science on estrogen and the brain before we would be signing up to pop pills for this purpose.

Relationships to Alzheimer's aside, researchers have repeatedly failed to find a connection between taking hormones and preventing memory loss. An article in the journal *Neurology* published in 2003 compared hormone users and women who did not take estrogen. The study found that "memory was unassociated with current or prior treatment with estrogen; memory did not vary with HT duration."[9] In other words, whether menopause plays a role in memory, it seems that ET does not. An exception to this may be in women who have gone through surgical menopause,[10] particularly those who have undergone oophorectomy.

That said, natural estrogen does have some significant role in brain function. While we don't think declining levels signal the end of the ability to retain and retrieve information (men have much lower levels of estrogen and a few of them are pretty bright), we do believe that the rapid hormonal changes probably cause some disruption to our systems and require some time and adjustments to get back to normal.

We don't deny that for many women, the timing of this adjustment can be spectacularly bad. Gayatri Devi of the New York Memory Clinic sees successful, brilliant women at the top of their careers as patients. She says, "What's happening to them freaks them out at a level where they definitely do not need to be freaked out. They're in the boardroom, and suddenly they just cannot find the right words, or they have no idea what has been said. It's alarming. It's humiliating at a time when their careers are really peaking."[11]

What can we do to help limit the odds that words will race from our brains or important facts, appointments, or dates head for the hills?

To answer this question, let's take a look at things besides estrogen that might be affecting your mental capacities. What are things that hurt your head, and what are some things that might help?

Like the Corners of My Mind

Getting a handle on memory loss is difficult because there are so many different regions of the brain, each responsible for different forms of memory. Scientists divide memory into two major categories: *declarative* and *procedural*. Declarative memory is then broken into two additional types, *episodic memory* and *semantic memory*.

Generally, declarative memory involves historical information, both public and personal. It's how you remember the dates of Civil War battles or the time when your family went to Hawaii together. Episodic memory holds our personal experiences and is most classically what we think of when we talk about "remembering." It's what happens when you call up the time your grandmother took you ice skating, or that song you loved in fifth grade. Semantic memory, as memory expert Rebecca Rupp writes, "stores the essential raw material that allows us to define, order and operate within the world: the definitions of bat and butterfly, for example, and the awful truth about poison ivy, the meaning of the red and green lights on traffic signals, the number of pints in a quart and the capital of Oklahoma."[12] In other words, if episodic memory stores our personal information, semantic memory stores our collective knowledge. Although these two types of remembering are related—you may know what you do about poison ivy because of that time you unwittingly rolled in some as a kid—they are distinct.

If declarative memory requires recall, procedural memory is all about unconscious learning. It is where we store things like how to ride a bike or type without looking at our fingers. Rupp explains, "Declarative memory in all its many human aspects is sometimes described as a process of know *that*. We know *that* Columbus, for better or for worse, reached the Caribbean in 1492; we know *that* we broke a leg by falling out of a tree at the age of ten. . . . Procedural memory, in contrast, is a process of knowing *how*. We know *how* to swim, *how* to dunk a basketball."[13]

There are many additional categories and alternate ways of thinking about memory; much like the only closet in a small apartment, we store all sorts of different bits of knowledge or experience in different corners and crevices of the brain.

There are nearly as many ways of forgetting as there are parts of the brain. Dr. Daniel L. Schacter, a Harvard University psychologist, has tried to document the various types of memory problems that many people encounter. He has created seven categories into which he groups our various slipups, misrememberings, and mental confusions.[14]

These seven categories are transience, absentmindedness, blocking, suggestibility, bias, persistence, and misattribution. Transience, absentmindedness, and blocking are familiar foes of middle-aged and older people.

Transience is what happens when you just can't learn and remember new things; it is a problem of the "working memory," the part of the brain that holds bits of information for short periods of time before they are transferred for long-term storage. This brain feature allows us to finish reading sentences and remember how they started. Most people naturally experience a little of this with age, and word and story recall slow down a little. It happens because of the effects of time on the temporal lobe or the hippocampus (significantly, these are also the parts of the brain that are earliest in revealing Alzheimer's-related damage). So next time you call your best friend because you just *have* to tell her something, only to find by the time she picks up the phone that you have forgotten what it was, you will know why.

The best way to reduce this problem is through mindfulness and the use of mnemonics. When you meet a new person, or you're trying to remember her name, think of her distinctive features and try to build connection with knowledge you already have. Come up with an elaborate or even a silly mnemonic: if you want to remember to tell your friend Ann about an idea for your children's school graduation, picture the ill-fated Anne Boleyn walking to her demise in a cap and gown. Make sure to visualize the scenario; this will help to fix it in your mind. This may seem ridiculous, but the sheer outlandishness of your image can help you to recall whatever you've associated with it.

Unfortunately, mnemonic devices take a lot of effort. It can be a pain to have to put so much thought and creativity into small details, even if it makes a big difference. If you are at a conference and are meeting many new people, it can be difficult to impossible to encode each one accurately in enough detail to insure remembering them.

Absentmindedness is different from transience; in this case information was properly stored but then couldn't be retrieved at crucial moments. This sort of problem usually arises when you aren't properly focusing your attention. This is a pretty easy problem to fall into when you are simultaneously trying to finish that presentation and making dinner and dealing with your mom's impending visit and trying to figure out why the cat is losing weight and (especially) coping with that particularly nasty hot flash.

Absentmindedness has to do with something called *prospective memory*. This concept has to do with remembering things to do in the future. Dr. Schacter writes, "Absent-minded errors of prospective memory are annoying not only because of their pragmatic consequences but also because others tend to see them as reflecting on credibility and even character in a way that poor retrospective memory does not."[15] When you stand your friend up at the coffee shop, she may assume you were selfish enough not to value her time. When you can't find important papers, it can seem as though you just don't have it together.

The best solution to this problem is to create concrete reminders that are both descriptive and accessible: make a note about things you need to do tomorrow and make sure that first, you put enough information in the note to remember what each item is, and second, you put your "to do" list in a place where you can't miss it—tied to your keys in your purse, perhaps, or placed next to your toothbrush.

As you age, it's more effective to convert time-based tasks into event-based ones.[16] For example, if you have to take a pill at 8 AM, and that is when you wake up each morning, think of it as something you do when you are getting up in the morning rather than trying to remember "8 AM."

Blocking, when you just can't remember an important word or idea, is particularly relevant to menopausal women. The most common form of this problem is forgetting proper names, even of people who have been close to you a long time. The hardest names to recall are those you haven't needed in a while. Studies have repeatedly shown that people will forget proper names with much greater frequency than other nouns and concepts.

There is no really good way to solve this problem, but when learning new names, you can try to turn the symbolic word into something more conceptual. Think "Barbara Seaman" and then "women's health author," and "Liam's grandmother." These latter concepts will be more readily available later on and can help trigger the more elusive name.

At other times, it's not names but words that just won't come to mind. Schacter calls this a TOT, or tip-of-the-tongue, situation. Here again, using alternative words is probably the best solution: rather than struggling to come up with the word *diabetes*, say "the illness where your body isn't using insulin correctly."

Memory Loss, Mild Cognitive Impairment, and Alzheimer's: A Slippery Slope?

Mild cognitive impairment (MCI) is a fairly common but vaguely defined condition that affects many older adults (and a few middle-aged ones as well). It is like a brain purgatory: your doctor would agree that you aren't functioning mentally at the level of a healthy person your age, but your condition isn't serious enough to suggest Alzheimer's or another really debilitating problem. As D. A. Bennett and colleagues at the Rush Alzheimer's Disease Center put it, "The condition represents older persons whose memory or other cognitive abilities are not normal, but who do not meet accepted criteria for dementia."[17]

While certainly not everyone living with MCI ends up developing full-blown Alzheimer's, enough do that doctors and scientists worry about what the connection might be. Catherine Arnst writes, "It is an ominous diagnosis, even though the condition doesn't interfere significantly with daily living, because it can be an early warning sign of something much worse. Every year some 15% of people with MCI go on to develop Alzheimer's disease."[18] As many as 22 percent of adults seventy-five and older have the problem.[19]

It is possible with expensive and somewhat new scanning technology to tell if a patient's memory problems are normal, related to MCI, or likely the first signs of Alzheimer's.[20] Cathryn Jakobson Ramin underwent both positron emission tomography (PET) and functional magnetic resonance imaging (fMRI) as well as a sophisticated battery of mental tests at UCLA's Neuropsychiatric Institute. PET scans use radioimaging to monitor brain metabolism, and fMRI looks at metabolism and blood flow. Ramin writes that a team led by psychiatrist Gary Small could "predict with 95 percent accuracy whether a patient would develop the symptoms of Alzheimer's disease within three years."[21] This kind of expensive, time-consuming testing just isn't an option for everyone, and although it can tell you with some certainty if you have Alzheimer's *now*, it cannot predict if you will have it in five years. The only way to know for sure if a patient has Alzheimer's is to perform an autopsy after he has died.

For the majority of women in their fifties and sixties, Alzheimer's isn't their problem.

One very significant cause of memory loss is the use of certain pharmaceuticals. The list of drugs that can cause your brain to falter includes antidepressants and antianxiety drugs prominently among them. Other potential culprits include certain cholesterol and diabetes medications, cough medicines, antihistamines, sedatives, beta-blockers, chemotherapy drugs, motion-sickness pills, steroids, and ulcer medications. Significantly, sleep aids, both prescription and over-the-counter, can have a negative effect on the brain. This is a frustrating situation: you want to do what's best for your brain, which would seemingly be to sleep, so you take a pill that in turn can have negative effects on memory.

We don't tell you this so that you will throw away all your drugs but rather so that if you are having memory problems and using medication to help you sleep, you may want to have a conversation with you doctor about whether this could be the cause.

Nutrition can have either a positive or a negative impact on your brain. If you are consuming a lot of alcohol, you shouldn't be surprised if it takes a toll on your thinking. While limited amounts of alcohol can have positive health benefits, drinking too much is always worse than drinking nothing.

While eating fish has classically been thought of as a head-healthy activity, recent concerns about the mercury content of popular fish such as tuna and swordfish have raised the possibility that eating too much fish may do more harm than good. On the other hand, getting the right balance of omega-3 fatty acids to omega-6 fatty acids may have benefits for the brain as well as the heart. The FDA provides updates on the mercury content of various fish, which you can find by logging on to its Web site (www.fda.gov).

The brain is an amazingly delicate thing, and even light head trauma can cause some level of brain damage. A mild concussion can be sustained without a loss of consciousness, and the effects of such a hit might not be evident for weeks or months to come.

A study on mice from the University of Pennsylvania School of Medicine demonstrated that mild, repetitive, traumatic brain injury hastens the onset of Alzheimer's disease.[22] Likewise a study of football players, who sustain a lot more head damage than most of us, found that pro ball players were 36 percent more likely to develop Alzheimer's.[23]

Frequent or serious head trauma can cause less serious memory problems than Alzheimer's, and if you engage in activities that make

cranial damage more likely (bike or motorcycle riding, rock climb-
ing, horseback riding, etc.) make sure you properly protect your
head.

Genetics and Environment

How good or bad your memory stays as you age may be a classic
study in both sides of the nature-versus-nurture debate. Both environment and genetics seem to play a role in how you weather the
tests of time, but one plays more of a role than you might expect, and
the other less.

When it comes to Alzheimer's, whether your family has a history
of the disease changes your odds of getting it yourself. There are two
different types of Alzheimer's: early-onset and late-onset. Early-
onset Alzheimer's tends to be associated with a genetic predisoposi-
tion. As with breast and ovarian cancer, there are genes that scientists
now recognize as being associated with higher risks of developing
the disease. In particular, the APOE gene is of continuing interest to
researchers.[24]

However, some scientists are concluding that Alzheimer's has
less of a genetic component than they previously thought. Investigators in the EURODEM analyses of studies, working with data pulled
from thousands of Europeans, found that "compared with the risk
reported in studies based on prevalent patients . . . the contribution
of family history to the risk of AD [Alzheimer's disease] may be
overestimated in studies."[25]

On the other hand, your environment both as a child and as an
adult can have a much greater role in how healthy your brain stays
then you might think. It seems that children who are exposed to
stressful conditions sustain a certain amount of damage to their
brain, hippocampal wear and tear that may not show itself until the
person is grown up and entering middle age.[26]

Getting more education during your younger years also seems to
put you at a long-term cognitive advantage, but if you think you
missed out in your early life, continuing to educate yourself is one of
your best natural defenses against both age-related cognitive decline
and Alzheimer's.[27] Although no one is sure why this is true, it is pos-

sible that highly educated or engaged people simply build up more brain cells. Another possibility is that they build more networks in the brain so that if one falters, they can fall back on an alternate route. Although many highly educated people have suffered and died from Alzheimer's and the ravages of the disease have been apparent—the late novelist Iris Murdoch, for one—there are examples of college professors dying of Alzheimer's disease and never having known they were ill.[28] Indeed, it often takes longer to diagnose highly educated people with Alzheimer's because they continue to do well on the battery of mental tests used to assess the illness.

We think engaging in challenging brain activities is one of the best ways to fight memory loss. Not only are there no side effects, but learning and trying new things will enrich your life and help you open up new possibilities of what you could know or who you could become. Menopause is a great moment to start learning things you have always wanted to try: take up a new language, learn to play an instrument, anything that is mostly fun and sometimes frustrating but in the end helps you to use your brain in ways that you haven't before. There's no need to invest too heavily in commercial programs that claim they will boost your brainpower; most of them have been shown to have limited usefulness.

Just as you can change your environment to help your brain stay active, there are many factors in our modern life that can work against your functioning at your best.

If having your attention divided makes it harder to encode things in memory and easier to suffer from absentmindedness, then the work world today is the enemy of a healthy brain. Computers, e-mail, cell phones, Blackberries, all these new aspects of work life have created an environment where concentrating on one thing is seen as bad and "multitasking" is considered optimum. Add these technologies to an increasingly global world, and you have a life that has lost its structure: you can work at midnight on a Saturday and grocery shop at 4 AM on a Tuesday. Ramin writes, "We are in shock, caught between the world in which we grew to adulthood, one that ran on conventional chronology, and the one we live in now which leaps over all boundaries . . . to be fractured has become a societal expectation."[29]

Remember, as you age, your response times slow. This is not to say that there is anything wrong with the older brain: it just works differently. Regardless, though, the do-everything-at-once and do-it-as-fast-as-you-can environment of today's work world ironically creates a terrible environment for working as efficiently as possible. Alison Motluk writes, "This 'always on' culture is taking its toll. . . . last year, Glenn Wilson at the Institute of Psychiatry in London found that being bombarded with emails and phone calls has a greater effect on IQ than smoking marijuana."[30] Perhaps as a result of this, many big companies have started deemphasizing multitasking. It's turning out that you get more done better if you work on one thing at a time.

Edward Hallowell says that this sort of multitasking, no-boundaries living is creating a condition he calls attention deficit trait (ADT). ADT is a lot like its cousin, attention deficit disorder (ADD); the difference is that ADD is a genetically based condition that persists over the course of a person's lifetime. ADT is a temporarily induced state that happens when normal people are trying to do too much.

He recommends more interaction and conversation with other people: "When you comfortably connect with a colleague, even if you are dealing with an overwhelming problem, the deep centers of the brain send messages through the pleasure center to the area that assigns resources to the frontal lobes. Even when you're under extreme stress, this sense of human connection causes executive functioning to hum."[31] Additionally, it can be helpful to break large tasks into smaller ones.

Somewhere in your home or office, you should have a space that is yours. Even if your desk is a little like a Mt. Everest of papers, create an area that is neat and maintained. Also, keep a journal for a week or two and record the times of day when you work most efficiently (and those when you are sleepy or more prone to anxiety or distraction.) Use this to decide when you are most alert, and leave the toughest tasks for those times.

Alzheimer's

In the fall of 1901, Dr. Alois Alzheimer, a neuropathologist practicing in Frankfurt, Germany, began treating a patient named Auguste D. Auguste was fifty-one years old, very young to be experiencing the type of senility the doctor associated with aged clients. Plaintively the woman explained, "I have lost myself."

When Auguste D. died five years later, Alzheimer examined her brain and found that it looked as if it were infected with measles or chicken pox and was sprouting weeds. He called the crusty brown clumps "plaques" and the weedlike growths "tangles." In 1910, his colleague Emil Kraepelin christened the condition "Alzheimer's disease." For the next half century, the illness was acknowledged, if at all, as a rare problem afflicting relatively young middle-aged people. Old-age dementia (the loss or impairment of mental powers) was attributed to other causes, including atherosclerosis, or fatty deposits that clogged the brain.

In 1952, Dr. Meta Neumann, the curator of the brain bank at St. Elizabeth's Psychiatric Hospital in Washington, D.C., discovered that Alzheimer's wasn't as rare as scientists believed, but her findings were largely ignored for many years. The final leap into full public awareness didn't come until 1987, with the publication of a government report entitled *Losing a Million Minds: Confronting the Tragedy of Alzheimer's Disease and Other Dementias.*[32] Meanwhile, in the first burst of enthusiasm, many people were misdiagnosed with Alzheimer's when in fact they had dementia owing to other conditions such as depression, thyroid disease, hypoglycemia, drug interactions, or chronic infection.

Though there are still many unanswered questions about the exact nature of the illness, what we do know is that Alzheimer's is responsible for between 55 and 60 percent of all dementia cases, and that around 25 to 30 percent of Americans over age eighty-five may suffer from it. Alzheimer's physically changes the brain. In the 1980s, researchers discovered that plaques that develop in the spaces between neurons and occur early in the disease process (sometimes as early as twenty years before symptoms emerge) were largely cell debris surrounded by beta-amyloid, a protein that is a by-product of a larger protein involved in cell membrane function. There is still debate today between scientists who believe the plaques act in Alzheimer's, causing some or most of the degeneration, and others who think they are merely a by-product of whatever is really going on.

It takes an average of eight years for the disease to regress a patient to a state that resembles infancy, but anyone who has nursed an Alzheimer's patient knows that dramatic transitions are not uncommon and can happen more quickly than eight years.

There are about 4.5 million Americans who have Alzheimer's and this number may triple in the next half century.[33] The current worldwide numbers are as high as 18 million.[34]

Besides head trauma, family history, and lack of education, being female puts you at an increased risk for the disease. This suggests that there might be a hormonal component to Alzheimer's, although there are other possible explanations for this statistic, including behavioral factors. The hormone theory led to the popular off-label prescription of HT for preventing dementia. When the Women's Health Initiative Memory Study (WHIMS) showed that sixty-one women taking estrogen and progestin were diagnosed with dementia, compared with only twenty-one in the placebo group, this belief went out the window.[35]

For those who do develop the disease, there isn't much that doctors can do for them. Although there are many experimental drugs and ongoing clinical trials, approved medications show only limited benefit. Most of the drugs approved to treat early Alzheimer's are acetylcholinesterase (AChE) inhibitors, medications that work through preventing the breakdown of neurotransmitters and prolonging their action on the neurons.[36] Some popular brand names of AChE inhibitors include Aricept, Exelon, and Razadyne. While there is some evidence that these drugs slow the progress of the disease for a little while at the beginning of the illness, they can't stop or prevent it. A newer drug, approved in the past few years, is called Namenda (memantine). It is the only drug currently approved for treating later-stage Alzheimer's. It works on NMDA receptors—parts of the brain that help with learning and memory—and, like AChE inhibitors, is able to provide better cognition for a very short time. Ultimately it has very little effect on disease progression. Namenda is sometimes being prescribed with AChE inhibitors, although the ultimate result of this cocktail is unknown.

Hopes were high when Elan Pharmaceuticals began trials of its experimental vaccine for the disease. In January 2002, however, human trials were halted when it was announced that some patients developed brain inflammations. The vaccine continues to be studied and may eventually hit the market. An experimental drug called Alzamed and other drugs that act on the beta-amyloid proteins that become Alzheimer's plaques are currently in phase three trials. This is a field that will most certainly see the entrance of several new drugs in the next decade. Whether any will offer substantial benefit to patients remains to be seen. Richard I. Hodes writes that ultimately, "solving its puzzle will require the involvement of scientists from multiple disciplines working on both Alzheimer's disease and normal aging."[37]

Drugs for Improving Cognition

For millennia, human beings have tried to improve their alertness with chemicals such as caffeine in coffee and tea. In the twentieth century, drugs like Ritalin and Adderall have become popular for both approved uses—the treatment of ADD—and off-label uses—improving focus in individuals without such conditions. Today there are as many drugs in development for brain enhancement as there are for brain illnesses and dementia. Many of these drugs raise ethical concerns as well as safety ones.

Ritalin, Adderall, and the more classic attention-deficit drugs are amphetamine or amphetamine-like stimulants. Amphetamines have great potential for addiction. They can also, ironically, make it harder to fall asleep and can contribute to high blood pressure and aggravate heart problems. Like antidepressants, these drugs have recently come under scrutiny for the unpredictable ways they can affect mood.

In addition to caffeine, amphetamines, and Aricept, the Alzheimer's drug, a pill called Provigil (modafinil) has been studied for its ability to increase alertness in tired or distracted people. It is currently approved for treating narcolepsy but is used off-label as an alternative for Adderall, Ritalin, and other drugs used to treat ADD and other attention problems. Although it was tested for use in military pilots, Walter Reed Army Institute researchers concluded "that there didn't appear to be any benefit to using modafinil over caffeine. Both drugs looked very similar."[38]

Common side effects include nervousness, headache, anxiety, and nausea. Less commonly, people experience serious side effects including chest pain, high blood pressure, and dizziness. People with heart problems shouldn't use this drug. Provigil is very expensive but less addictive than Adderall and Ritalin.

Stephen S. Hall writes, "Despite an incessant media drumbeat about the coming revolution in what one magazine has dubbed 'Viagra for the brain,' smart pills are not around the corner."[39]

Certainly the use of any miracle drug for the brain would bring along with it some serious ethical quandaries. Would you give such drugs to children? (Let's hope not.) To what extent would taking them as a healthy individual be akin to using steroids as a professional athlete? Certainly steroids help people hit more home runs, but as recent congressional hearings show, we aren't ready to accept such enhancements as either natural or morally acceptable.

If there seems to be an increasing number of prescription drugs available for brain building, they are dwarfed by the available herbal alternatives. Vitamin stores and health-food stores devote entire sections to pills promising to stave off memory loss or prevent cognitive decline. Ginkgo biloba is an herb that got a lot of press in the late 1990s for its supposed ability to sharpen mental skills and treat Alzheimer's "naturally" in forms from teas to tinctures. Although most clinical trails have shown it to have little or no effect, some doctors believe it holds promise in treating Alzheimer's and represents an improvement over pharmaceutical alternatives in terms of side effects.

With drugs both of the natural and pharmaceutical variety, it is worth asking how much memory is too much. While it is an advantage to have excellent recall, our minds forget for reasons of mental health. We encounter so much information on a daily basis that if we were to hold onto all of it, we wouldn't be able to distinguish useful from useless detail. James L. McGaugh writes, "More is not better. At the extreme more is worse."[40]

The Mount Sinai School of Medicine notes, "Dementia can be a symptom, sometimes temporary, of dozens of diseases and disorders. These include poisoning, reactions to medications, viral infections, malfunctioning glands, benign brain tumors and severe nutritional deficiencies."[41] About 10 percent of cases of dementia are due to a cause that can be partially or completely reversed: the effects of a prescription medication. Vascular dementia, caused by stroke or heart attack, is the second most common cause. It is estimated that up to 42 percent of heart-surgery patients suffer measurable mental deterioration during the five years after surgery, and up to 40 percent of strokes result in some degree of dementia.[42]

Type 2 diabetes can significantly raise a woman's chances of experiencing cognitive problems. A study published in the *British Medical Journal* analyzed data from the Nurses Health Study and found that "women with type 2 diabetes had poorer cognitive function . . . than women without diabetes, especially if they had had diabetes for more than 15 years."[43] The good news was that when the disease was managed, women's brains functioned at the same levels of those without diabetes.

For treating both these conditions, exercise and weight control are essential. Like education, it is never too late to start being physically active or making smarter food choices.

Thinking Things Through

Cognitive health is an area that will certainly change completely in the next decade, and many new drugs will undoubtedly flood the market. We are hopeful that scientists will find ways to preserve our brains and in particular prevent the ravages of Alzheimer's. At this time, though, there is no pill that can prevent Alzheimer's, and nothing you can take that will make your memory function better. Given the side effects of the available drug options, we would caution you to be wary of false hope in quick fixes.

Instead, if menopause is making your mind a little uneven, have patience with yourself. Find ways to make small changes that will ease the situation until your hormones can balance out and things will return to equilibrium.

In Western culture we have a bad attitude about aging brains. Altering that would cause more radical changes than the most cutting-edge drug. Rebecca Rupp writes of a study performed with aging deaf and hearing populations of Americans and Chinese. The deaf populations, who had less exposure to negative stereotypes of aging, performed better on cognitive exams, as did their hearing Chinese counterparts, who lived in a society with more positive associations with being elderly.[44] Other studies have found that elders in cultures that value older people consistently perform better on brain tests.

If you are sitting around waiting for your mind to fail, chances are you won't be disappointed. While there are very real biological changes in the brain as you age, and some amount of memory loss is normal, your ideas about how your memory works will have a huge impact on how it actually does.

16

loving the skin you're in
skin, hair, and midlife beauty

Beauty—be not caused—It is—
Chase it, and it ceases—
Chase it not, and it abides—
—EMILY DICKINSON

The fountain of youth is not a myth. Just watch late-night info-mercials or read pretty much any women's magazine—the fountain of youth is alive and well and living on the tips of advertisers' tongues. All you need is a certain cream, wash, lotion, vitamin, supplement, laser treatment, or surgery.

Of course we all know, if we are honest, that there is nothing—not something we can put in or on or do to our bodies—that will change the fact that we get old. The amazing thing is that despite this knowledge, we all keep trying things "just in case." So in the way we might knock on wood or throw salt over our shoulders, we try this beauty treatment, that supplement, or this new exercise.

Our culture is obsessed with staying young. Every day the evening news runs hand-wringing stories about women getting Botox at thirty or plastic surgery at twenty-five. When the show *Desperate Housewives* became a runaway hit in 2004, magazines ran gushing headlines exclaiming, "Sexy at 40!!??" Clearly forty is not even close to being old enough for anyone to be asking that question incredulously, and twenty-five is obscenely young to be enlisting surgical knives in the service of a quest for longer youth. Things like this betray a dangerously unhealthy attitude toward aging that is unfortunately part of American life.

We all know the expression "aging gracefully." We do this by making the transition between being a young woman to a middle-aged woman and eventually to an older woman confidently and smoothly. If we are going to start to change our culture's bad attitude about getting older, we need to be aware of the prejudices and negative myths we carry around. One way to do this is by understanding rather than resisting the way our bodies change with age.

As women, we have had to work and fight hard to have the power we do in our lives. We guard it closely and realize what a fragile thing it can be. It is unpleasant to believe that any of it came from something as out of our control as our sexual attractiveness.

Although most of the changes we will talk about in this chapter begin happening at midlife, they are not the result of menopause. This is important to say up front, because for years women have been taught to associate menopause with aging and try to reverse menopause chemically as a means to avoid getting older.

In 1966, Dr. Robert Wilson wrote *Feminine Forever*.[1] It sold a hundred thousand copies in the first seven months of its publication.

If you thought you had a healthy outlook on getting older, you didn't by the time you'd finished reading Wilson. If you had some concerns about taking hormones, when you were finished with *Feminine Forever* you ran out and got some: whatever the risks, they must be better than slowly turning into a man-hating zombie incapable of performing basic tasks.

In some ways, the story of hormone therapy (HT) is the story of a wrong turn on the map in the journey toward the fountain of youth. The idea seemed like a simple one: if you ascribe many of the changes in the body that occur as women age (be it deterioration in the heart or the skin) to hormone decline, then perhaps by maintaining youthful estrogen levels, the aging clock could be stopped. The problem is that this still identifies young bodies as normal bodies and sets up an unnecessary and unrealistic standard for older women.

To what extent does estrogen decline play a role in changes in skin, hair, nails, and other parts of the body? What is normal aging, and what are some less common things that might happen?

Skin Deep?

For years, forty-seven-year-old Molly had been proud of the fact that she looked years younger than her driver's license revealed her to be; the only hint that she was getting further out of her thirties had been tiny lines in the corners of her eyes and small lines tracing the outline of her wide smile.

Suddenly those little lines seemed to deepen, and new ones appeared. Molly found herself spending more money on lotions and peels and microdermabrasion treatments. She wondered why this was happening so fast. Could it have to do with the irregularity of her periods, which were becoming further and further apart? Or was this just the way that getting older happened?

When Wilson included skin aging among the menopause problems that could be cured by HT, he was participating in a long tradition that didn't end until the Women's Health Initiative (WHI) revelations of 2001 to 2003. Well into the 1990s, doctors were advising women to "be aware that hormone replacement therapy can help firm the skin."[2]

Skin: A Primer

Although the old adage "Beauty is only skin deep" uses our largest organ as a metaphor for superficiality, there is nothing simplistic about skin. Ever notice how your healthy body temperature is always the same whether you're hiking through the Arctic or sitting in the burning summer sun? Well, this is largely because of the skin. Weighing in at around 15 percent of our entire body weight, it contains about a thousand nerve endings and hundreds of sweat glands in a single square inch.

The outermost layer of your skin is called the *epidermis*. It is thin, about the width of a sheet of paper.[3] It sits on top of the dermis like the icing on a wedding cake, bolstered by small, column-like cells called *basal cells.* These cells are responsible for producing *keratin,* a protein that provides protection against bacteria, infections, and fungi.

The inner layer (which makes up the majority of the skin) is called the *dermis.* This part of the skin is full of blood vessels, nerve fibers, oil and sweat glands, hair follicles, and muscle cells."[4] The dermis is made up of two tissues: *collagen* and *elastin.* The strands of these two substances weave tightly together, with the white collagen fibers giving strength and support and the yellow elastin allowing flexibility. There is a bottom layer to the skin called the *subcutaneous layer.* It is responsible for holding in heat and also for protecting the internal organs.

When we are young, the skin is stretchy and firm, like a new skirt that fits snuggly around the body, accenting the curves. As we age, the body begins to produce less collagen and elastin. The effect is like the elastic in that new skirt giving a little. It still fits, but it doesn't have the perfectly tailored look anymore, becoming prone to looseness in inconvenient places. Another natural change, says Dr. Richard D. Granstein of the Weill Medical College at Cornell University, is that oil and sweat glands don't work as well, allowing skin to become drier and less able to keep cool.[5] Yet another problem is that skin loses fat and doesn't have as much plumping it up. This is part of why we get lines in the forehead and around the mouth and eyes.

Collagen loss impacts lots of other parts of the body: it can dry out the hair and scalp, be involved in hair loss, receding gums, and brittle nails, and may even cause vision problems.[6]

We all know, if we are honest, that one of the simplest, cheapest ways to slow skin aging is to stay out of the sun. It's hard to do: nothing feels better on an early summer day than lying out and letting the rays dance across our noses and shoulders. Unfortunately, sun exposure directly contributes to weakening elastin fibers, which make the skin more likely to sag.[7] When skin gets this masklike quality, it is the result of a condition called *elastosis,* a sort of more serious version of the loss of elastin that happens in most people as they age and is worsened by sustained sun exposure. In addition to decreasing skin flexibility and adding to wrinkles, sun exposure can create pigmented spots that are technically called *solar lentigines* but are usually (and not coincidentally) known as *age spots.*

One Manhattan dermatologist says bluntly, "The most effective strategy for improving the tone and texture of your skin is to use SPF 15 sunscreen and moisturizing facial creams every day."[8]

Like everything else in life, this issue isn't cut and dried. We aren't suggesting that women hide indoors in the hope of remaining eternally youthful. Rather, we are saying that for safety's sake, good sense and a lot of sunscreen should be used. Another thing to consider here is that the sun offers some benefits, perhaps most significantly the creation of vitamin D in our bodies. Vitamin D is important for many reasons, but one of them is that proper calcium absorption is difficult without it. Remember: everything in moderation. Realize and be honest about the havoc sunlight can wreak, but don't forget the positive things it does either.

If you get a lot of sun and like it that way, be sure to be diligent in checking for signs of skin cancer and discussing suspicious moles, skin discolorations, or growths with your doctor. The average person has somewhere between ten and forty moles.[9] Those with larger numbers and those with fair skin are at an increased ristk for skin cancer, and in particular the most dangerous variety, melanoma. Melanoma is rare, but if untreated, potentially deadly. Joan Liebman-Smith and Jacqueline Nardi Egan suggest using the "alphabet" method of assessing whether a mole is dangerous: look for a) asymmetry, b) border is irregular, c) multicolored, d) diameter larger than a pencil eraser, e) evolving (meaning the size, shape, or color changes noticeably).[10]

You already know you shouldn't smoke. Just so you have another good reason to quit, however, there have been several studies that show that this nasty habit interferes with collagen metabolism and causes vasoconstriction that basically smothers that skin.[11] Want to look older faster? Keep puffing away.

Chemically Speaking: A No-Nonsense Look at Common Antiaging Ingredients

We all live under the laws of gravity and biology, which both unfortunately extract a yearly tax on us. But is there anything we can do—

any product we can buy, supplement we can take, or procedure we can undergo—that significantly curtails this process?

Let's start by looking at some of the more common ingredients in skin-care products. The idea is not to endorse products—marketers do quite well on their own without our help—but rather to help you understand what these chemicals actually do.

Alpha and *beta hydroxy acids* are found naturally in fruits and are created synthetically for skin-care products. They are exfoliants, which means they help to strip away dead skin cells and help new ones grow, as well as stimulating collagen production.

If you use products with alpha or beta hydroxy, be careful; they can cause skin sensitivity (they are acids, after all), and you probably want to be extra careful to avoid the sun for a few days. Doctors at the Mayo Clinic conclude that these chemicals may contribute to "modest improvements" in small wrinkles.[12]

Another acid product that is becoming more popular is *alpha lipoic acid* (ALA), which works partially as an exfoliant but also works as an antioxidant, which prevents or limits damage caused by oxidation. While there is some evidence that ALA diminishes fine lines and spotting, it also, like other acids, causes inflammation. Scientists are unsure if this puffiness itself isn't responsible for the lessening of wrinkles.[13]

A very popular variety is *vitamin A derivatives* such as tretinoin and retinol. Tretinoin is available in prescription brands such as Retin-A. Like the other preparations we discussed so far, retinol can cause redness and irritation; it works by shedding the top layer of skin cells and encouraging the growth of collagen in the emerging cells.

Consumers should be wary when purchasing nonprescription products containing retinol. A bottle of face cream may list it as a key ingredient, but this doesn't really tell you how much retinol may (or more likely may not) be in the product. The FDA warns that many over-the-counter preparations "may contain almost no retinol."[14]

Coenzyme Q_{10} (CoQ10) is a compound that the body produces to encourage cell growth and promote proper cell functioning. CoQ10 levels seem to decline with age. Supplemental CoQ10 is being tested for its ability to cut side effects in cancer patients and is also sold as a cardioprotective agent. It is one of the main ingredients in several popular heart-protecting vitamin supplements. It is also taken as a skin strengthener. The compound is thought to be an antioxidant. There is no long-term data on CoQ10, although two clinical trials suggest that at least in the short term, CoQ10 reduced wrinkles around the eyes and was able to curtail sun damage.

Soy has recently been touted as a skin-saving ingredient. However, whether in cream or supplement form, soy works on the same chemical principles as estrogen and should carry the same cautions. *Vitamin E* has been a home remedy for scarring and wrinkling for years. It is the major antioxidant found in human skin and has been shown in animal studies to reduce wrinkling. Since vitamin E levels steadily decline in the skin as it ages, it is thought that perhaps supplementing it will slow aging.

Like most antiwrinkling agents, it is possible that vitamin E products will cause swelling and redness. In some cases a more serious allergic reaction called "contact dermatitis" may occur. This skin inflammation can cause itchiness and redness.

One reason more trials are needed is that it is unclear what kinds of vitamin E are most readily absorbed into the skin. It is possible, for example, that tocopherol and tocopherol acetate (the forms of vitamin E most often found in beauty products), may be poorly absorbed.[15] This is important to think about with all vitamins. Because they are often derived from different sources, certain varieties of a given nutrient may be more effective in the body than others. Another consideration is that it is unclear whether vitamin E is effective alone or more useful when partnering with other vitamins and antioxidants.

Vitamin C, for example, is often touted as a wrinkle remedy because of its ability to help maintain and reuse vitamin E. There are many (rather expensive) vitamin C preparations available. Again, there is not enough research to feel very confident in most of them. Another reason for the buyer to beware: vitamin C deteriorates very quickly. Dr. Deborah Jailman explains that this can often leave consumers with "little more than a moisturizer."[16] If you do invest in vitamin C products, be sure to store them carefully: use airtight containers and make sure they aren't exposed to the sun.

Copper peptides are a popular class of ingredients that aid in the action of other antioxidants. Like vitamin E, they have long been thought to aid in the healing of wounds. There is very little research on this option.

Face creams respond to trends: certain ingredients will be in vogue, and suddenly every cosmetics line will have its own version. A few years ago a popular middle-end cosmetics company introduced a line of products touting tea as a major antioxidant ingredient. *Tea products* have been shown in animal studies to protect against sun damage and maybe even to help prevent skin cancer. They seem to have fewer negative side effects (such as reddening), which means that even if they don't help as much as we hope, they don't seem to hurt either. Like vitamin C, tea products may deteriorate over time, so store them properly.

Growth factors such as *kinetin* are another minimally irritating variety of product enhancers. If a product is not known to have significant or distressing side effects, we feel much more confident recommending it.

It would be wonderful if we could supplement a biochemical that's been lost through aging simply by smearing some on the skin. Unfortunately, this doesn't always work. Collagen creams are a great example of this. Deemed "possibly ineffective," doctors at the Mayo Clinic explain, "collagen isn't absorbed through the skin and doesn't increase the body's production of collagen." They add, "Applying a collagen cream may give the sensation of firmness, but it's probably due to skin hydration that could be achieved by using any moisturizer."[17]

Feeling tired reading through this list? Let's perk you up: a final and extremely popular face cream ingredient is none other than that beverage classic, *caffeine*. While as Dr. Orly Etingin of Cornell University wisely says, "No product can actually lift the skin—only plastic surgery can do that," when applied topically, caffeine can tighten the skin for several hours. We would also suggest you remember some other effects of caffeine: it is dehydrating. So if dehydration is implicated more generally in skin aging, it is worth asking whether employing a notoriously dehydrating chemical in the service of preventing skin aging is perhaps doing as much harm in the long term as it is good.

HT and Skin: More Questions than Answers

The Daily Show, Comedy Central's wildly popular "fake news" program, did a segment in 2005 that featured a beautiful sixty-year-old woman who claimed the secret of her preternaturally preserved looks was to generously apply vaginal Premarin cream to her face. The commentator made merciless fun of the notion that "vagina cream" could make you young. The woman was so stunning, however, that we began to worry that women were taking notes.

Estrogen has long been rumored to revitalize and preserve skin. In pill, cream, or patch form, ET and HT have long been looked to with almost mystical hope to prevent wrinkles and preserve skin tone. This is not a notion that has disappeared in light of the WHI findings. A review in the *American Journal of Clinical Dermatology* in 2001 argued that estrogen provided a variety of benefits for the skin;[18] it could prevent a decrease in skin collagen that seemed to happen after menopause and provide additional moisture by increasing natural acids. Finally, the authors claimed, it was possible that estrogen would speed in wound healing. An article published in 2002 in *Experimental Dermatology* was less assured. It said that although the presence of estrogen receptors in skin had long made it clear that there is a significant relationship between estrogen and skin, "studies on estrogen action in skin have been limited."[19] It seems it is possible that skin collagen rates decline slightly more sharply around and right after menopause.[20] Indeed, we have found in recent years that women who undergo oophorectomy suffer accelerated skin aging.[21] This again would seem to affirm the role of estrogen decline in looking older. What this *doesn't* mean is that taking estrogen—or unsafely using vaginal cream incorrectly on the face—will counteract menopausal skin changes.

But be careful: many articles assume something we don't think is really true—that women "appear to be at a greater risk of developing wrinkles with age than men."[22] While our culture has a lot more baggage for aging women to carry when compared with aging men, we don't really think the extra weight is on the face. It is worth remembering that men, who don't have to worry about their estrogen levels plummeting, worry plenty about their skin aging.

Something else worth thinking about is that it is very difficult to map wrinkles scientifically; they can't be weighed or measured. And sometimes study methods are a little suspect. One study offered as evidence of the role of lowered estrogen in wrinkling the fact that women ten years after menopause had more wrinkles than women five years after menopause. Well, almost everyone has more wrinkles after a longer period of time.

Indeed, at the height of estrogen fever in the mid-1990s, even otherwise pro-ET doctors cautioned that antiwrinkling properties were not alone a "sufficient reason to take" the drug, [23] and others put estrogen's skin-preserving abilities on par with, not ahead of, topical treatments such as tretinoin and alpha hydroxy acids.[24]

Bottom line: although we think there is enough evidence of an important relationship between estrogen and skin to warrant significant further research, there is too much that we *don't* know. Remember, making a choice to use HT or ET is not like putting tea extract lotion on your face. It is a serious drug with health repercussions in both the long and the short term, a known carcinogen. We would seriously warn you against believing that uneven evidence about its skin benefits is any sort of reason to enter into long-term usage of such a powerful and possibly dangerous chemical.

The First Cut Is the Deepest: Medical Treatments for Aging Skin

So what about more aggressive actions to improve the skin? Well, as no-nonsense women, we don't really like the idea ourselves, but if you're thinking about pursuing surgical or less drastic cosmetic options, we want you know about the safety risks involved in different choices.

Remember that with all of these treatments, we are talking about cosmetic choices, not health choices. None of these procedures are performed because they make you a healthier person. They are done because they make you look different. In fact they are often undertaken even though they can hurt your health and subject you to unnecessary dangers.

Injectable substances such as collagen are extracted from cow tissue or even from human cadavers and are injected under the skin around the eyes or lips to plump wrinkles and give the targeted areas more fullness. This procedure lasts somewhere between three and twelve months[25] and can cause swelling and allergic reaction. If you get cold sores, this procedure can cause outbreaks. Because many of these products are derived from animal tissue, they carry the risk of spreading disease.

Hyaluronic acid fillers such as Restylane and Juvéderm provide a nonanimal alternative but carry the same risks of allergic reaction, redness, and swelling. They last for between six months and a year. If you are prone to allergies or have a history of anaphylaxis, you shouldn't even consider this kind of procedure.

Another popular and heavily advertised treatment is Botox, which is the commercial name for a weak form of the bacteria that causes botulism. It works to eliminate some wrinkles by simply freezing the muscles in the forehead or around the eyes. Botox makes furrowing or scrunching impossible. We were shocked to see a segment on a local news station discussing Botox parties, increasingly popular for thirtieth birthdays.

This procedure doesn't last very long—about three to six months—and can cause headaches, bruising, burning at the injection sight, and nausea. It seems strange to us to spend days with bruises to reap benefits that will last only months, let alone incur the other potential side effects. Because this is a relatively new procedure, we don't know much about its long-term health implications.

Another injection option involves taking fat from other parts of the body—the legs or buttocks, for example—and injecting it into the chin, forehead, and other facial creases. This procedure lasts a lot longer than Botox or collagen, possibly one to three years, but requires more injections because the body slowly absorbs the fat.[26] A sort of comical side effect of this procedure is that our old friend the fat cell likes to lump up. You know how bumpy and uneven your butt can look? Well, the fat can do the same thing in your face.

Chemical peels, dermabrasion, and microdermabrasion are all popular procedures and are increasingly available not just in doctor's offices but at beauty salons and spas. A *chemical peel* uses various chemicals and acids to remove layers of skin, revealing newer, smoother skin underneath. Strong peels should be performed only by a doctor and should be considered a medical procedure. Even a mild peel can have side effects such as persistent redness, blisters, swelling, even infection and scarring. Chemical peels can permanently change the color of your skin and lead to brown spots on the face, particularly if you use birth control pills or HT. One popular cosmetics line recently created an entire group of products designed to help the skin recover from the effects of these procedures.

Dermabrasion uses a spinning device with an abrasive surface similar to sandpaper to grind away layers of dead skin.[27] The difference between dermabrasion and microdermabrasion is similar to the difference between a nail file and a nail buffer. While the latter produces a more polished result, it may take multiple treatments to achieve it. Dermabrasion can be serious business: it can cause swelling, infection, scarring, and excessive bleeding. We would suggest that incurring scarring for something so temporary isn't a good plan. *Microdermabrasion* seems to be much milder in its side effects.

Laser resurfacing and photorejuvenation both involve using light beams and lasers to stimulate collagen production and remove dead skin. As with dermabrasion, *laser resurfacing* is a more serious procedure and is used for the treatment of deeper wrinkles. For every action there is an equal reaction, and in this case, that means more serious side effects including scarring, swelling, sensitivity to makeup, and skin redness that can last a long time, perhaps up to six months. *Photorejuvenation* is a newer procedure, and there is much that isn't yet known about it. Side effects may include blistering, abnormal skin coloring, and redness.

Plastic surgery is a hot-button issue in our culture. The authors of this book really don't want to get involved in it and would really discourage you from pursuing this option, but again, we know that some of you will.

The two most frequent procedures for the face are face-lift and forehead lift. *Face-lift* involves lifting the loose neck and face skin by removing fat and tightening face muscles. It is meant to target the entire face and will last between five and ten years. There will be bruising and swelling following the procedure, and possible bleeding and scarring as well. A *forehead lift* is similar, removing excess skin to tighten the brow. With both of these procedures, you should be aware that there can be nerve damage and loss of motion in the face.[28]

While there are enough cosmetic procedures and products to fill several books, we want to urge you to nourish the body you have and help it grow beautiful as it ages, rather than trying to pinch, beat, force, and discipline it to become something it once was and never will be again. If you think an attractive body is synonymous with a young body, you will never understand or appreciate your body as it is today and as it will be in the future.

The Red and the Brown of It: Some Common Skin Problems

On a less cosmetic note, as you get older and your skin thins and becomes more fragile, you are much more likely to injure it, and those wounds will be slower to heal. Also, the blood vessels right under your skin become more delicate, which means you may bruise much more easily.

There may be a nutritional component to this, and chronic illnesses like diabetes, liver disease, heart disease, and blood vessel problems can all play a role. So can stress, which most of us tend to wear on our faces regardless of how old we are (or aren't).

Making sure you get enough water is particularly important as you get older. The skin craves moisture, and given the more sensitive nature of aging skin, letting it get low on hydration increases the chances of injury.

Chloasma is a skin problem characterized by light brown spots and blotches on the face. It can show up if you use birth control pills or during the hormonal ups and downs of pregnancy and childbirth. It can also happen early in menopause, although on the whole it is most common in women between the ages of twenty and forty.[29] If you start having this problem, make sure to stay out of the sun, use a good sunscreen every day, and think about getting off hormonal birth control if you are on it. Same goes for HT. Oddly, some facial care products can also exacerbate it. We know this because men generally don't get the problem, but those who use a lot of toiletries sometimes do. This is probably because the chemicals in the products interact with the sun.

Rosacea

Many people now know that comedian W. C. Field's famously red, bulbous nose was not the result of drinking, as was long thought, but rather a chronic skin condition called rosacea. Approximately 14 million Americans experience this disease, made visible by redness in the face, particularly around the nose, pimples or bumps on the face, watery, irritated eyes, and thickened skin.

The most common sufferers of this condition are adults between the ages of thirty and sixty. The good news is that Field's nose—a particular and advanced manifestation of the disease called rhino-phyma—is extremely uncommon in women. The bad news is that significantly larger numbers of women have rosacea, and it seems particularly pronounced around menopause.[30]

Unfortunately there is still no particularly good solution to their problem. While we know the condition seems to get perceptibly worse around menopause, the relationship to hormones is ill understood. In fact, no one knows what actually causes it. While anyone can get it, the disease seems to occur more frequently in fair-skinned people who flush or blush easily. The National Institute of Arthritis and Musculoskeletal and Skin Diseases provides this relatively unhelpful explanation: "Doctors do not know the exact cause of rosacea but believe that some people may inherit a tendency to develop the disorder. . . . Some researchers believe that rosacea is a disorder where blood vessels dilate too easily resulting in flushing and redness."[31] Rather confusingly, the National Institutes of Health (NIH) tells us that "researchers have not established a link between rosacea and bacteria,"[32] but the primary treatment method for the condition involves the use of topical or systemic antibiotics. In earlier stages, rosacea is most frequently treated with topical drugs such as metronidazole applied right to the affected areas of the skin. In later stages, or if the eyes are involved, oral drugs may be used, including tetracycline, minocycline, erythromycin, and doxycycline.

It should be emphasized that these treatments are designed to lessen the symptoms of the condition; there is no cure. The bumps, pimples, and pustules will probably respond to treatment, but general redness and flushing may persist unaffected by medication.

Recently, new laser technologies are showing great success in treating rosacea. The same procedures are being used to combat precancerous skin cells.

What might cause flare-ups of rosacea for one person might not affect another at all; keeping a diary of your experiences can help you identify your personal triggers.

If your eyes are affected, you may need to take more aggressive action. While the first line of treatment will probably be oral antibiotics, your doctor may also prescribe a regimen of eyelid-scrubbing with a mild cleanser, applying warm compresses to the eyes several times a day, and perhaps steroid eyedrops.[33]

Some simple things you should be sure to do if you have this condition include wearing sunscreen of 15 SPF or higher each day, since sunlight is a major trigger for a lot of folks. Also using a mild moisturizer can be a good idea, but make sure it is fragrance- and

Types of Rosacea

TYPE OF ROSACEA	CHARACTERISTICS
Papulopustular rosacea	Includes redness, bumps, pimples, pustules or "plaques," raised red patches.
Erythematotelangiectatic rosacea	Involves flushing, redness, and possible visible blood vessels.[34]
Phymatous rosacea	Skin thickening, possible rhinophyma or enlarging and swelling of the nose.
Ocular rosacea	Swelling and redness in the eyes, dry eyes, tearing, potential vision loss or corneal damage.[35]

irritant-free. The same thing goes for makeup if you decide to wear it; make sure it doesn't have too many perfumes or chemicals that could add to inflammation.

Formication

A skin problem that has nothing to do with appearance is a disorder called *formication*. This happens when nerve endings in the skin deteriorate. The result is itchiness and the sensation that bugs are crawling on your skin. Actually, that's where the name comes from: *formica* means "ant" in Latin. In a study of five thousand women, one in five suffered from formication within twelve to twenty-four months after their last menstrual period. About one in twelve women continue to suffer from formication for more than twelve years after menopause.

Hair

We all expect to get gray hair. This happens because pigment in hair follicles (melanin) decreases with age. Beth is a schoolteacher who lives just outside New York City. Slowly over the last decade, gray hairs have begun to weave through her thick, mahogany-colored hair. When her son was getting married in the summer of 2006, friends pressured her to dye her locks. "I thought about it, but in the end I decided I like the way it looks," she explains. "It's distinctive. And besides, I hear that gray is the new blond." We think this kind of outlook is fantastic—when women start to redefine beauty, culture will follow close behind. For too long we've been trying to do things the other way around.

One thing women *don't* expect is to lose their hair, but some of us do experience thinning as we get older. It's estimated that around 30 million women in America experience some kind of hair thinning.[36] If you take a look at your hairbrush, you know that you lose hair every day—potentially 100 to 150 strands a day.[37] At any given moment you have about 100,000 to 150,000 hairs on your head in various states of regrowth. Hair has an active phase, when it grows at a rate of about half an inch a month, and a resting phase. Generally, individual hairs alternate between the two for about five years before falling out.

There are two major types of hair: *vellus hair* is the fine fuzz that covers your arms and torso; *terminal hair* is the kind we have on our heads, over our eyes, under our armpits, and in our pubic areas (most women also have some terminal hair on their arms and legs).

The main difference between male and female hair loss is that in women, hair follicles are rarely damaged, which means when the cause of the hair loss is addressed, hair can often regrow. Women also tend to lose hair all over the scalp, which makes it less noticeable than in men, who will have uniform recession or a patch in the back.

The most common type of female hair loss is *androgenetic alopecia* (*alopecia* is the medical term for hair loss). It is caused by an excess of male hormones and is often accompanied by facial breakouts and an increase in facial hair. This kind of hair loss happens when hair's growth cycle gets shorter and shorter and the hairs don't have a chance to grow very long before they fall out. The easiest treatment for this problem is topical Rogaine, but unfortunately this drug must be continually taken to keep seeing results, and (like any drug) it comes with side effects. During the menopause transition, your levels of testosterone may be significantly higher in proportion to your levels of estrogen than they were when you were premenopausal. That could lead to this kind of hair loss.

Telogen shedding (hair lost during the resting phase) happens when hormones shift dramatically; when it happens, you lose a lot of hair in a short time. This kind of hair loss wouldn't be a big surprise during the ups and downs of perimenopause. This is also the kind of hair loss that happens when you are malnourished or sick. Most hairs lost this way will grow back after whatever imbalance caused it is resolved. For menopausal women, this means that once your hormones settle down, hair should grow back.

If you find your hair falling out in patches or clumps, you may be suffering from an as-yet-unexplained condition called *alopecia areata*. When this happens, small patches of hair will completely fall out in the course of a short period of time, such as a single day. This problem tends to recur, and sometimes those patches of hair won't grow back. This leads some doctors to theorize that this condition is caused by an autoimmune problem in which your body accidentally attacks the roots of your hair.

When hair follicles are damaged, hair will not grow back. This can happen as the result of an illness such as lupus, because of a bacterial infection, or because of physical damage to the scalp from something like a burn. This means you need to be careful not to hold your blow-dryer too close to your head—this could actually burn the scalp.[38] Also, make sure to cover your hair when you go to the beach, and generally protect it from sun damage. Be careful not to pull your hair too harshly or brush it too hard. Be gentle on your follicles and be careful about what chemicals—hair dye and permanents included—you put on your head. Washing hair regularly will help limit bacteria.

Your diet can play a role in this problem, especially if you're not getting enough protein or iron. Finally, stress can take a toll on your scalp.

If you are losing hair, you may want to consult a dermatologist to see what sort of treatment options might be available. Your doctor will be able to rule out an underlying problem, such as a thyroid disorder, that could be causing your locks to languish. Keep in mind that there are more than 290 medications that can cause thinning hair; tell your doctor what drugs you are taking, so she can rule out this possibility.

As you get older, hair on the body and face may naturally thin, but the ones that stay may be thicker.

"I know this sounds silly." Joya is looking down at her hands as she and Barbara share lunch. "But something that really bothers me are all the little hairs on my face that didn't used to be there. And on my neck, too." Joya is in her early fifties with dark curls and striking brown eyes. "I feel like I could spend my life plucking and bleaching."

While some of what Joya is experiencing might be the result of too much testosterone, it could also just have to do with genetics. Much of how your hair will grow—or not grow—has to do with your heritage.

Nails

If your face is a map of the life you have lived, your nails are an indication of your health at this moment. Because of this, identifying certain problems of the nail can be a red flag for potentially serious health problems.

Your nails are made up of dead tissue, which is why you can cut them and not feel pain. The areas under the cuticle and the nail are alive. There are normal changes in the nails that happen with age. They can grow more slowly and become a little more thick and brittle. You may be more likely to have uncomfortable problems like ingrown toenails and fingernails that split.

If you love getting manicures and pedicures, be careful that your salon uses sterile equipment. Fungus and bacteria can be passed on the equipment used to do nails, so you need to be cautious and aware. Be assertive with nail technicians; tell them to push back the cuticle, not to cut it.

Fungal infections are the most common nail problem, accounting for up to 50 percent of all problems.[39] It happens usually when a white, black, green, or yellow fungus builds up under or at the base of the nail. Often called *onycholysis* or *tinea unguium*, this problem can be characterized by nails that become loose and may actually separate from the nail bed. Detaching nails can indicate a number of problems, including thyroid disorders, drug reactions, and psoriasis.[40]

Psoriasis is an extremely common nail (and skin) problem that can show itself in a number of different ways, including small depressions called *pitting* and discoloration. It is caused by problems with the immune system and it can be treated if addressed early.

Significant nail discoloration can be a sign of bigger health problems. Yellow or green nails can indicate lung problems and chronic bronchitis. Clubbing happens when your fingertips get bigger and your nails start to grow around them. This problem is often caused by a lack of oxygen in the blood.

If you see a black streak under the nail, it could be a bruise or an injury, but it might be something much more serious. *Subungal melanoma* is a type of cancer that is much more common in nonwhite patients.[41] If you see a nail streak that doesn't seem to go away, ask your doctor about it.

Voice

Strange as it seems, changing hormone levels can affect the voice. As estrogen and progesterone decrease, testosterone levels stay a little higher, and the result of suddenly having more testosterone can be that the voice gets lower—just like in men.

Be careful though! If your voice starts dramatically changing, it can be a sign of other things, such as a thyroid problem. See your doctor if you are experiencing other changes in the body such as weight gain or tiredness.

Part of the menopause transition involves reconsidering your identity and doing some serious thinking about who you have been in the first half of your life and who you want to become in the second. Such a moment is a privilege; like adolescence before it, the menopause years are an opportunity to redefine yourself, both mentally and also physically. This includes finding beauty in your changing body and finding ways to reconcile your hopes for the future with the physical vessel that will take you there. You are on a journey from which there is no turning back. We hope you will look to the future with promise, eyes set firmly ahead, rather than constantly turning your head to reflect on what came before.

17

the great pretender
thyroid disease and menopause

You must be careful. People in masks cannot be trusted.

— The Princess Bride

Let's play a game: it's called "Is It Menopause?" We'll give you a series of symptoms, and you can tell us if you think the woman experiencing them is about to go through the transition:

- Erratic periods and bleeding
- Hot flashes
- Mood swings and irritability
- Memory problems
- Skin changes
- Vaginal dryness and libido problems
- Trouble sleeping

This seems like an easy game, doesn't it? Of course it's menopause! Unless it's not. All of the problems mentioned above can be caused by a thyroid that isn't functioning properly.

The thyroid is like a great mimic: it can capture the appearance and manner of other problems so convincingly that even the best doctors may not be able to tell the difference without some very sophisticated tests.

Shortly after turning forty, Rosa was diagnosed by her doctor as being hypothyroid. Several years later, she started to have some erratic bleeding. Rosa didn't know what to think: her mother didn't go through menopause until her later forties. When Rosa returned to her doctor for her bleeding problems, he was at a loss: he told her it could be her thyroid causing the problems, or it could be perimenopause.

A lot of women are in Rosa's position, and many more have undiagnosed thyroid problems. They are struggling with symptoms they think are caused by menopause and aren't receiving treatment for the real source of their problems.

The thyroid gland is a part of your endocrine system, as are your ovaries and the parts of your brain that command them, the hypothalamus and the pituitary gland.

Located at the lower part of your neck and appropriately shaped like a bowtie, the thyroid produces chemicals that help to regulate how quickly or slowly your cells can use the energy from food. The more of the thyroid hormones (thyroxine and thriiodothyronine) that are in the blood, the faster your body will use the energy. Like most parts of the endocrine system, the thyroid is a team player; it depends on other glands to work properly. The pituitary gland makes a hormone called thyrotropin (thyroid-stimulating hormone, or TSH), which signals the thyroid to produce thyroid hormones and helps to control their levels in the blood.

Thyroxine is also called T4, and it is the most plentiful of the total thyroid hormone, comprising about 80 percent. Triiodothyronine is called T3, and it makes up about 20 percent. The *4* and *3* come from the number of iodine atoms in each molecule of hormone. This is the reason that table salt has iodine added: to reduce the chance of iodine deficiency and make sure that your thyroid can produce enough hormones. If it doesn't, the thyroid gland can grow and become a goiter. Although your body has more T4, it's T3 that is actually able to accomplish most of the things that thyroid hormones do in the body. Your thyroid produces small amounts of T3, and your body also converts T4 to T3.

Because of the similarity of thyroid disorder to menopause, it's not a bad idea to ask your doctor to check your thyroid during routine physicals, especially if you are having symptoms like those described at the beginning of this chapter. Generally getting thyroid levels checked every five years is a good idea after age forty, but if you think you are entering perimenopause, that might be a time to double-check.

The two most common thyroid problems occur when the body produces either too much thyroid hormone or not enough. When your body has too much thyroid hormone, either because your gland is making excessive amounts or for some other reason (a common one is taking too much pharmaceutical thyroid hormone), you are *hyperthyroid*. When your body isn't making enough thyroid hormone, you are said to be *hypothyroid*. Both of these conditions have a number of different causes and occur in mild, moderate, and severe forms; each can echo menopause in certain distinctive ways. When you have normal thyroid levels, you are said to be *euthyroid*.

According to the American Association of Clinical Endocrinologists, approximately 27 million Americans are either hyper- or hypothyroid; eight out of ten of these are women.[1] This is a strikingly high number, but there is no way to know why thyroid problems are so ubiquitous in our culture. We are finding more genetic components of the problem all the time. It may also be that our lack of consistent standards combined with sensitive measurement tests are leading to overdiagnosis and treatment. Or maybe it's a more complicated set of endocrine issues involving the interaction of other hormones. Only time will tell.

Moving in Slow Motion: Hypothyroidism

Hypothyroidism is a fairly common health problem, especially in older women. It's possible that as much as 10 percent of the population suffers from it, and the number might be as high as 25 percent in people over sixty.[2] Hypothyroidism is characterized by a general slowdown in the body; you feel tired, your digestive system doesn't work as well, you gain weight and lose interest in sex. Your memory may decline, your injuries take longer to heal, your pulse actually slows down, and your reflexes can become unresponsive.

Primary hypothyroidism can be caused by disease (a virus or bacterial infection), an autoimmune response, or external factors such as radiation therapy or hyperthyroid treatments. Lithium, a common treatment for bipolar disorder, can also cause certain thyroid problems to show themselves. In addition, several other drugs, including "corticosteroids, dopamine, calcium supplements, some antacids and aspirin can affect the results of thyroid function tests."[3] In 1969, Barbara noted that birth control pills might impact thyroid hormone readings. It is an interesting question if the lower-dose pills used by women today still have this effect, and if so, whether HT and ET preparations might have similar outcomes.

Secondary hypothyroidism usually occurs when a problem with another organ, particularly the pituitary gland, stops the reception of TSH by the thyroid gland.

Mild, or subclinical, hypothyroidism is very common; it occurs when levels of thyroid hormone are lower than the normal range that labs use but high enough that patients may have few or no symptoms. Doctors have started to diagnose patients this way more frequently since more sensitive tests have become available, and this has caused some controversy between those who think subclinical women should be treated and those who think it is unnecessary. A large analysis published in the *Journal of the American Medical Association (JAMA)* in 2004 concluded that "the consequences of subclinical thyroid disease are minimal and we recommend against routine treatment of patients with TSH levels in these ranges."[4] Most medical professionals lament a lack of information and real data on this subject, as well as inconsistent markers for determining who is or isn't hypothyroid. When compiling available data for the *JAMA* study, authors observed "a striking paucity of evidence bearing on the major clinical questions examined."[5]

What happens if you don't treat a subclinical thyroid condition? According to the information we have, not very much. The most common outcome is a progression to a more significant thyroid condition. A more serious concern is heart problems, which have been associated with untreated hypothyroid. While unaddressed subclinical thyroid does seem to be related to more atrial fibrillation, studies have suggested it doesn't cause more cardiovascular disease or heart attack deaths.[6] As with bone density, thyroid levels are variable between individuals, and what is normal for one person may be unhealthy in another. It is more likely, therefore, that doctors are simply seeing a normal thyroid hormone range for that patient, rather than an actual problem in the making. If you decide not to treat subclinical hypothyroidism, be educated about thyroid disease and, along with your doctor, continue to watch for changes that could indicate a worsening condition.

Depression is a major indicator of a hypothyroid condition and can often be confused with either depressive disorder or the mood swings of the menopause transition. The relationship between mood and thyroid isn't clear, but it seems to work both ways: a significant number of depressed people, around 15 percent, develop hypothyroidism.

Another common midlife problem associated with both the thyroid and perimenopause is weight gain. When the basal metabolic rate (BMR—the rate at which we turn food into energy) slows as part of a thyroid problem, packing on pounds is a common result.[7] While menopausal women often complain that they don't have to eat as much to gain weight as they used to, a patient who is hypothyroidic will often literally be eating significantly *less* (appetite loss is another symptom) and still be packing on the pounds.

Muscles and joints can become sore, and coordination is affected; an increase in clumsy behavior may be noted.

Hair loss is a problem of aging that is sometimes wrongly associated with menopause. It does, however, have to do with hormones. Hypothyroidism often causes hair loss and also changes in texture, causing individual strands to thin and become dry. As with most female hair loss, this problem is usually reversed when hormone levels return to normal.

Hypothyroidic women, like their menopausal counterparts, are often excessively tired. The big difference is that women who are hypothyroidic will sleep for long periods and still feel exhausted, while menopause-related tiredness is usually very much the result of a lack of sleep. Hypothyroidic women may be unable to enter slow-wave sleep, which means that even though they are putting in the hours of shut-eye, they aren't seeing the physical benefits.

The memory doesn't work as well as it did for hypothyroidic

women and can even mimic early symptoms of dementia. A big difference between menopausal women and hypothyroidic women is that the latter are usually cold, even in hot weather. Women going through the change, on the other hand, are always stripping off clothes and searching for the nearest air conditioner as though it were the fire exit in a crowded theater.

A final symptom that might seem to be related to menopause but may in fact be thyroid related is heavier, more frequent periods. This is a particularly tricky symptom, because as menopause comes closer, the menstrual cycle shortens noticeably.

Iodine: How Much Is Too Much?

One of the best-known bits of nutritional trivia is that a lack of iodine in the body will result in the swelling of the thyroid gland, causing a goiter. Before the second half of the twentieth century, iodine deficiency was still very common in America and the Western world. The addition of iodine to salt was one of the first large-scale nutritional campaigns in the United States in the 1920s.[8] Although in many parts of the world iodine deficiency is still a major problem, it has been virtually eliminated in North America.

It might seem, then, that more is better when it comes to iodine consumption, but that is not the case. While a lack of the element as a cause of hypothyroid problems has all but disappeared in the United States, cases of hypothyroidism due to autoimmune problems have gone way up. Dr. Kenneth Ain and Dr. M. Sarah Rosenthal write that this may well be because of an excess of iodine, which can stimulate immune responses in the body.[9] For this reason, doctors advise patients against taking kelp, a naturally high source of iodine.

Diagnosing and Treating a Sluggish Thyroid

If you have outward signs of a problem, including a goiter, your doctor will perform blood tests to understand better the particularities of your disorder. A TSH test measures how much thyroid-stimulating hormone is in your body. Checking T4 levels will show how much of those hormones actually got made. By comparing these two measures, doctors can tell which variety of thyroid problem you are suffering from. In the case of hypothyroidism, high TSH levels can be a tip-off. Like a diabetic making too much insulin, the brain of the hypothyroidic person will try to respond to the failure of the gland to answer its messages with an overproduction of TSH. Cross-checking between the TSH and the T4 is important because a low T4 level in combination with a low TSH level might indicate a problem with the pituitary gland and secondary hypothyroidism.

The most common treatment for the problem is taking thyroid hormone supplementation with pharmaceutical T4, which your body converts to T3. There are several popular brands, most notably Synthroid; the chemical taken is levothyroxine sodium. All brands work similarly and about as well as the others; don't be afraid to take generic levothyroxine if it works for you. However, patient reactions to different brands can vary, so don't switch back and forth; make sure your doctor checks the "Fill as Written" box on the prescription slip.

Kenneth Ain and M. Sarah Rosenthal explain that lab standards for what constitute high or low thyroid levels were set based on research in men. There have been recent movements to create standards for women, who would have naturally lower levels than their male counterparts. If your lab uses a standard range of 0.5 to 5.0 for TSH, that is the norm for men; Ain and Rosenthal believe that a more realistic estimate for women would be 0.5 to 2.0.[10] What is so complicated about this is that like all hormone levels, thyroid varies tremendously from individual to individual, and it is difficult to impossible to set a standard of "normal."

Because of this, it is equally difficult to get the doses of thyroid hormone medication right. Prescribe too much, and a person can become hyperthyroidic. Give a patient too little, and their symptoms will persist.

Some evidence shows that thyroid tests can vary widely depending on when they are performed. The Australian doctor Ralph Faggotter writes, "If you measure someone's thyroxine (T4) levels regularly for a while, you will notice that the readings bop around, sometimes quite markedly."[11] This means, among other things, that many of us will have T4 levels that traverse the boundaries of normality and then head back again. The problem, as Faggotter sees it, is that once you start taking T4, it changes your thyroid, and it is hard to discontinue use. For these reasons, we would urge caution. If you have a diagnosis of hypothyroidism, perhaps ask your doctor if she thinks it is safe to wait a few weeks or months before beginning treatment and retest the thyroid before doing so.

Although there are no herbs that have been shown to be effective for treating the thyroid, some women take an older "natural" thyroid hormone made from pig glands called Armour, which contains both T3 and T4. This preparation works, but dosage may be less precise than in synthetic drugs.

If you are a menopausal woman and are taking thyroid hormone, be sure to swallow your daily multivitamin or any other mineral supplements five hours before or after your medication. If you are taking iron for anemia, which menopausal women who are having heavy bleeds often do, the same rule applies. Not putting some space between your thyroid meds and your vitamins can cause the body not to absorb thyroxine properly.

Hashimoto's Disease

One of the most common causes of hypothyroidism is an autoimmune response in which the body's natural defense mechanisms are wrongly triggered to attack the thyroid gland.

No one is sure why this happens: there is most likely a genetic component.[12] Nancy Ross-Flanigan writes that "half the children, parents and siblings of people with thyroid disease are susceptible to it."[13] It may also be the result of environmental factors such as stress, smoking, and infection. Like heart disease, doctors theorize, the immune system activates to fight a real infective agent and then progresses to attack the tissues. This may be because the thyroid tissue resembles the original infective agent or it may be caused by something else.

The most common form of this is called Hashimoto's disease; it was first recognized by a Japanese doctor of that name in 1912. As many as 20 percent of women may eventually develop the problem. If you don't treat Hashimoto's disease, the white blood cells may eventually destroy the thyroid, as well as causing heart problems, depression, and a rare condition called myxedema that can lead to lethargy and coma.

Other autoimmune problems are often seen in combination with thyroiditis, including anemia, diabetes, rheumatoid arthritis, and Addison's disease.[14] If you have any of these problems, it is a good idea to get a thyroid check.

Fatigue is one of the first symptoms of Hashimoto's, along with goiter. In general, any swelling in the lower neck is a good reason to talk to your doctor. Because the problem seems to run in families, check to see if your older female relatives have had it, and make sure your kids know that you do. Your doctor can check for Hashimoto's by looking for antibodies like thyroid peroxidase (TPO) and anti-thyroglobulin (TG) in the blood.

Hyperthyroidism and Thyrotoxicosis

When your body has too much thyroid hormone, you are said to be thyrotoxic. This can be because you are actually making too much thyroid hormone or because of another cause, such as taking excessive amounts of pharmaceutical thyroid hormone.

When you are in this state, you may feel jumpy and you may have a racy, rapid heartbeat. This is because too much thyroid hormone creates more receptors for the chemical adrenaline. While you might think this would be accompanied by high energy levels, in fact women experiencing this feel exhausted and agitated, the way you might after an all-nighter with no sleep. Even though you are tired, you will have trouble sitting still and concentrating on anything for very long will be a challenge.

Thyrotoxic women feel hot all the time, and may even experience hot flashes. Combine this with the racing heartbeat, and you can see how many doctors might assume women with these symptoms are experiencing menopausal symptoms.

Like menopausal women, those with hyperthyroidism can be irritable and have trouble sleeping. This can mimic depression as well as menopause, and a misdiagnosis of either can lead to a lack of proper treatment. Sexual desire can take a dive, and symptoms like breast tenderness echo the hormone chaos of the change. Perhaps the most similar symptom is that periods become light and irregular and fertility is challenged or even lost. Skipping periods is common.

A big difference between the two states is that thyrotoxic women will often lose weight—not usually a problem for those of us in menopause. The association of hyperthyroidism and weight loss led many women to unwisely use thyroid medication off-label as a weight-loss drug for many years (this still occasionally goes on). This is a dangerous course of action that could actually result in real thyroid problems as well as damage to the heart and bones.

If you were hypothyroid, have been taking medication, and start to experience these symptoms, talk to your doctor about the possibility of lowering your dose.

Some women with Hashimoto's disease initially leak thyroid hormone into the body, becoming thyrotoxic. Once the hormone is gone, it can't be replaced, and the patient becomes hypothyroid. If this happens to you, don't start taking T4 until the first stage is over and symptoms of hypothyroidism begin to appear.

To diagnose hyperthyroidism, your doctor will test T4 and T3 levels and TSH levels. It can be hard to treat this problem, and doctors often take extreme measures. If your condition is mild, the doctor may suggest using antithyroid drugs and hope the problem resolves on its own. Some common medications are Propylthiouracil and methimazole. Beta-blockers, a popular class of blood-pressure drugs, may be prescribed to alleviate the racing heartbeat and problems caused by excess adrenaline receptors.[15]

Sometimes patients may opt for either surgery or a treatment called radioactive iodine therapy. In the latter procedure, radioactive iodine is injected into the body and slowly destroys the thyroid. If you take either of these two courses of action, you will need to take thyroid hormone for the rest of your life.

Graves' Disease

Graves' disease is to hyperthyroidism what Hashimoto's disease is to hypothyroidism: a form of the disorder caused by an autoimmune response gone wrong. Unlike Hashimoto's, Graves' disease is rare: only around five of ten thousand people in the United States will be diagnosed with it."[16] In this condition, the body makes a chemical called thyroid-stimulating antibody (TSA) that leads the thyroid to go into overdrive, producing huge amounts of hormones.

Among other things, such as skin problems on the legs and feet, Graves' disease is characterized by an eye condition that causes bulging, itching, watering, and general discomfort behind the eyes. It can also lead to double vision and sensitivity to light. Goiters are another common warning sign.

This problem often becomes evident for the first time when women are consciously dieting and losing weight, particularly if they are trying to drop pounds quickly. Remember that the thyroid produces a hormone that regulates the body's metabolism. Your doctor can test for antibodies in the blood as well as using the TSH, T3, and T4 tests, and should also perform a physical exam, looking particularly for eye bulging and other signs of the eye condition.

Too Darn Hot: Thyroid Nodules

Thyroid nodules are lumps found in the lower neck area. This common problem (as many as half of us may have one at some point in our lives and many never know it) can be discovered as part of a thyroid self-exam or a friend's observation about your appearance, or your doctor may find them during a routine physical. They will have a different texture from the firm, smooth tissue of a healthy thyroid gland.

Because of concerns about cancer, most thyroid nodules will be biopsied. The first step, however, will be for your doctor to decide if the nodule is "hot" or "cold." A "hot" nodule is usually an autonomous toxic nodule (ATN), a growth that makes its own non-pituitary-controlled supply of thyroid hormone. An ATN is one of the few nodules that doesn't need to be biopsied because it isn't associated with thyroid cancer. First your doctor will check to see if your levels of TSH are low: if your thyroid nodule decides to freestyle and overproduce its own hormone, the pituitary will respond by lowering its orders for the chemicals by reducing output of TSH. If your TSH is low, the doctor may perform a test using radioactive iodine. If your nodule is hot, it will use the radioactive iodine. Your doctor will then discuss possible treatment options with you and continue to observe your nodule for the months and years ahead to make sure it doesn't grow or change. If the nodule doesn't use the iodine, it is pronounced cold, and biopsy may be required before you and your doctor can decide how to proceed.

Thyroid Cancer

Thyroid cancer is extremely rare, accounting for as few as 2 percent of the total cancers in the United States. The other good news is that it is usually a very treatable cancer. It is often discovered as part of an exam for a thyroid nodule or a lump in the neck area.[17]

Recent demographic information shows a sharp increase in thyroid cancer in the past three decades. While this may be the result of an actual increase in the disease, it is more likely because screening methods that allow early detection have improved.[18]

Self-Help Thyroid Care

According to Drs. Kenneth Ain and M. Sara Rosenthal, you can perform a thyroid self-examination at least once a year to check for lumps or nodules.

Just as men and women are different when it comes to thyroid problems, so the elderly may require different treatment criteria. One study published in *JAMA* suggests that older adults with hyperthyroidism may actually have longer life spans.[19] Like so many issues involving the elderly, we just don't have enough clinical evidence to truly understand their unique concerns.

If you are beginning to have symptoms you believe are those of perimenopause, ask your doctor to check your thyroid gland. A 2001 poll conducted by the American Autoimmune Related Diseases Association found that of five hundred women with "serious autoimmune diseases," all had visited approximately four doctors in four years without a proper diagnosis of their problem.[20] Forty-five percent of the women surveyed had been accused of hypochondria and had their health concerns dismissed.

The need for thyroid screening is an even better idea if problems

how to do a thyroid self-exam [21]

1. Sit looking into a mirror and hold your chin out. Put your right hand on the middle of your neck, and gradually work your fingers down your neck until you hit your breastbone. Feel the rings of your esophagus and stop when you get to one where there is a soft, fleshy bit on top of a ring. That is the middle of your thyroid.
2. Move your fingers gradually to the left of the middle. This will allow you to feel your left thyroid lobe. If it is enlarged, it will extend toward the upper-left side of your neck.
3. With your fingers on the left lobe, swallow. The tissue should feel smooth and firm. Any nodules or lumps are good reasons to call your doctor.
4. Repeat this process but move to the right in step two.

run in your family, but we would recommend it to everyone approaching menopause. If thyroid conditions go untreated, they can hurt your heart and lead to other serious health problems. We have real concerns about overtreatment, particularly in women who have subclinical thyroid hormone levels, and hope that if serious interventions such as radioactive iodine therapy are undertaken, they are truly necessary. However, you might also end up taking drugs unnecessarily to treat menopause symptoms and not receive the care you need. Know what sort of health problem you are dealing with and you will make better decisions throughout your menopause and your life.

18

taking heart
menopause and heart disease

Sweet Skepticism of the Heart—
That knows—and does not know—
And tosses like a Fleet of Balm—
Affronted by the snow.
—Emily Dickinson

You would have to be completely hidden from medical information on television, on the Internet, or in print in the past few years not to have heard the news: contrary to popular perception, heart disease is the number one killer of women in the United States, not cancer, as many people think. According the U.S. Department of Health and Human Services, "Almost twice as many women die from cardiovascular diseases than from all forms of cancer combined."[1] Although men have more heart attacks and strokes, women are more likely to die when they do have them.

This message is getting out: "red dress" events are becoming almost as common as pink breast cancer ribbons, and celebrity campaigns have helped to raise awareness about how common heart problems are among women.

Preserving heart health is one of the major reasons many started taking and stayed on estrogen before the Women's Health Initiative (WHI) results reversed long-held beliefs that taking hormone therapy (HT) was good for your ticker. Since then, many midlife and older women have turned to a powerful new class of cholesterol-lowering drugs called statins, now the best-selling class of drug in the United States. Although these pills are revolutionary and have the potential to save many lives, they are also understudied, particularly in female populations.

How did heart disease become intertwined with menopausal health? And since the WHI, what can women do to create their best odds of preserving heart health into old age?

Menopause and the Heart

One of the reasons we think of heart attacks as a men's issue is because women don't start having them until they are considerably older than the typical age for risk of heart attacks in men. While men's chances of heart attack and stroke increase dramatically after age fifty-five, women won't catch up with them until after age sixty-five.[2] For a long time, doctors have theorized that this is because the extra estrogen women have throughout their lives keeps their hearts stronger and younger. Even so, it is estimated that 20,000 women in the United States under sixty-five die of coronary problems each year.

No matter when a woman has a heart attack, she is more likely to die from it than her male counterparts, according to the Centers for Disease Control and Prevention (CDC).[3] While deaths from heart disease have gone down across the country, female deaths have remained constant or even gone up.

Historically women have faced a lot of bias in heart medicine. The vast majority of trials were performed on men; heart drugs were tested in either exclusively or predominantly male populations; doctors failed to identify crucial warning signs, which are different in women, and make potentially lifesaving referrals for treatment less likely. Older adults were similarly understudied. This has been changing slowly, but research still has a long way to go.[4]

Dr. Sharonne Hayes of the Mayo Clinic writes, "The danger is that if you have no hard evidence for women, you may undertreat or overtreat them, or simply not understand their unique risks."[5] Case in point: a study published in the journal *Circulation* in 2005 found that doctors were more likely to identify female patients as having low or moderate risk of heart problems and fail to make crucial recommendations about diet and lifestyle changes.[6]

If women do have and are lucky enough to survive heart attacks, they are less likely than men to be put in rehabilitation programs. In one study a whopping 68 percent of male patients went through rehabilitation, compared with a paltry 38 percent of women.[7] Exclusions like this are probably part of the reason that not only are female patients more likely to die of a heart attack in the first place, they are much more likely to die in the months immediately following one.

One new theory about women and the heart comes from the results of a federally funded trial called the Women's Ischemia Syndrome Evaluation (WISE).[8] Researchers have theorized a different kind of heart disease that they are calling "coronary microvascular dysfunction," or "CMD"; women with CMD have arteries and smaller channels feeding the heart with blood that fail to dilate normally. Although CMD patients may have chest pains like those suffering from more documented forms of cardiovascular disease, they don't have blocked arteries and other risk factors for predicting coronary artery disease (CAD). This theory helps explain why women have such different (and often milder) symptoms from men before a heart attack and why cardiac events can be so much tougher to anticipate.

Heart Diseases

As you may remember from middle-school biology, the heart is a fist-sized muscular pump that sends blood carrying oxygen and nutrients around the body. The veins and arteries, which carry the blood, are like pipes that over the years can become blocked. This happens very slowly, like one hair catching in a shower drain at a time, with cholesterol, fat, and other cells gradually piling on each other until the passages become too narrow for blood to pass through, and a heart attack happens.

Heart disease and cardiovascular disease are different conditions. While they are both problems of the heart and the blood vessel system, heart disease refers only to problems within the heart rather than problems with the heart and blood vessels.[9] It is important to make distinctions between the different types of heart disease and cardiovascular disease because it may make a difference in determining what problems you are at a higher risk for or which are treatable in certain ways.

Cholesterol

Cholesterol is a waxy, fatlike substance found in all parts of the body. Your liver makes most of the cholesterol your body needs; the rest comes from food. Cholesterol helps to form cell membranes, some hormones, and vitamin D.

Because cholesterol is a fat, it doesn't dissolve in the blood; it must be carried through the body by something called a lipoprotein, a biochemical that contains both proteins and fats. Low-density lipoprotein (LDL) and high-density lipoprotein (HDL) are the two types of lipoprotein that function in the blood. LDL has a higher amount of fat than protein. As a result, it is a much less efficient carrier of cholesterol and is more likely to allow sticking and clotting. For this reason it is sometimes called "bad" cholesterol. HDL has an equal amount of fat and protein and is good at carrying cholesterol away from the arteries and dropping it in the liver, where it is reprocessed. This is why HDL is often called "good" cholesterol.

There is a lot of debate about what constitutes "high" cholesterol. The American Heart Association defines total cholesterol levels under 200 in which the HDL cholesterol is above 40 as "optimum." Other risk factors for heart and cardiovascular disease make a difference; for example, if you have no other risk factors (no high blood pressure, for example) then a level of 230 or lower is considered near optimal. If you do have risk factors, levels around 230 begin to be seen as high. Levels above 240 are considered dangerous, raising your risk of heart attack and serious illness.

Some doctors disagree with this system of evaluation, claiming that it is more important to have a correct ratio of HDL to LDL than to have numbers that fit into specific parameters. But most argue that cholesterol has to be kept below certain thresholds. Like so many areas of science we have talked about in this book, researchers are still trying to understand exactly how cholesterol works.

We've been groomed in the past two decades to view cholesterol as "bad." The truth is probably much more complicated. Harriet

Rosenberg and Danielle Allard write, "Cholesterol has come to represent a virtual disease state itself rather than one risk factor among many and has distracted from grappling with other risk factors which are strong indicators of cardiovascular disease and cardiovascular risk."[10]

For example, it seems that for older people—people in their seventies, eighties, and above—somewhat higher cholesterol may be a good thing. A study of older Italian women found that those with higher cholesterol levels lived longer. It seems only fair to mention that these women were probably eating what we have come to think of as a traditional Mediterranean diet. Still, the idea that cholesterol might play different roles at different moments in our lives is intriguing and food for thought in an era that assumes lowering cholesterol at all costs is desirable.

On the flip side, data from the Framingham Heart Study suggest that up to 35 percent of heart attacks occur in people whose cholesterol is clinically considered optimal, that is, *less than* 200.[11]

Women's cholesterol levels begin to rise when they are in their twenties and make a notable jump when they hit menopause. This upward trend seems to stop in a woman's sixties. So you should expect to see a rise in cholesterol as you are going through the menopause transition; on average "total cholesterol generally rises by about 6 percent, low-density lipoprotein (LDL) cholesterol [so-called bad cholesterol] by 10 percent and triglycerides by 11 percent."[12] Triglycerides are fats that, like LDL cholesterol, are associated with increased risk for heart disease. Levels less than 150 are considered optimal, 151 to 199 borderline, 200 to 400 high, and above 500 dangerously high. Lipoprotein(a)—Lp(a)—is a genetic variation of LDL. High levels are a risk factor for prematurely developing blocks in the arteries. Scientists aren't sure why this happens; one theory is that lesions in the artery walls have chemicals that interact with Lp(a).

Cholesterol guidelines are constantly under revision. In 2001 the National Cholesterol Education Program (NCEP) released new standards that widened the fence around high and moderately high cholesterol. Not surprisingly, many health professionals concluded, based on the new standards, that general adherence to the new recommendations would cause the number of patients taking cholesterol-lowering drugs to explode from 13 million to 65 million in the United States alone.[13] The standards were revised again in 2004. If 2001 built a bigger tent for potential heart disease sufferers, 2004 started a revival movement, advocating the aggressive treatment of people with both high and moderately high risk for heart attack.

Among other things, the NCEP recommends that people have a lipid profile performed every five years. It also advocates pharmaceuticals for prevention.

You can take a drug to treat a current illness (for example, if you have had heart attacks and want to use drugs to manage your cardiovascular disease) or to prevent a future problem. The first course of action is uncontroversial: when people are sick and need medicine, they should take it. The second is more debatable. Prescribing patterns for statin drugs provide a striking example of "pills for prevention," and one that should be of particular interest and concern to midlife women and older adults.

Statins

In recent years, the first line of pharmaceutical defense against dangerous cholesterol have been a class of pills called *statins*. These drugs caused a revolution in cardiovascular medicine and today are some of the most frequently prescribed long-term medications in the world. Some popular brand names include Lipitor (atorvastatin), Zocor (simvastatin), Pravachol (pravastatin), Crestor (rosuvastatin), Mevacor (lovastatin), and Lescol (fluvastatin).

It all began with the work of two Japanese scientists, Akira Endo and Masao Kuroda.[14] In the 1950s and '60s, cholesterol-lowering drugs had been developed that could cause LDL and triglycerides to tumble but unfortunately also caused pretty unpleasant side effects. Drs. Endo and Kuroda began experimenting with molds and microbials that might block the action of HMG-CoA reductase, an enzyme that plays a key role in the making of cholesterol.

After years and six thousand microbes, the scientists found a new compound called ML-236B, which later became known as Mevastatin. In extremely early tests of the drug, mevastatin was administered to a seventeen-year-old girl with exceptionally high cholesterol. Her lipid levels went down, but after two weeks "muscular weakness at the proximal part of the extremities similar to muscular dystrophy was observed."[15] Doses were adjusted and the side effects were curtailed, although not eliminated.

In the late 1970s Merck developed lovastatin, which in 1987 would become the drug Mevacor, and the ball was rolling.

These drugs have undoubtedly worked wonders for many people living with heart disease. Today it is estimated that around 150 million people take these drugs alongside their cornflakes each day, and many doctors love them so much that many rhapsodize about "putting them in the water."

Women and Statins: A Lack of Evidence

Although we believe that statins are important drugs that save many lives, we see that there is a critical lack of evidence regarding their safety and efficacy in women and the elderly.

By 2004, Lipitor was the embodiment of a drug company's grandest hopes: it was making $10 billion a year around the world and it had recently been approved for preventing heart attacks based in part on the ten-thousand-patient ASCOT trial. Taken as a whole, the data were good; there was indeed a general reduction in total heart attacks. Up close, though, things weren't so rosy. Indeed, when you examined the numbers on female patients, those who had never had heart attacks before the study actually experienced 10 percent *more* attacks when compared with the placebo group.

Although there is a dearth of specific information on this class of drugs and female patients (some key trials have completely excluded women, and others have failed to disclose independent results for male and female populations), the science we have suggests that very low cholesterol, already known to be less healthy for older adults, may not be the safest thing for women either. An Austrian study humorously titled "Why Eve Is Not Adam" looked at more than eighty thousand women for fifteen years. They found that not only was high cholesterol not an efficient predictor of cardiovascular problems for women over age fifty (it was for those under fifty), but that having low cholesterol after fifty was correlated with higher death rates from cancer and liver problems.[16] Harriet Rosenberg and Danielle Allard explain that this trial confirms similar findings in "five previous studies (including the Framingham heart study) which found that high cholesterol was not a strong predictor of cardiovascular problems in older women."[17]

A massive meta-analysis of women and statins was performed in 2004 by Judith Walsh and Michael Pignone. Amazingly, they found that out of 1,500 articles published, there were only twenty-one clinical trials on cholesterol-lowering drugs that included women. Of those, a paltry nine studies revealed sex-specific data (the others lumped male and female results together). It turned out that while statin drugs might lower the frequency of cardiovascular events, they didn't lower the death rate from heart attacks.[18]

A ratio that can be helpful in understanding how well a drug works is something called *numbers needed to treat* (NNT). This is the number of healthy women that would need to take a drug without any heart attacks or cardiac events before one heart attack could be prevented. It's basically asking how many healthy people would need to suffer the side effects of a long-term prescription drug before one sick person's health would benefit. In the case of statins, that number is high (not nearly as high as bone drugs like bisphosphonates, as we will see). It is estimated that 140 women would need to pop their pills each day to prevent one coronary event from happening.[19]

Secondary prevention is another matter. It seems that women who have had heart attacks and strokes may see some benefit from the drugs. Some studies have questioned how significant that boon might be: Walsh and Pignone found that in trials that revealed enough data to understand the differences between primary and secondary statin users—that is, between women who have never had heart disease (primary users) and those with existing cardiovascular problems who take the drugs to prevent future events (secondary users)—102 women who were using the drugs died from cardiac events, compared with 103 deaths in the placebo group. Not exactly a compelling statistic. It may turn out that statins provide the same benefit in secondary prevention that they do in primary; that is, fewer "incidents" but roughly the same number of deaths. Still, some women in this group may benefit from the drugs, and the NNTs are much smaller than in primary prevention.

Despite the lack of evidence that these drugs work for primary prevention in women, it is estimated that 75 percent of those taking statins haven't had any cardiovascular incidents.

For older people (men and women alike) the news about statins is worse. Although there have been no randomized trials specifically looking at the drugs in individuals over seventy-five, researchers at the University of California, San Diego (UCSD), note, "Low cholesterol may be a risk factor for heart arrhythmias, which are the leading cause of death if heart attacks occur. And in the elderly, a heart rhythm abnormality called atrial fibrillation that may be increased with low cholesterol is a particularly important risk factor for stroke in the older elderly."[20] In other words, statins don't seem to help—and may hurt—the type of problems more common in older people.

Reading Between the Lines: Statin Side Effects

Beatrice Golomb is a professor at the UCSD Medical School. Along with colleagues at UCSD, Golomb has created one of the best Web sites about the statins and their potential benefits and side effects (http://medicine.ucsd.edu/ses/).

Regardless of what future science will tell us about whether women should or shouldn't be taking statins, the reality is that many do. It is important, then, to know the potential side effects; however, this is easier said than done. In her powerhouse newsletter *Health Facts,* consumer advocate Maryann Napoli quotes Canadian analyst James Wright of the University of British Columbia: "It is crucial," Wright says, "to understand that ten of the major 12 statin trials have not reported their data on harm. These data were collected but have not been published or released to research scholars despite explicit repeated requests to do so."[21] We wouldn't pretend to understand all their reasons, but drugmakers don't think you need to have basic information about bad reactions to their wares. This means we have some idea about what serious adverse reactions are happening (situations where patients needed to be hospitalized or worse) but we just don't have much data on the more common problems (which may be serious even if extremes like hospitalization aren't involved).

One of the most common side effects of statins is problems with liver function; most doctors will monitor a patient's liver health with blood tests on a regular basis, just to be on the safe side.

Frequent but less acknowledged side effects of cholesterol and lipid-lowering drugs are muscle pain and other muscle problems. These range from aches and pains that you might barely notice or might attribute to something else to serious muscle-wasting conditions such as rhabdomyolysis and peripheral neuropathy (muscle problems are often called "myopathy").

In 2000 a popular drug called Baycol was pulled from shelves after thirty-one patients died from rhabdomyolysis, a problem characterized by the breakdown of muscle tissue into the blood. The reason this happened is because along with blocking the stuff that makes cholesterol, the drug stopped other important activities in the cells, including some responsible for muscle maintenance.

While not all statins cause this kind of problem, there are concerns that as new higher-dose varieties are pushed to meet increasingly stiff national guidelines, serious complications may become more common. Greg Critser writes that more recently, "Crestor has come under attack by the same researchers and public-health advocates who blew the whistle on Baycol for causing a similar reaction while providing no better results than existing, proven statins. . . . It is at higher doses of statins that problems are more likely."[22]

In addition to higher doses, taking other cholesterol-lowering drugs in combination with statin therapy makes muscle problems more likely to occur (in particular, fibrates such as TriCor, Lopid, and Atromid-S, which work on triglycerides).[23] Grapefruit and antibiotics can interact poorly with many statins, so if you are taking statins, avoid this fruit, and if you have to take antibiotics, remind your doctor that you are on the drugs.

To check for muscle problems, your doctor can test for creatine kinase (CK), a muscle enzyme. CK levels are often monitored to check for muscle damage. Sometimes patients with normal CK levels have nevertheless sustained statin-related muscle damage,[24] so be aware that even if your doctor has given you a clean bill of health, persisting muscle pain may be a red flag to check back with your health care professional and reconsider your situation.

It seems that when patients discontinue therapy, muscle pain goes away. Muscle wasting, on the other hand, isn't always reversible after discontinuing statin use, although it usually is with time.

Peripheral neuropathy is a rare but serious problem that involves nerve damage and muscle wasting. Its symptoms can be as mild as simple tingling and numbness or they can be far more serious. Long-term statin use makes this problem more likely.[25]

Because of the lack of good data on side effects, it's hard to say how common these problems are, but they are more frequent than drugmakers concede. Many people who aren't hospitalized experience real changes in their lives and what they feel they can do because of muscle aches and pains.

Aside from the more serious problems with muscle wasting, a real concern is that pain and fatigue will compromise people's ability to exercise and maintain a healthy lifestyle. We know that being able to maintain some level of physical fitness is key, in terms of not just the heart but the bones and brain as well. Muscle problems show up more frequently in professional athletes, who have trouble staying on the drugs as a result.[26] This is particularly a concern for women because some studies have suggested they are more likely to suffer this side effect than their male counterparts.[27]

Statins and Memory Problems

One absolutely essential thing that cholesterol does is to help the brain work properly. Beatrice Golomb explains, "Cholesterol is the main organic molecule in the brain and constitutes over half the dry weight of the brain."[28] It makes sense, then, that eliminating large quantities of lipids from your system could affect the way your mind functions.

Complaints of memory loss from patients taking statins are less common than complaints of muscle problems but still far more frequent than much of the available information on statins would suggest. Dr. Matthew Muldoon studied patients taking statins for six months and found that they performed poorly on cognitive tests when compared with the placebo group.[29] Dr. Muldoon concluded, "given the wide use of these drugs, any adverse cognitive effect might be interpreted as important."[30]

The Statin Effects Study describes how this problem appears in patients: "They may have trouble finding the right word, may forget tasks they started to do; and may have trouble following conversations. Some people describe 'holes in their memory.' Some people worry that they are developing Alzheimer's."[31]

There is something of a conundrum in these findings: on the one hand, some middle-aged folks and many seniors already struggle with memory challenges, so to add any pharmaceutically induced ones seems counterproductive. On the other hand, cardiovascular events are a major cause of memory problems and even dementias. Indeed, some studies show a reduction in Alzheimer's and other dementias with use of the drugs. Until more research is done to assess what statin drugs really do to the brain, it is hard to know whether they ultimately provide more benefit or harm.

There is also a chance that statins can encourage depression and mood changes in some patients. One study found an association with use of the drugs and severe irritability.[32]

Coenzyme Q_{10}

Coenzyme Q_{10} (CoQ10) is a substance produced by the body that is needed for cells to work properly.[33] As people age, their bodies naturally have lower levels of this substance, and this can cause problems. It is possible that statins lower CoQ10 levels, and this may be part of the reason side effects persist for some people after they discontinue taking the drugs. Because of this, taking CoQ10 supplements may help side effects abate.[34] Even if you are still taking statins, using supplements may not be a bad idea, although we don't really have enough data on CoQ10 to prove that it actually helps. Long-term safety data about CoQ10 use aren't yet available.

Big Questions about the Big C: Cancer and Statins

Questions about cancer and statin use are particularly relevant for women. Although some studies have dismissed links between the two, other trials (particularly those that differentiate female results) have found an increase in breast cancer among users. The Cholesterol and Recurrent Events (CARE) trial found a statistically significant increase in breast cancer in women whose average age was sixty-one.[35] One result of these findings (the results were published in the late 1990s) was that people with histories of or predispositions to breast cancer were excluded from subsequent trials. If you fall into a high-risk category for breast cancer (if you have had the disease or have a family history of it) you may want to take this into consideration when making a decision about these drugs.

The Prospective Study of Pravastin in the Elderly at Risk (PROSPER), which looked at older people (over seventy), found that using statins seemed to raise your risk for cancer generally and breast cancer specifically.[36] The *British Medical Journal* notes, "If statin treatment is carcinogenic, it should be seen first in people at high risk such as smokers and old people."[37] The result of the increase in cancer seen in the PROSPER trial is that it basically counterbalanced the benefits of reduced heart attacks.

Cancer takes a long time to show up as the result of drug therapy gone wrong; it can take years to develop, and proving a conclusive connection to a given drug is difficult. Because of the dearth of long-term trials, and in particular long-term studies of women and statins, it is hard to know the truth about this connection. There are some data suggesting the link between the two is tenuous, and others that offer enough support for this theory to make us nervous. We probably won't know the truth for some years to come.

High-Dose versus Low-Dose Statins: What Does the Evidence Say?

Americans tend to like extremes: we want our meals supersized and our cars to be the biggest on the block. We want the thinnest bodies and the least amount of downtime. This kind of all-or-nothing attitude permeates the way we think of health too. A powerful example of this ethos in action has been the recent debate about high-dose statins like Crestor and higher-dose Lipitor. The argument for such drugs goes like this: cholesterol is bad, therefore low cholesterol is good, and the lowest possible cholesterol is best. Since the release of the 2004 cholesterol-guideline revisions by the NCEP, this theory has increasingly become a drumbeat urging doctors to get as many patients as they can onto the highest possible dose.

The problem with this way of thinking is that it ignores the fact that side effects, rare in low-dose statin therapy, become increasingly common when you up the ante. Also, to date, high-dose pills haven't been shown to provide significant benefits over lower-dose ones. As Jay Cohen, an associate professor of family and preventive medicine at the University of California, San Diego, puts it, "Seventy-five to 80 percent of all side effects are dose-related. . . . When you double the dose, not only do you see an increase in muscle pain and memory problems and abdominal problems, but also liver toxicity doubles."[38]

In March 2005, Pfizer released the results of a study called (without any irony) "Treating New Targets." Of the one hundred thousand patients studied, those on higher-dose Lipitor had fewer cardiac events and strokes. They also had a lot more side effects and no fewer deaths. It also seems that the higher the dose, the longer a patient takes to recover from problems after discontinuing drug use.

If you are having an adverse effect, don't suffer in silence—let your doctor know. Contrary to popular mythology, you can go off a statin, although, as with many powerful drugs, you should seek guidance to do so. If you aren't sure whether your symptoms are caused by your pills or some other problem, you can try stopping the drug for a period of time or reducing your dose under your doctor's supervision. Then try taking it again. If the side effect resumes, you will know with some certainty that the drug is the cause.

Because your doctor may or may not know about some of the problems associated with these drugs, check out the "Statin Effects Study" Web site at http://medicine.ucsd.edu/ses/ and print out any relevant information; it always pays to go a doctor's visit prepared.

High Blood Pressure

If you are alive, you have blood pressure. This is the force created by your heart beating and moving blood through the arteries. With each beat, blood travels far and wide along its corporal highways, spreading nourishment as it goes. High blood pressure happens when it becomes harder for the heart to move blood along its necessary path. The result is strain on our hearts that can eventually lead to heart attack, stroke, and other very serious problems. Although we're not really sure why many cases of high blood pressure develop, we know that if left untreated, it can have very serious consequences.

Have you ever wondered why guidelines about cholesterol or blood pressure are always changing? There are a lot of reasons, but one of the most disturbing is because of a drug company marketing strategy that the Australian journalist Ray Moynihan calls "selling sickness." One of the surest ways that drug companies have found to build new markets for drugs is to redefine illness standards (such as what constitutes "high blood pressure," for example) to include larger and larger populations of people or to rename health conditions that weren't previously thought of as sickness with medical names.

The debate over blood pressure standards provides examples of both tactics. First, the limits of what is considered normal, healthy blood pressure were made tougher in 2003. While for many years, a systolic pressure under 130 was considered healthy, suddenly 120 could be considered unhealthy.[39] In fact, pressures between 120 and 139 were put into a new category of illness "prehypertension."

This might seem like a simple case of scientists realizing that with a problem as serious as high blood pressure, they hadn't been stringent enough in their guidelines. In its excellent "Selling Sickness" series, the *Seattle Times* reports that the story was actually a little more complicated. The 2003 changes were the result of recommendations from panels in the World Health Organization (WHO) and the National Institutes of Health (NIH), seemingly reputable organizations. As it turns out, a sizable majority of panel members had relationships with pill makers: "Nine of the eleven authors of the [NIH] guidelines had ties to the drug companies."[40] The *Guardian* newspaper in 2003 obtained memos from WHO that admitted "undue influence" from pill makers on guideline panels.

Why would drug companies take measures as extreme as infiltrating government health panels and altering the very definitions of diseases? Because blood pressure drugs alone are a nearly $17-billion-a-year industry in the United States. Like estrogen, blood pressure drugs tend to be long-term medications that patients stay on for years and even decades.

Ray Moynihan and Alan Cassels write that when a massive government study, the Antihypertensive and Lipid-Lowering Treatment to Prevent Heart Attack Trial (ALLHAT), was performed, it was discovered that new blood pressure drugs were less safe and no more effective (and obviously more expensive) than older pharmaceuticals such as diuretics: "The study found that lisinopril and amlodipine . . . were no more effective than water pills in preventing deaths. On the other had, lisinopril was linked to 60 percent higher frequency of strokes. Amlodipine . . . was linked to increased rates of suicide and depression."[41] It is not uncommon to discover after adequate testing has been performed that old drugs are just as good if not better than new ones.

Risky Business: Things That Might Increase or Decrease Your Risk of Heart Problems

With cardiovascular disease, there are a few things you can't change—nonmodifiable risk factors—and a lot that you can—modifiable risk factors.

There is nothing you can do about genetics: if heart problems are sprouting everywhere on your family tree, you can't just pull out a giant eraser. You can't stop the clock and not get any older.

There are many choices you make every day, though, that can have a giant impact on your chances of having heart problems. In fact, the *biggest* risk factors are things that you have control over: smoking, eating too much salt and animal fat, gaining weight, and not exercising.

Blood Pressure Drugs

DRUG TYPE	POPULAR BRAND NAMES	WHAT IT DOES	SIDE EFFECTS
Thiazide diuretics	Diuril (chlorothiazide), Esidrix, Ezide, Hydrocot, HydroDIURIL, Microzide, Oretic (hydrochloro-thiazide), Lozol (indapamide), Aquatensen, Enduron (methyclothia-zide), Mykrox, Zaroxolyn (metolazone)	Often called water pills. Help the body get rid of excess water through the kidneys.	Diuretics can increase blood sugar and uric acid levels. They can cause high levels of sodium, magnesium, and calcium in the blood. You may feel con-fused and weak; rarely, patients can experience abnormal heart rhythms.
Beta-blockers	Tenormin (atenolol), Lopressor, Toprol-XL (metoprolol), Inderal LA (propranolol)	Shown in Stanford Medical School trials to be the best medications for following up with angina patients. Work by lowering blood pressure and helping the heart not to work so hard.	If you take beta-blockers and are exercis-ing, don't overdo it; these drugs slow your heart rate, so your pulse won't rise to target rates. Common side effects include fatigue and insomnia.

Angiotensin converting enzyme (ACE) inhibitors	Vasotec (enalapril), Prinivil, Zestril (lisinopril), Accupril (quinapril), Altace (ramipril)	Help to cut heart attacks by potentially relaxing blood vessels, inhibiting blood clots, and stabilizing plaque deposits.	Side effects can include ankle swelling, cough, headache. The dry cough associated with these pills leads a lot of patients to pursue different drugs.
Angiotension II receptor antagonists	Atacand (candesartan), Teveten (eprosartan), Avapro (irbesartan), Cozaar (losartan), Benicar, Olmetec (olmesartan) Micardis (telmisartan), Diovan (valsartan)	Cause vasodilatation and reduce blood pressure.	Side effects can include headaches, dizziness, liver problems, rash, diarrhea, insomnia, muscle cramping.

(continued)

DRUG TYPE	POPULAR BRAND NAMES	WHAT IT DOES	SIDE EFFECTS
Alpha-blockers	Cardura (doxazosin), Minipress (prazosin), Hytrin (terazosin), Flomaxtra (tamsulosin)	Help muscles relax and small blood vessels remain open, which reduces pressure.	Typically not the first treatment option. You may experience pronounced low blood pressure when starting the drug. Be careful of dizziness or faintness when rising from a reclining or seated position. Side effects can include headaches, pounding heart. According to the ALLHAT trial, may increase the risk of heart failure with long-term use.

| Calcium channel blockers | Norvasc (amlodipine), Plendil (felodipine), Cardene, Cardene SR (nicardipine), Procardia, Adalat (nifedipine), Nimotop (nimodipine), Sular (nisoldipine), Cardif, Nitrepin (nitrendipine), Motens (lacidipine), Zanidip (lercanidipine) | Act on the heart to reduce contraction force. | More expensive than older beta-blockers and believed for a long time to have fewer side effects, but this has recently been shown not to be true. Should be used for angina only when beta-blockers aren't an option. If calcium channel blockers don't work, try long-acting nitrates before resorting to surgery. |

Diabetes, Obesity, and Exercise: Metabolic Syndrome?

In the past few years an ill-defined condition called *metabolic syndrome* has started to make the news. This controversial constellation of symptoms is being hotly debated in the medical community.

In July 2005, the Mayo Clinic estimated that 47 million adults in the United States and 40 percent of those over age sixty might suffer from this problem, also called *syndrome X*, *dysmetabolic syndrome*, and *insulin resistance syndrome*.[42] It was first identified in the late 1980s by a Stanford University endocrinologist named Gerald M. Reavan.[43]

The Mayo Clinic explains, "Metabolic syndrome isn't a disease, but a cluster of disorders of your body's metabolism—including high blood pressure, elevated blood sugar, excess body weight and abnormal lipid levels."[44] If you suffer from metabolic syndrome you are at higher risk for type 2 diabetes, heart attack, and stroke.

Doctors aren't exactly sure why the cluster of symptoms occurs, but they think it has to do with insulin resistance, the same thing that causes type 2 diabetes.

Whether metabolic syndrome actually exists or whether it is an artificially assembled collection of distinct conditions is still undecided. While we believe that scientists may yet find an underlying association between these conditions, any time someone tries to suggest that a near majority of a population has something that could be termed a "disorder," we get suspicious. That sounds to us like marketing rather than scientific evidence.

P. A. Tataranni studied the Pima Indians of Southwestern Arizona, who have high obesity rates but not the associated problems of high blood pressure and cardiovascular disease. Tataranni concludes, "Based on the lack of support from our studies, one could conclude that the metabolic syndrome is an artificial construct and that clinical treatment and prevention strategies based on the 'metabolic syndrome' may prove suboptimal compared with treatment of the individual components."[45]

This said, you do need to address the individual components of the syndrome if you have them, including blood sugar problems, being overweight, and having high blood pressure.

Diabetes

In one San Francisco study, scientists set out to identify what, if anything, might predict heart failure in women. They found diabetes, particularly when it was uncontrolled, to be the most reliable clue that a woman's heart would give up suddenly.[46] Unfortunately, diabetes can eliminate the natural heart attack protection women under sixty-five seem to enjoy and make the chances you will get heart disease equal to a man's. According to the *New England Journal of Medicine*, people with diabetes are more than twice as likely to develop heart disease and 20 percent more likely to die without warning from a heart attack.[47] This risk goes up if you are a woman.[48] If you do survive a heart attack, having type 2 diabetes will make it more likely that you will be disabled. The good news is that, according to the journal *Circulation*, women who manage their blood sugar properly have less heart failure and potentially less overall heart trouble.[49]

Exercise

One of the simplest ways to cut your risks of developing diabetes and hypertension is to exercise. The United States Department of Health and Human Services estimates that "about 60% of American Women do not engage in the recommended amount of physical activity needed to maintain health."[50] *Cardiovascular* exercise is called that because running, biking, or vigorous walking will get your heart pumping. A study from the University of Florida that was published in the *Journal of the American Medical Association (JAMA)* in 2004 found that exercise was more important than weight in terms of the prevalence of heart attack and stroke, but noted that "while it's possible to be both fit and fat, it's healthier to be fit and not fat."[51]

If you've already had a heart attack, you fall into a different category when it comes to exercise, even though it has been shown that some exercise following a heart attack can increase your survival odds. Definitely talk to your doctor about what is safe for you, and don't let anyone pressure you into doing anything that makes you uncomfortable. Especially if you are older, you need to be careful.

Polycystic Ovary Syndrome and Heart Disease

If you are among the estimated 5 to 10 percent of American women who suffer from a condition called *polycystic ovary syndrome*, a disorder characterized by erratic or nonexistent periods, high androgen (testosterone) levels, and small ovarian cysts, you may be at a higher risk for heart disease. Researchers at the University of Pittsburgh compared women with polycystic ovary syndrome to women without and found that women with the problem were at higher risk for narrowed carotid arteries and other cardiovascular problems: 21.6 percent compared with 15.5 percent.[52]

Hearts Aflame: Inflammation and Cardiac Health

About twenty years ago, some scientists first theorized that inflammation—the kind you get when your cut is healing or your throat is sore—plays a role in heart attacks.

It would be one explanation for why women's heart attacks are so different from men's and also why so many people who have heart attacks don't have notably high cholesterol. Men tend to build up plaque in the arteries in chunks, while women are more likely to lay down plaque evenly along the blood vessels. Cholesterol in the artery can act as an irritant: when the body senses the problem, it sends out an alarm to the immune system, which responds by sending white blood cells called *monocytes* to clear out the intruder that is causing trouble. The result is inflammation, part of the way the body tries to heal many different types of injuries.

At first, the body is effective in breaking down the plaque, but as Mount Sinai School of Medicine explains, "Over time—the process can go on for decades—as more and more cholesterol continues to be deposited on the arterial wall, the monocytes become overwhelmed."[53] When this happens, the immune system raises the white flag and deserts the battleground. Two potentially bad things happen: chemicals from the white blood cells can make the plaque more likely to rupture and enter the bloodstream, and these chemicals also make blood more likely to clot. Some doctors believe inflammation can occur in the blood as well, which would account for the lack of plaque as a factor in some heart attacks. Though this model is still considered theoretical, inflammation's role in heart problems increasingly seems to be real.

Doctors have developed several tests for inflammation. The most common, and the one doctors think might tell them the most, is for something called *C-reactive protein* (CRP). High CRP levels are detectable in women with normal cholesterol, so this test can be a good companion to a lipid profile in a physical exam.[54] Although no one is sure if CRP is actually part of the inflammation process or a by-product of it, recently scientists have been leaning toward the former.[55] Regardless of the role it plays, "when the body tissue becomes injured or infected, blood levels of CRP can increase 10,000 times as your immune system jumps into action."[56]

Scientists are exploring the potential of other inflammatory markers, including fibrogen, Lp(a), and homocysteine.

The theory that high homocysteine levels could adversely influence the heart was first proposed in 1969.[57] In 1997, the *New England Journal of Medicine* published a study suggesting again that homocysteine levels had a relationship to heart disease. Like so many things in the body, homocysteine is a naturally occurring protein that in small amounts helps to keep tissue healthy. When you get too much, though, it can turn destructive. In the study, with 587 subjects, those with higher homocysteine levels had a four-and-a-half-fold increase in heart-attack deaths.[58] Since then, this amino acid has come to be considered, along with CRP, to be another, if slightly less reliable, inflammatory marker.[59] Making sure that you get enough vitamin B is one way to control high protein levels. Vitamins B_6 and B_{12} helps to convert excess homocysteine into other aminos.[60] Food sources include green leafy vegetables, beans, liver, grains, and certain meats.

Tests

Your doctor should take a complete medical history and do a physical exam. Did one of your parents die of a heart attack? Other family members? Grandparents? Aunts and uncles? Make sure to tell your doctor.

Besides a lipid profile (cholesterol test) and checking for certain inflammatory markers, your doctor may want to perform additional tests. These tests aren't a starting place for diagnosing heart disease; they are used if your doctor feels there is cause for concern or if more information is needed to make a conclusive diagnosis.

An *electrocardiogram* (EKG) measures electrical activity in the heart by applying small sensors to the skin. Taken either while resting or exercising, this measure helps to understand irregular heartbeats better or to see the potential damage done by a cardiac event. If your doctor has you exercise while performing an EKG, it's probably because she is hoping that certain problems that might play coy while you are resting will make an appearance. Among other things, this test can help your doctor decide how much exercise is safe for you. Unfortunately, women experience more false positives than men (and false negatives), meaning the test is more likely to give an inaccurate result—suggesting, for example, that you've had a heart attack when you haven't.

An *echocardiogram* uses ultrasound to create images of the moving heart. It shows the size and shape of the heart chamber, the activity of the chambers and valves, and how much blood is ejected with each contraction. It's used for diagnosing heart valve disorders and several ventricular and muscular problems with the heart and even to find blood clots and evidence of scarring.

Nuclear imaging involves injecting a short-life radioactive substance into a vein and using computer assisted tomography (CAT) scanning or other technologies to make images. It can reveal blockage in blood vessels, show the extent of heart damage, and even help predict the likelihood of future heart attacks. It may be a more accurate diagnostic approach for women and is usually prescribed for people who can't exercise while being tested because of frailty, arthritis, vascular disease, or other conditions, but also involves more unpleasant side effects.

Coronary angiography (also called *coronary ateriography*) is the gold standard for diagnosing coronary blockages. It provides an X-ray of the blood vessels or the heart chambers. A dye, called a contrast medium, is injected into a selected site. Some recent research suggests that this may be a more accurate way to look at women's hearts, and we hope that more information on this will be forthcoming. This is an invasive procedure and carries with it some fairly serious risks, including triggering a heart attack or an adverse reaction to the dye.

Signs of Heart Attack

Almost everyone is familiar with the classic symptoms of a heart attack: discomfort or uncomfortable pressure in the chest; a feeling of fullness; squeezing or pain in the center of the chest that lasts longer than a few minutes or comes and goes; spreading pain to one or both arms, back, jaw, or stomach. So why are women's heart attacks often misdiagnosed or even ignored by the women who suffer them?

The problem is that women may experience these symptoms differently: the chest pain may be less overt and other signs may be more dramatic. They may be more likely to have shortness of breath, or nausea and vomiting, or feel unexplained pain in the back, shoulders, or jaw. Some 30 percent of heart attack patients experience no chest pain at all, and women are more likely than men to experience this. Kathleen King of the University of Rochester School of Nursing says, "I would discourage trying to give women a list of symptoms that would cause them to sit at home and self-diagnose. Symptoms of heart attack are more unique than most people realize."[61] Dr. Bruce A. MacLeod, chairman of emergency medicine at Mercy Hospital in Pittsburgh, Pennsylvania, says, "To put it bluntly, the Hollywood heart attack is totally misleading."[62]

Still, if you feel pain in your chest, seek attention: "The pain may feel like crushing, squeezing, burning or a fullness in the center of the chest. It may radiate to the neck, one or both arms, the shoulders or jaw. It may go away and return."[63] Keep in mind that this feeling may be more accurately described as discomfort than pain; just because you're not howling in agony doesn't mean it's not serious.

Women often don't seek treatment or delay treatment for heart attacks because they don't realize what is going on. On average, they take an hour longer than men to go to the emergency room and sometimes wait days. Sometimes it is their doctors who don't identify the signs. This is in part because most research and writing about heart attacks is done on or about men. Elizabeth Agnvall explains that for women, heart attacks may not be discovered until later medical tests are performed: "When they go for their yearly physical, the doctor hooks them up to an EKG, takes a look at the result and asks, 'When did you have your heart attack?'"[64] The shocked patient replies that she didn't know she had one, let alone when it might have happened.

When women do manage to get themselves to emergency rooms, gender still seems to make a difference in the quality of treatment. Appallingly, research shows that women wait more than two hours longer than men between arrival in the emergency department and

what to do if you are having a heart attack

1. Call 911. Don't hesitate because you aren't sure, and don't try to drive yourself to the emergency room.
2. Chew one uncoated aspirin.
3. When emergency crews arrive, give them a detailed list of your symptoms: when they started, what has happened, and anything else that might be relevant.
4. The *New England Journal of Medicine* recommends that you ask to be taken to a high-volume hospital: "Data based on 100,000 heart attack victims treated at hospitals across the country show that within 30 days of admission, patients were 15% more likely to survive at a high-volume hospital—that is, a hospital that treats lots of heart attack patients—don't necessarily ask for the closest hospital if you live in an area where the difference between the two isn't significant."[65]
5. Ask to see a cardiologist. According to the *Journal of the American College of Cardiology*, patients who see a cardiologist in the hospital are nearly 20 percent more likely to survive.
6. Most of all, don't let anyone push you around or make you feel your situation isn't important. Too many women have suffered unnecessary problems because they were being polite.

admission to the coronary care unit. So be assertive: if you think you're having a heart attack, tell the ER personnel and insist that you be seen right away.

Signs of Stroke

A stroke happens when there is a problem in the system that gets blood to the brain. When deprived of the nutrients traveling in the blood, the brain cells begin to die within minutes. According to the Mayo Clinic, strokes account for a third of deaths in America and the majority of disabilities.[66] Strokes have the same major risk factors as heart attacks: high cholesterol, high blood pressure, smoking, obesity, and inactivity.

Symptoms of a stroke include sudden numbness in the face, arm, or leg. This is especially true if the lack of sensation happens on one side of the body. You may be disoriented, unable to understand the speech of others, or unable to speak yourself, and may have a severe headache that comes on suddenly accompanied by a stiff neck or pain in the face, vomiting, and dizziness. Other signs include blurred or double vision.

If you think you are having a stroke, call 911. Just as with a heart attack, don't try to drive yourself to the hospital.

If you are with someone you think might be having a stroke, ask her to smile, and look to see if one side of the face droops. Ask her to repeat a simple sentence and see if she can manage it. Have her raise both arms, watching to see if one arm slowly travels down while the other remains in the air. One or all of these symptoms could indicate stroke. If your companion exhibits them, don't hesitate—call 911 and get her emergency care. Remember, sometimes the outward physical signs of a stroke will subside; this doesn't mean the person no longer needs medical care.

Nutrition

Preventing heart disease has always been a driving force in national dietary policy. After World War II, heart attacks and strokes (as well as obesity) shot up all around the nation. The government began to raise alarms, suggesting dietary changes such as lowering meat and dairy consumption. In the more than six decades since then, we've gone through more national diet crazes than we have presidents, and still obesity rates climb.

John Abramson, a Harvard Medical School professor and fierce drug company critic, believes that our medical technology has been, in this case, our worst enemy. He notes that between 1970 and 1990, government warnings about saturated fat and meat consumption were having an effect. People were getting less cholesterol and fewer calories from fat, and slowly but surely heart attacks and strokes were

changes you can make in what you eat to help your heart

1. Cut down on high-fat meats and dairy foods. Try to think of meat as a food you eat two or three times a week rather than two or three times a day. If that's not a possibility for you, try to eat lower-fat meats and cheeses most of the time.

2. Eat more vegetables. Although we associate heart-healthy omega-3 fatty acids with fish, they are also found in green leafy vegetables along with a host of other valuable nutrients. And while adding a salad or a bowl of broccoli to your fried-chicken dinner is better than not eating vegetables at all, it would be better if you made a vegetable-chicken stir-fry with a side of string beans.

3. Drink that glass of wine with dinner; just don't have more than that. Any benefit that one or two glasses of wine confer is lost and actually far outweighed if you start knocking back the drinks.

going down a little: "Largely as a result of these lifestyle changes and improved blood pressure control, the death rate went down by half between 1970 and 1990."[67]

The reasons this trend began to reverse itself, Abramson argues, are statin drugs and the false impression that medically lowered cholesterol counterbalances bad eating and inactivity. Statins were *too* effective: they brought cholesterol numbers low enough that people forgot cholesterol is only *one* risk factor for heart attacks and cardiovascular incidents; they began pigging out on bacon cheeseburgers and weren't working so hard to make it to the gym regularly. If you are on a statin, keep in mind that eating healthfully is still a top priority for you.

The government has several suggested diets for increasing heart health, including the Heart Healthy Diet, the Therapeutic Lifestyles Changes (TLC), and the DASH eating plan. For more information

4. Eat fish once or twice a week. Fish are high in omega-3s because of their diet of plankton and ocean greens. Farm-fed fish, which often eat corn just as cows and chickens do, will be full of omega-6 acids, the kind that already dominate our Western diet. For online updates on the mercury content of specific fish, you can go to the FDA Web site (www.fda.gov) or check out the Monterey Aquarium's "Seafood Watch" Web page (www.monterey bayaquarium.org).

5. Start using omega-3-rich oils and incorporating omega-3-rich foods such as flax and walnuts into your diet. Sprinkle ground flax seeds on your morning cereal or use a nut oil to dress your salad. These oils break down and lose their benefits when heated, so they should not be used for high-heat cooking.

6. Make sure to get your fiber: replace your breakfast bagel or English muffin with a whole-wheat version or oatmeal and fruit.

on these regimens, check out the National Women's Health Information Center Web site (www.4women.gov) and look in the section called "Heart Healthy Eating."

Taking a regular aspirin each day has been shown to help post-menopausal women prevent heart attacks. This benefit needs to be weighed against the risks of stomach damage that can happen with overuse of aspirin and other painkillers. To counterbalance this, take a coated aspirin but have some uncoated ones on hand in case of a heart-related emergency.

Having your ovaries removed and other kinds of gynecological surgeries that can cause early or medical menopause can raise your risk for heart problems. This is probably because the ovaries continue to produce heart-protective hormones into and after the menopause transition.

Finally, despite the findings of the WHI, there continues to be controversy about estrogen and the heart. In an April 2007 article in the *Journal of the American Medical Association,* the WHI study leaders conclude, "Women who initiated hormone therapy closer to menopause tended to have reduced CHD risk compared with the increase in CHD risk among women more distant from menopause."[68] This information seemingly provides support for a popular theory that suggests that if women were to initiate HT at younger ages it would be good for their hearts after all. This is a tenuous notion, especially considering most support for it is based on WHI data in which the benefit did not meet statistical significance. We would say that until more evidence is available, women shouldn't consider taking hormones for the heart, regardless of their age. Even if this benefit is real, it is insignificant when compared with lifestyle changes such as diet and exercise—changes that don't carry an increased risk of cancer. These new WHI data do suggest that younger women who want to take HT in the short term for other reasons—to curb severe hot flashes, for example—don't have to worry so much about damaging their hearts.

19

close to the bone

osteoporosis, bone density, and menopause

It is one of the defining memories of Laura's childhood and the worst-case scenario for many aging women. Laura's stylish, dynamic grandmother, Grace, was caring for her young grandchildren. It was a rainy evening, and the two children started chasing each other down the driveway. Grace, worried they would run into the street, went after them. She hit a bit of slick driveway and fell, sustaining a broken hip that required hospitalization and several subsequent surgeries. In many ways, Laura's grandmother never fully recovered.

Many of us have older relatives who have had their mobility limited, their lives interrupted, and their health threatened by a bad fall, and we fear having this sort of accident ourselves. In the past several decades, menopausal women have increasingly been told that bone health is "their" issue and that the cessation of bleeding is a warning signal that osteoporosis and other serious problems are looming on the horizon. Is this true? How worried should we be and what can we do to insure our bones have the best possible chance of staying healthy?

A Family Crisis Becomes a Public Crusade

In 1994, the New Zealand health educator and author Gillian Sanson received a phone call: her sixteen-year-old daughter Camille had broken her wrist while skiing and was told by clinicians at a local hospital that her bones were excessively weak for someone her age. "I have the bones of an eighty-year-old," she told her mother matter-of-factly. Sanson's siblings, husband, and son were tested; several members were found to have osteoporosis, and others had osteopenia, conditions in which the bones become porous and more prone to breaks.

Sanson began to furiously research every study she could find on the subject. She writes, "The more I read, the more I was convinced that women and their doctors were misinformed. I uncovered an increasing amount of evidence that well women were being frightened into unnecessary testing, handed questionable diagnoses, and urged to undergo long-term treatments for a disease that they probably didn't have." The result of her reading was a devastating and thorough book called *The Myth of Osteoporosis* that documented point by point the ways that the very real concerns of aging women and the pain of those who have experienced disabling falls were being exploited by drug and medical device makers.[1] Well-meaning doctors were being drawn into this situation, prescribing dangerous and undertested drugs. Women themselves were changing and limiting their lives to protect against fractures they might never experience.

In this chapter we will look at some of the big questions raised by Sanson: Who is really at risk for fracture and who isn't? Which treatments are the best and which are the safest? How can all of us, young and old, work to keep our bones healthy and safe?

Bone Basics

We think of bone as being solid, stable, and unchanging. The truth is that living bone is in a constant state of building and tearing down, modeling and remodeling. The human frame is sort of like New York City: it has to adapt to ever-changing needs and it has a limited amount of space in which to do so. The solution to the problem is to rebuild constantly.

Like other living matter, bones need a lot of water: far from being solid, our bones are about half fluid. Collagen, the same protein responsible for making your skin pliable, is another major component, and of course calcium and other minerals, which are what make our bones strong.

There are two types of bone; hard or compact bone and spongy or cancellous bone. Compact bone provides structure and protection for the internal organs, while spongy bone cushions the impact of movement, protecting the body from stress and damage. Think about a skyscraper that has to be strong enough to stand but needs just a little bit of bend to ensure that it doesn't snap too readily.

Compact bone is made up of canals of cells that grow around individual blood vessels. These canals are called *osteons*. Two other important types of bone cells are called *osteoblasts* and *osteoclasts*.

An osteoblast helps to make new bone and an osteoclast gets rid of old bone by helping it be reabsorbed into the bloodstream. One easy way to remember the difference—an iconoclast is someone who tears down or seeks to destroy traditions or accepted truths. An osteoclast is something (a cell) that tears down or seeks to destroy bone.

This constant conversation between the creative and the destructive is what animates our skeletons and helps keep them dynamic and healthy. Indeed, everything with bone health seems to come back to keeping a good balance between different forces—biological, nutritional, and environmental.

What Our Bones Do

Bones have a number of important jobs besides giving the body shape and support: they protect fragile internal organs from damage, they anchor the muscles allowing the body to move, they produce blood cells, and they store energy and minerals.

Of all the minerals our bones store, the one that gets the most attention is calcium. It is hard to underestimate the importance of calcium. Without calcium, your brain wouldn't work right and your muscles couldn't contract—and of course you wouldn't have bones to hold your body upright.

The bones store and manage 99 percent of the total calcium in the body: at any given time, if you are an adult woman, you are carrying around about two and a half pounds of calcium. When receptors in the parathyroid glands sense that blood calcium is getting low, they send a message to the osteoblasts to free more of the nutrient from the bones.

It's ironic that midlife women are pressed to believe that their bone decisions are the most crucial. In fact, what a young woman chooses to eat and how she chooses to use her bones are much more important. It is a somewhat clichéd metaphor but one that bears repeating: your bones are like a bank where deposits and withdrawals are constantly made. You want to be sure that you are putting in as much as you are taking out.

Unfortunately, unlike your bank balance, it is harder to account later in life for the mistakes you make—the nutritional accounts you overdraw—when you are young Most of our bone building is done early, during childhood and young adult years, when new bone is created faster than old bone is removed. By our late thirties, we may start to remove more bone mass than we lay down. Pregnancy and breast-feeding can have dramatic effects on our bones. This is one time where bone withdrawals can definitely exceed deposits. There is even a condition called pregnancy-related osteoporosis. It is rare but involves developing bones that break too easily during or after childbearing.

What Happens at Menopause

After years of basically ignoring your bones, doctors suddenly get very interested in them when you hit menopause. The National Osteoporosis Foundation recommends bone mineral density (BMD) testing for all women sixty-five and older, as well as for all postmenopausal women who have had a bone fracture, have been taking hormones for a prolonged period of time, or have additional risk factors.[2] The idea, of course, is to identify and treat that dread disease, osteoporosis.

What exactly is osteoporosis? And why has it got so many doctors in such a frenzy? The truth is that the definition is unclear, and some of the professionals who aspire to prevent and treat it have an incomplete understanding of the condition, the medical definition of which has gone through several variations. In general, osteoporosis is considered to be diminished bone mass that raises the likelihood of *fragility fracture*, when the bones break in situations where most people's wouldn't. Historically, and still in some parts of the world, this means that if a woman starts to experience fragility fractures, doctors become concerned that she has osteoporosis—while of course U.S. doctors still respond to excessive fragility fractures. In the United States since the mid-1980s, we define *osteoporosis* as existing in relationship to bone density, established by tests usually performed at a certain age, whether or not a woman has experienced bone breaks.

What is the big difference? As Dr. Robert P. Heaney puts it in a *Journal of the American Medical Association* (*JAMA*) editorial, "the problem is that fragility is not measurable, while bone mass is."[3] Historically, and still in many parts of the world, osteoporosis is defined, like menopause, in retrospect. In the United States, Canada, and many parts of the Western world, osteoporosis is determined ahead of time.

For most physicians, an osteoporotic patient is identified through BMD and bone measurement tests. The score is expressed as a standard deviation above or below the bone density of a normal young adult of the same sex. The more negative the number, the greater the risk of fracture. A patient with a score between 1 and -1 is considered normal, while a patient with a score between -1 and -2.5 is considered to have osteopenia, or diminished bone. A score lower than -2.5 marks the point at which physicians say a patient has osteoporosis. Using this definition, it is estimated that more than 20 percent of postmenopausal women have osteoporosis, and some researchers estimate the number to be closer to 50 percent. It only takes a little common sense to figure out that 50 percent of women age forty-five and up aren't suffering from a disease. As Gillian Sanson reasons, "How do we get such figures, and are they true? Surely our hospital beds should be full of people with fractures and most elderly women afflicted by a dowager's hump."[4] This isn't the case, so what is really going on here?

This radical shift in the way medical professionals and patients understand osteoporosis was cemented in 1994 at a World Health Organization (WHO) conference. Not coincidentally, this meeting happened right around the time BMD testing was becoming available and just a year before a powerful class of new drugs would hit the pharmacy shelves.

Most doctors will tell you that osteoporosis is a disease. We want to encourage you to consider that it might be merely a risk factor. What difference does it make how we define osteoporosis? Well, a risk factor is one variable among many that may or may not increase your chances of a certain outcome, just as long-term use of birth control pills may increase your risk of breast cancer but is not the only or even the primary determining factor in developing the disease. According to the National Women's Health Network, "Although preventing osteoporosis is one of the things we should be trying to do to prevent fractures, it is not—as the pharmaceutical industry would have us believe—the only thing."[5]

Low BMD and fracture are two different things. So are low BMD and osteoporosis. They have a well-defined relationship, but one doesn't guarantee the other. In between having your bone density decline slightly and ending up in the hospital with a hip fracture are a number of things that can affect your probability of being injured or disabled as much or more than your bone density. As Gillian Sanson writes, "Calling low BMD osteoporosis is like calling elevated cholesterol heart disease, or calling high blood pressure a stroke."

How Our Bones Age

As we get older, not only do we lose more bone than we replace, but the mineral content of individual bones declines, as does the amount of water in the bones. Our ligaments can lose flexibility, and the amount of cartilage (a dense connective tissue that adds strength) can be reduced. Keep in mind, though, that as the American Academy of Orthopaedic Surgeons explains, "Many of the changes in our musculoskeletal system result more from disuse than from simple aging."

Bone Density versus Bone Quality

One problem with most of the measurement tools we have is that they take only bone density into account and ignore bone quality. An equally important factor in how likely bones are to break, bone quality cannot be quantitatively measured. Because of this, the medical community has for years erroneously seen bone density and bone quality as one and the same. Think about heavy ceramic dishes and fine china. One may be heavier and seemingly tougher, but when dropped, the china stands up better. That is how bone density and bone quality square off.

Birds, Bees, and BMD: Men, Women, and Skeletal Health

Do women have lower bone density than men? The answer is complicated. It seems that as young people, women actually gain more bone per gram than men. This might be an evolutionary change that prepares women's bodies for the bone "withdrawals" made during pregnancy and nursing. After menopause, the situation reverses, and men are able to maintain bone density better than women. This certainly doesn't mean that every man has stronger bones than every woman: both men and women experience natural and expected reductions in bone density as they age, and plenty of men are now finding themselves squarely in the marketing sights of bisphosphonate and bone-drug makers. To understand bones as a women's issue is like understanding heart attacks as a men's problem: just because women experience certain declines at menopause earlier than their male counterparts doesn't mean that both sexes don't have to consider the problem and struggle with it as they become older adults.

Interestingly, in BMD testing, 50 percent of men are found to have osteopenia—roughly, the same number as the female population. And yet men have only 35 percent as many hip fractures as women.[6] How can this be?

We think there could be several answers, all of which underscore the limitations of using BMD as a sole predictor of fracture risk. First, men are built differently from women; their bone structure comes together at different angles and alignments. This means their balance is different, as is the way they put on and carry weight in the body. Second, men tend to be bigger than women; they have more fat and muscle padding them if they do fall. Third, men tend not to wear balance-inhibiting footwear such as high heels and platforms that make taking a tumble all too likely.

DXA and Measuring Bone Density

Chances are that if you are a forty- or fifty-something woman and you have health insurance, your doctor is going to recommend a BMD scan. The most popular scan (though not the only one) is called a dual energy X-ray absorptiometry, or DXA.

Although not even a majority of women are undergoing BMD measurements (the *Journal of the American Geriatrics Society* puts the figure at about 23 percent for women sixty-six and older[7]) the procedure is becoming pretty standard among younger generations of women.

While BMD scanning is a great technology and has probably alerted many women to dangerously thin bones, there are some serious reasons to question what kinds of knowledge we can get from them. BMD scanning machines do not test for osteoporosis in the sense that a throat culture test for strep or a blood test can confirm HIV. What they do (and some machines do this more accurately than others) is measure bone density, *not*—and this is important—bone quality. From those measurements doctors can determine if, based on WHO guidelines, a woman falls into a density range deemed osteoporotic or osteopenic.

What BMD can't tell us is whether a patient will break bones, particularly in the hip and spine. As the British Columbia Office of Health Technology Assessment writes, "Even the most favorable reports on the effectiveness of bone mineral testing reveal that BMD testing does not accurately identify women who will go on to fracture as they age."[8]

Reasons to Question BMD

In an article frankly titled "The Fallacy of BMD," the Danish doctor S. Pors-Nielsen outlines several good reasons to assess BMD testing with a grain of salt.

First, bones are three-dimensional, while BMD happens in two dimensions. This means BMD can't take into account very significant issues such as bone size and shape. The angle of a woman's hips, for example, can make a difference to her chances of breaking one of them. And having more fat around your bones provides important cushioning that doesn't show up in a DXA measurement.

DXA measures bone loss in selected sites, which can include the hip, spine, and wrist. Bone loss in one place has been shown to be inconsistent with loss in another; just because your wrist is weak doesn't mean your spine is. Even within the same site—for example, the hip—measurements can vary widely from one part of the bone to another.

All of this is not to argue that BMD isn't a useful measurement but rather to point out that it isn't the only answer to the questions of skeletal health. Bones are as complicated as the human beings they animate, and no one measure can untangle the factors that lead one person to fracture and another to remain healthy.

Another reason to question BMD machines is that they can yield notably different measurements from one piece of equipment to another. Gillian Sanson describes an episode in which a healthy fifty-year-old woman was sent to have her bones measured by two different major brands of DXA machines. One machine estimated her bones to be almost normal, while another put her perilously close to a diagnosis of osteoporosis.[9] The extent to which you can trust the measurement of an individual machine may be in question, and the error in measuring bone can be up to 8 percent. That means that when you get a score, your bone density could be 8 percent higher or lower than what you see on the page.[10]

When you get the result of your BMD test, it will most likely be expressed as a T score and a Z score. The T score shows how you stack up against the bones of a young person. The Z score compares you with your peers.

Although the WHO guidelines set osteoporosis and osteopenia boundaries as densities above or below a normal bone, they don't say what "normal" is.

Who decides what a normal range is? DXA machines aren't standardized, so each manufacturer is left to determine for themselves what constitutes "normal young bone." In one study, doctors compared a manufacturer's guideposts with ones developed by the researchers and concluded that without standardization, WHO guidelines are difficult to interpret and apply, and BMD manufacturers are left to set standards that lead to overdiagnosis of problems in otherwise healthy women.

In general, when you get the results of a BMD test, put the accuracy and significance of the test in perspective. Also, we would suggest paying more attention to your Z score: why *should* your bones look like they did when you were twenty-five? In general our culture seems to locate normalcy in youth, to the detriment of the rest of us. The changes in our body should be understood and honored, not labeled as "abnormal" or "disease." Trying artificially to maintain "young" bones is a losing game: it prevents us as a society from making the necessary changes in thinking and lifestyle that could really lead to fracture prevention.

Why Not Have a BMD Test?

Many women make serious changes in their lives based on results suggesting a lowered BMD.[11] Once you find out you have lowered bone density, let alone osteoporosis, your immediate response may be fear, which can lead you to do things that may not actually improve your health. For example, you may be more likely to take bone drugs, hormone replacement therapy, or calcium supplements.[12] We are all for the calcium, but many of the pharmaceutical alternatives for bones have been shown to be either unsafe or are simply untested. While women with severely compromised bones may definitely want to explore pharmaceuticals, there is no reason for otherwise healthy women to take drugs.

Even more distressing is evidence that women with lowered bone mass are less likely to exercise and engage in physical activity, when that might be the best thing they could do to improve skeletal health. The *Journal of Gerontology* found that fear of falling led to a significant restriction in physical activities among a group of African-American adults aged forty-nine to sixty-five.[13] What is particularly interesting about this study is that it points out that even in a middle-aged population, fear about breaking bones leads people to be less active. And fear of fracture—not just experience of fracture—leads to significant and negative alterations in lifestyle.

Exercise is one of the best things you can do for your bones, as well as the rest of your body. If you are worried about falling, talk to a doctor (or a personal trainer, for that matter) about exercises that are safe for people with frailties. Don't ignore low BMD, but don't let fear keep you from living the best life you can.

Other techniques for measuring bone include quantitative ultra-sound, which measures bone primarily in the heel. It costs less money but has the same drawbacks as DXA. Its measurements are limited to a specific site in the body, and because density is inconsistent from site to site, the relevance of measuring just one part of the body may be limited. Doctors can also test for chemical by-products of bone formation and breakdown in the blood and urine. Doctors are still largely unsure how to understand these measurements, which, like DXA, don't give an accurate measurement of bone strength. This kind of testing is promising but a long way from being as useful as DXA.

Menopause and Teeth

A study from the University of California, Los Angeles, published in 2005 found that dental X-rays could be analyzed for evidence of osteoporosis.[14]

Menopause can be, dentally speaking, a difficult time. When the body is going through big changes hormonally, oral health can suffer. During pregnancy women are prone to gum inflammation and infection, among other problems. Hormone shifts can make us more vulnerable to gingivitis and gum problems, but bone loss at menopause can make us more likely to get cavities and have problems with our teeth. Make sure to get frequent dental checkups and maintain a good brushing and flossing routine. Be aware of the fact that you may be more likely to have teeth and gum problems while you are changing.

What About Osteopenia?

Many women have been frightened by diagnoses of osteopenia, a nebulous condition that women are increasingly being told they have after BMD testing. Basically it means that your bones have thinned a little, but many doctors paint the diagnosis as the first step on a potholed road to osteoporosis. However, many of these women will find that this potentially ominous sign comes to mean little or nothing at all.

Doctors are as confused as women about the meaning of this newly popularized problem. Dr. Ethel Siris of Columbia University Medical School explains, "Most people would agree that if someone has osteoporosis, you should treat them . . . but no one knows what to do about the woman who has quote unquote osteopenia."[15]

You probably won't be surprised to learn that this is a relatively new problem: the condition of osteopenia was defined at the same WHO conference in 1994 that radically altered the boundaries of bone disease. In theory the idea was to create a boundary to help doctors identify at-risk populations who could benefit from early intervention. In practice it has become an invitation for drugmakers and some doctors to push bone drugs on otherwise healthy women. As Dr. Stephen R. Cummings of the University of California, San Francisco, says, "More than half the population is told arbitrarily that they have a condition they need to worry about," a condition the doctor says has "no basis, no biological, social, economic or treatment basis."[16]

Let's be clear about this: osteopenia is *not* a disease. It may not even be a "condition."

We would argue that all women (and men) should be taking care of their bones, but we would caution women to be very slow to take bisphosphonates and certain other bone drugs. The truth is that while we can debate the usefulness of such drugs for people with osteoporosis, there is no evidence to suggest they help prevent fractures in patients with osteopenia. This is partially because the fracture rate in these patients is already so low that showing improvement is tough. If a population already has a low fracture rate, it seems unnecessary to treat them with drugs shown to make only modest improvements for seriously at-risk people.

So Who *Should* Worry about Osteoporosis?

While we are asking women to wrestle with some serious questions regarding the received wisdom about osteoporosis, we are in no way suggesting that many women don't struggle with debilitating bone problems. The issue becomes deciding who really is at risk for fractures.

Women with histories of breaking bones continue to do so later in life. If your bone quality is already susceptible to breaks and cracks, this becomes only more true as bones naturally thin with age.

Genetics play a huge role in fracture risk; your family history may be one of the best predictive tools you have in assessing your personal fracture risk. Women whose mothers broke their hips are much more likely to do so themselves.

Nutrition and Bone Health

It is perhaps obvious to say that proper nutrition both before, during, and after menopause is essential to bone health. But after that seemingly simple statement on which everyone agrees, things become more complicated.

Another thing everyone agrees on is calcium: it's important, and not getting enough of it can cause big problems, but it's not as simple as popping a supplement or drinking a glass of milk, unfortunately, and doctors are still puzzling over some big questions raised by this nutrient.

Calcium doesn't work alone to protect osteocytes; it needs other nutrients, chief among them vitamin D and magnesium, to be properly absorbed. Without these nutritive partners, calcium is powerless to protect you.

Vitamin D is a fat-soluble vitamin that works as a hormone in the body. Its primary source has traditionally been sunlight, but as people increasingly try to protect their skin against damaging (and potentially deadly) UV rays, they have also blocked the production of vitamin D by the action of sunlight on bare skin. Milk is another source of vitamin D, but a person would have to consume huge quantities of milk to get enough of the vitamin.

A study of 2,310 adults published in the *Journal of the American Medical Association (JAMA)* concluded that getting enough vitamin D reduced the need for calcium, adding, "Our study suggests that vitamin D sufficiency may be more important than high calcium intake in maintaining desired values of serum PTH [parathyroid hormone]." [17]

In 1998, researchers at Massachusetts General Hospital in Boston discovered that 57 percent of the adult study population ages eighteen to ninety were deficient in vitamin D; it may be that Americans are getting enough calcium but not enough of this partner nutrient to use it properly. The recommended daily intake for vitamin D (DRI) is 600 IU. Fish and milk are good food sources. Don't take more than 800 IU a day: like many potentially beneficial nutrients, too much vitamin D may cause as many problems as too little. [18]

It is estimated that Americans get about 70 percent of their total calcium from dairy products; the benefits of dairy were an unquestioned assumption for years before milk mustaches started gracing celebrity mugs. But why is it, some ask, that the nations that consume the most dairy in their diets—the United States among them—have some of the world's highest osteoporosis rates? [19] If dairy is the cure, then why do we struggle disproportionately with the problem?

The answer may be that dairy isn't the great source of calcium we thought it was. Evolutionarily speaking, dairy is a new food. For most of human history, only nursing young have relied on milk, and many cultures still exclude dairy from their diets, notably in Asia and Africa. In China, where dairy plays little to no role in the traditional diet, hip fracture rates are some of the lowest in the world, although as the nation continues to Westernize, this is changing. [20] One reason might be that in order for your body to process calcium, magnesium must also be present. Fruits and vegetables are high in magnesium, so when they serve as primary sources of calcium, calcium/magnesium ratios are pretty even, around 1:1. When dairy is the primary calcium provider, as it is in the West, calcium is favored over magnesium in ratios closer to 12:1.[21]

It's all about balance; if you get too much magnesium, calcium absorption would also be affected. You can take calcium/magnesium supplements, but be careful—many women find that magnesium supplementation can cause diarrhea and uncomfortable loose stools. The best thing is probably to work at eating more natural food sources of the nutrient. We recommend eating magnesium-rich foods such as dark-green and leafy vegetables, nuts, legumes, and brown rice.

Not all dairy foods are created equal. Milk may be better and safer than processed cheese or acid-curd products such as cottage cheese.[22] This is probably because these products are high in both sodium and acid, both of which influence calcium release and absorption. If you consume a lot of milk, we recommend you opt for organic, because the cows producing organic milk are raised without unnecessary antibiotics and other undesirable chemicals (organic milk is, unfortunately, more expensive and not accessible to everyone).

Beyond how you take in calcium, there are other controversies. Some people argue that calcium intake has been overemphasized and definitive evidence is lacking that either taking in a lot of it from food or supplementing it with pills provides any benefit. Gillian Sanson calls the belief that calcium alone can save bones "the myth of the magic bullet," and she writes, "Because the amount of calcium in the blood is so carefully regulated, increasing calcium does not necessarily mean that the body will build more bone."[23] She adds that cultures with low calcium intakes haven't been shown to have problems with bone formation, suggesting that perhaps only seriously calcium-deficient diets pose a problem. So while getting extremely small amounts of calcium may well cause bone problems, megadosing on the nutrient will not necessarily prevent or fix them.

Bantu women of Africa consume only about 350 mg of calcium a day. Compare that with our recommended average of 1,200 mg to 1,500 mg, and you would expect these ladies to be disabled and fractured in disproportionately high rates. Not only is this not the case, but Bantu women tend to lose a strikingly small number of teeth and break few bones.[24]

Although no one is sure why this is, one theory is that the vegetable-based diet that Bantu women consume is low in animal protein as well as calcium. Although protein is necessary for building bone,[25] excessive meat consumption of the sort rampant in the United States may cause higher acid levels in the blood and urine, which the body tries to balance out by releasing calcium. This may be increasingly true as we age and our kidneys are less able to handle high acid loads.[26] Consuming protein through vegetable sources, like consuming calcium, seems to have advantages over animal foods. We aren't recommending you give up steak or hamburgers, just that you balance your diet to include more vegetables and less meat.

Not everyone thinks losing calcium in the urine will hurt your bones. A Canadian study tested high-protein (from vegetable sources) diets and found that although greater amounts of calcium were excreted, there seemed to be no negative impact on the balance of calcium in the bones.[27]

Another element of the Western diet that may hurt bones is our high salt intake. Kidneys have to let go of calcium in order to get rid of salt from the body. This might be a reason early humans, who ate very little calcium, had such good bone mass.

Many studies of older women and calcium have yielded disappointing results. In 2005, the Women's Health Initiative (WHI) calcium and vitamin D trials found that women who took a calcium regimen prescribed by the National Institutes of Health (NIH) over a ten-year period showed no statistically significant improvement in their bone mass or reduction in their fracture rates.[28]

Most of us accept as gospel that calcium will improve our bones, so were the WHI findings a radical revision of conventional wisdom? Or was the design of the study itself flawed?

There were some significant problems with the WHI study. For starters, it excluded women who had been taking calcium their whole lives. Researchers were really testing to see if calcium intervention at a later stage of life—postmenopause—would make a difference. Remember: all the WHI women were postmenopausal. Since we know that much of your bone mass is laid down in your teens, twenties, and even thirties, one thing the study may reinforce is the importance of getting calcium as a young woman. Some other problems: there were concerns about the length of the study—it might have been too short to show reliable results—and it wasn't careful about whether participants were also taking bisphosphonates or estrogens in addition to calcium, two things that could have had major impacts on bone mass.

The Nurses Health Study, which looked at various health patterns in 121,701 women, found that neither milk nor calcium consumption seemed to make a difference when it came to preventing broken bones. Intriguingly, the Nurses Health Study investigators also determined that milk and calcium consumption as a young woman didn't significantly reduce their risk for fractures (although there was a nonsignificant reduction found in hip fracture rates; again, it may or may not have been a coincidence).

So why should older women bother with calcium? Among other reasons, because we know that the nutrient is important for so many reasons, and there are still too many unanswered questions. The Nurses Health Study results showed that continuing to drink milk and take calcium seemed to counteract the bad effects that a lifetime of caffeine drinking could have on the hip and spine.[29] Also, the *Archives of Internal Medicine* reported that calcium and vitamin D intake were associated with reduced PMS.[30] We know that women who have PMS are more likely to suffer from bad menopausal mood swings. Perhaps getting adequate amounts of calcium and vitamin D can help your mood.

We say get your calcium: eat lots of calcium-rich foods, particularly vegetables. Just remember that, as Joel S. Finkelstein writes in the *New England Journal of Medicine*, "One message is clear: calcium with vitamin D supplementation by itself is not enough to ensure optimal bone health. . . . Even if a woman is receiving adequate calcium with vitamin D supplementation, she may still be at risk for fracture."[31]

And remember, getting calcium from food is better than from supplements. Dr. Robert Heaney, an endocrinologist and internist at the Osteoporosis Research Center at Creighton University in Omaha, Nebraska, says, "The five best sources of calcium are food, food, food, fortified food, and supplements in that order."[32]

If you are taking calcium supplements, remember that calcium citrate is a more easily absorbed form of the nutrient than the also popular (and less expensive) calcium carbonate. The FDA recommends 1,000 mg of calcium each day for women between the ages of thirty-one and fifty, 1,200 mg for ages fifty-one to seventy, and 1,200 to 1,500 mg per day for women older than seventy.

Some other important nutritional factors to consider: if you are partaking too heavily of the unholy trinity of alcohol, cigarettes, and caffeine, you could be hurting your bones. All three have been shown to have a negative effect in excess on skeletal health. In particular, soda can be bad, perhaps because of some issue with its chemical composition—its phosphorus or its combination of carbonation and caffeine—or because it simply replaces milk and water in the diet.

One French study found that while excess alcohol consumption can hurt bones, moderate drinking of one to three glasses of wine per day might be good for bone mass.[33] Take this with (no pun intended) a grain of salt: any amount of alcohol can inhibit balance and make falls more likely.

Recent studies have suggested that perhaps a better balance of omega-3 and omega-6 fatty acids may improve bone density. A study from Indiana University School of Medicine found that diets where the two fats were represented in equal proportions seemed to be connected with less bone loss. This information is far from conclusive but does provide another reason to eat more omega-3-rich foods.[34]

It was discovered in the 1960s that a mutation in a specific gene could lead to unusually high concentrations of the amino acid homocysteine in the blood. Although no one is sure why this is tough on your skeleton, one theory is that it stops collagen from properly connecting and forming tissue. Some of the first information about homocysteine came from the massive Framingham Heart Study (also one of the first trials to offer negative information about HT and the heart). Framingham found that men with high concentrations of homocysteine were more likely to break their hips.

In 2004, the *New England Journal of Medicine* reported on a

Dutch study analyzing levels of homocysteine in both men and women. The study found that even though people with high levels were more likely to fracture, their bone densities were pretty much the same as those with low homocysteine.[35]

Both vitamin B12 and folate seem to help with this problem by lowering levels of homocysteine in the blood.

A Capsule a Day: What About Drugs for Stronger Bones?

Estrogen

In 1982, a San Francisco radiologist named Harry Genant performed a study that would both revive estrogen, the use of which had declined in the 1970s, as a best-selling drug and change public perceptions of osteoporosis forever. Genant's study showed that in women who had undergone oophorectomy, taking estrogen helped to prevent some of the bone loss previously associated with the procedure. Genant wasn't the first to suggest that ET and HT could help protect bones; that honor goes to Fuller Albright, a Harvard doctor who was an early proponent of estrogen as a pill to keep women young and had been one of Genant's influences. Albright's theory hadn't really caught on until Genant's paper was published in the *Annals of Internal Medicine*, but then it spread like wildfire.[36]

When the bad news from the WHI began to emerge in the early 2000s, many women were concerned that if they gave up their estrogen, as so many felt was the right thing to do, what would keep their skeletons safe? Many ran for bisphosphonates and others started megadosing on calcium.

The WHI confirmed that, indeed, HT and ET could build bone and decrease fractures.[37] All that benefit was lost, unfortunately, when hormones were discontinued. While many results of the WHI are debatable, one thing the trial clearly showed was that HT and ET in the long term aren't a good idea. The older you get, the harder these hormones are on your body. For this reason, we would discourage you from choosing hormones to strengthen bones except in the case of extreme skeletal weakness.

Laura's mom was on Premarin very briefly before she started

having side effects, and her doctor switched her to Evista (raloxifene), a pill from a pharmaceutical class called selective estrogen-receptor modulators, or SERMs. These drugs act like estrogen on some receptors and have antiestrogenic effects on others. Because they don't accomplish the things that traditional estrogens do—they actually increase hot flashing and don't seem to help vaginal problems— marketers have primarily targeted SERMs at patients with cancer sensitivities and for the purpose of building bone. Trials have shown that the drugs help build bone in the spine and femoral neck and cut the likelihood of a spine fracture.[38] While SERMs don't carry the same cancer risk as estrogen, they still cause many of the other problems associated with hormones, including blood clots. Indeed, because these are newer drugs, real safety data will probably take many more years to amass.

Bisphosphonates

When Barbara and Laura were writing *The Greatest Experiment Ever Performed on Women: Exploding the Estrogen Myth* in 2002, a new class of drugs called bisphosphonates seemed like a promising option for women who were worried about bone health.

This class of drugs includes Fosamax (alendronate), Actonel (risedronate), and more recently Boniva (ibandronate sodium) and Zometa (Reclast or Aclasta). The drugs work through inhibiting the activity of osteoclasts (the cells that break down bone) and the reabsorption of bone into the blood. Specifically, bisphosphonates attach to the surface of the bone and create a barrier against osteoclasts.

In 1995, the drugmaker Merck launched what would become the blockbuster Fosamax. Before the company had even gained FDA approval, it was spending tons of money to subsidize BMD-scanning machines. Why? Most obviously to help build a client base. If more women received screenings, they could be put in the osteopenic and osteoporotic categories, both groups of people to whom Fosamax could be heavily marketed. Doctors could be given continuing medical education that advised writing prescription slips for all patients whose BMD fell outside certain limits.

A year before Fosamax came to market, the definition of osteoporosis was rewritten by the WHO, "a definition that automatically made the bones of many older women 'abnormal' . . . and automatically defined 30 per cent of all post-menopausal women as having a disease."[39] John Abramson compares this large-scale creation of a disease with the medicalization of menopause that occurred in the 1960s: "This reframing of normal aging into a pathological process is reminiscent of Dr. Robert Wilson's successful campaign to convince women and their doctors that menopause was not a natural event but a hormone-deficiency disease."

The difference, Abramson points out, was that while Wilson was an individual being heavily compensated by drug companies, the WHO was a trusted organization seemingly in the public service. Closer scrutiny, however, reveals that if Wilson was a pharma-bought individual able to stage an impressive change in public opinion, the WHO committee responsible for the new standards was no less influenced by drug company dollars. In fact, the WHO study group that produced the final standards for diagnosing osteoporosis was funded by at least three pharmaceutical groups, all of which were developing new bone-building drugs.

Early journal articles on the drug provided further support. The Merck-sponsored Fracture Intervention Trial announced that Fosamax could reduce a woman's risk of hip fracture by 50 percent. What did this mean? In this case it simply meant that two women participating in the placebo trails had hip fractures, and one person taking Fosamax did. And this was a group of "high-risk" women—those who had histories of fractures—not normal menopausal or post-menopausal females.

According to John Abramson, a study published in *JAMA* in 1998 showed that for women with osteopenia, hip fracture risk actually went up on Fosamax. That's right: it went *up* by 84 percent. What does this mean? Well, among other things, it means that bisphosphonates may not be so great for women who do not have severe bone loss (but this was in such a small study that significance was hard to determine, and again, that is a relative risk).[40]

In 2004, it seemed as though some definitive evidence about the benefit of bisphosphonates was finally on the way. The first long-term, double-blind, placebo-controlled clinical trial of the drugs was published in the *New England Journal of Medicine*. The study looked at the effects of Fosamax on a population of women over ten years. The news reports sounded like good news both for women worried about bone density and for Merck stockholders: Fosamax increased density in the spine and the hip, and more of the drug created better density.[41] To add a bit of poetry to the good news, the head doctor on the trial was a man named Henry G. Bone.

A closer examination of the data, however, revealed something that didn't seem to be making the evening news reports: even though women taking the drug had greater bone mass, they had about the same number of breaks as those in the placebo group. In a letter written to the *New York Times* responding to the study, Abby Lippman, the cochairwoman of the Canadian Women's Health Network, said that while "it may be reassuring to some" to be told in a study funded by Merck that Fosamax was safe and bone-building, "what is not underlined in your report is that there seems to be no real difference in fracture or height loss, the 'outcomes' that matter most to women, between those on the drug for up to 10 years and those in the placebo groups." Lippman cut through the rosy news stories, saying, "The question for women remains: so what if bone density doesn't fall off, if the medical and cosmetic outcomes are not affected? More profits for the drug and bone density measurement machinery manufacturers, true. But what about the 'bottom lines' for women's health?"[42]

What does all this mean to you? First, it means that bisphosphonate drugs haven't been proven to seriously help reduce the risk of fracture. Second, because, like estrogen, the drugs' benefits are lost when treatment is discontinued, you would have to be on bisphosphonates for a long time to see potential benefits. Gillian Sanson explains that based on Merck's own study claiming a 50 percent reduction, ninety women would need to take the drug to prevent one hip fracture. That means eighty-nine women who wouldn't benefit would need to deal with the side effects for every one woman who stopped a bone break. And this, remember, was a study of high-risk women. For women with osteopenia, it is possible that hundreds of women in their fifties would need to take the pill for one to prevent fracture.

It's also important to note that this class of drug has some serious safety questions surrounding it that have yet to be answered.

When bones remodel, they remove what are called "microfractures" and "microdamage," tiny, nearly imperceptible flaws that could compromise bone quality. Bisphosphonates limit remodeling and therefore can also prevent the removal of microdamage. This means that what starts as an almost imperceptible problem has the chance to develop into something bigger. Dr. Satoshi Mori and his colleagues studied the effect of long-term suppression of remodeling in dogs and found the dogs sustained greater microdamage over time.[43] They didn't find, however, that it made a difference in spinal fractures. Still, this problem needs further exploration. Recent information has suggested that bisphosphonates can cause osteonecrosis of the jaw, particularly in patients using the drug as part of their cancer treatments. In this rare but very serious condition, the very drugs being used to help rebuild bones being compromised by anticancer treatments end up causing the breakdown of bone in the jaw. The condition begins as a painful tingling or burning but may develop into actual bone disintegration and disfigurement.[44]

A more common side effect is gastrointestinal disturbance and stomach pain. As many as one in three women taking these drugs may have stomach problems ranging from burning and pain to actual "ulceration of the esophagus."[45] Dr. Alan Cassels writes, "Fosamax is relatively useless and harmful but boy is it ever marketed . . . it is well known for its ability to burn a hole in your esophagus. Some scientists I know call it Tub'n'tile cleaner because it has a chemical structure not unlike a popular household cleaner."[46] Indeed, the chemicals in bisphosphonates were used for "making soap and descaling boilers."[47] If you're having severe heartburn, chest pain, or other signs that you might be experiencing this side effect, discuss your symptoms with your doctor.

In a sad irony possible only in our culture of creating pharmaceutical stew, many bisphosphonate patients have turned to taking a class of stomach drug called a proton pump inhibitor (PPI), whose brand names include Prilosec, Prevacid, and Nexium, to counteract stomach problems. Researchers at the University of Pennsylvania recently reported that long-term use of PPIs resulted in a 44 percent increase in hip fractures.[48] So if you take the drug to save your bones, you get stomach problems. If you take the drug to fix your stomach, you hurt your bones.

It's worth mentioning that if you are taking nonsteroidal anti-inflammatory drugs (NSAIDs) for pain—particularly ibuprofen or naproxen sodium (Advil, Motrin, or Aleve)—your chances of developing ulcers are increased.

If you do break a bone while taking bisphosphonates, it may be harder for you to heal. Bone remodeling, the process that is suppressed by these drugs, is required to heal breaks and cracks. Because the drugs have a long half-life, their effects will be felt in your body potentially for years after you discontinue use and there is no way to speed up the process. Other observed side effects of bisphosphonates include joint pain, abdominal pain, visual disturbances, and spontaneous fracture.

A study published in the *New England Journal of Medicine* randomized women between the ages of seventy and seventy-nine to receive either Actonel or a placebo. They concluded that even women with severe osteoporosis "derived only small benefit from these drugs."[49] John Abramson writes that "hip fractures were reduced only in the women who already had a spine fracture when the study began (40% of the women in the study). . . . For the other 60 percent of women in the study without a preexisting spine fracture, Actonel did not significantly reduce the risk of hip fracture. Moreover, the drug appeared to have no beneficial effect on their overall health. There was no difference in the number of serious illnesses, including fractures, that occurred in the women who took Actonel compared with those who took the placebo.[50]

An attempt on the part of Procter & Gamble—the makers of Actonel—to prove their product superior to Fosamax proved disastrous. In the summer of 2002, P & G hired the British doctor Aubrey Blumsohn and his colleagues at Sheffield University to oversee a comparative trial of the two drugs. The pharma giant paid the doctors and their university a hefty sum of money—180,000 pounds—for their services. Blumsohn assumed, wrongly, that they actually expected him to be involved in the research and analysis. He asked early in the trial to see the data. Time went on, and it still didn't arrive. Blumsohn grew more persistent, demanding to see the results coming in from the trial. Amazingly P & G refused. They expected to "ghostwrite" a report, employing staff authors to draft a paper that would eventually bear Blumsohn's name for a prestigious medical journal. After more than a year and much heated conversation, Blumsohn was eventually allowed to see limited data. What he saw convinced him that what he wasn't seeing (around 40 percent)[51] showed that Actonel was not better than Fosamax and potentially less effective. Blumsohn, feeling used and fed up, blew the whistle on the drugmakers' dubious practices.

Most bisphosphonates are taken once a week (originally they were taken every day) and are available in regular and "+D" formulas. Boniva (ibandronate sodium), a once-a-month treatment, is available as an injection as well as a pill. The drugs have been found to have similar benefits and limitations in men as in women.[52] Some other brand names include Didronel (etidronate) and Bonefos (clodronate). These two early bisphosphonates aren't approved in the United States but are available in other parts of the world. Aredia (pamidronate) and Zometa (zoledronate) are intravenous drugs injected once a year.

Parathyroid Hormone and Calcitonin

Like estrogen, parathyroid hormone and calcitonin are hormones that naturally occur in the body. Parathyroid hormone is made in the parathyroid glands and it helps to regulate the amount of calcium in the blood. When these levels get low, parathyroid hormone is the repair crew sent out to restore calcium to normal levels.

A type of pharmaceutical parathyroid hormone, teriparatide, is sold under the brand name Forteo. Administered daily by injection pen, this drug seeks to build bone rather than preventing reabsorption, as the bisphosphonates do. It was approved in 2002, but there is a certain amount of caution surrounding this drug because early trials of it in rats found that it increased the risk of getting bone cancer. It's too soon to tell if this will be true in the human population, although there was at least one documented case of bone cancer in a patient being treated with Forteo. The drug is expensive; a twenty-eight-day supply can run you around $700 if you are paying out of pocket.[53] Side effects include rapid heartbeat (especially when first taking the drug), dizziness, leg cramps, and nausea. If you have certain kinds of bone problems (Paget's disease, a remodeling disorder where normal bone is replaced by soft, porous bone), have had radiation or bone cancer, or have high blood-calcium levels, you probably shouldn't take this drug.

Calcitonin helps to regulate calcium and phosphorous levels. It prevents the reabsorption of bone and prevents the kidneys from getting rid of too much calcium in urine. It may not have as big a role in humans as it does in animals like fish and mice.[54] Pharmaceutical calcitonin (Miacalcin, Calcimar, and Fortical) is usually prescribed to postmenopausal women who are at least five years past the transition. It can be taken by injection or as a nasal spray. Side effects include nasal inflammation, facial flushing, skin rash, urinary frequency, backache, bloody nose, and headaches. If you are allergic to fish, you probably want to skip this drug—it is made from salmon.

Statins

Recently some scientists have suggested that statins, anticholesterol medications such as Lipitor, may be able to reduce fractures. A study published in the *Annals of Internal Medicine* performed an observational trial using data from the WHI observational study. Researchers found that "statin use did not improve fracture risk or bone density," adding "the cumulative evidence does not warrant use of statins to prevent or treat osteoporosis."[55]

No matter what drug you take for bone health, studies show that you aren't likely to stay on it. A study published in the *Archives of Internal Medicine* looked at adherence rates for patients prescribed an array of bone drugs including Fosamax, estrogen, calcitonin, and raloxifene. Only one year after receiving a prescription, researchers found that 45.2 percent of patients were no longer filling them. Five years after, this number had risen to 52.1 percent.[56] This is yet another reason that working to maintain bone health through diet and exercise are important even if you are taking drugs.

Things That Can Hurt Your Bones

Although we often think of postmenopausal status alone as a huge risk factor for lowered bone density, the truth is that there are a number of conditions and health problems that can hurt our bones.

Drugs

When you go to pop a pill to help some other part of your body, make sure you aren't hurting your bones in the process. Several commonly prescribed medications can really damage your skeleton. Steroids, specifically glucocorticoids such as prednisone, hydrocortisone, and dexamethasone, taken to treat serious conditions such as asthma, lupus, arthritis, and Crohn's disease, are a major and well-documented factor in thinning bones. Bone loss from steroid use can be seen as soon as six months after starting a drug.

Inhaled steroids became the standard treatment for asthmatics more than a decade ago. At that point, it was thought that steroids posed little to no risk to bones. However, an October 2001 *New England Journal of Medicine* study, which looked at 109 asthmatic women, revised that finding. The women were divided into three groups: one that didn't inhale steroids, another that took four to eight puffs a day, and a third that inhaled eight or more puffs a day. The results were startling: not only did inhaled steroids cause bone loss, but they specifically "caused bone loss at the hip, the most serious site of fractures." Despite such findings, the study concluded that "inhaled glucocorticoids . . . remain among the most effective and safest medications for the treatment of asthma."[57] However, the report suggested switching to the lowest possible dose and getting BMD testing to monitor for possible losses.

The effects from inhaled steroids for the treatment of asthma are similar to those from oral steroids taken for arthritis, estimated to be used by 30 million Americans.

Another class of drugs that may be hazardous to bones is antidepressants. A Canadian study from McGill University found that people over fifty who were taking selective serotonin reuptake inhibitors (SSRIs) had double the risk of having fractures when compared with a placebo group.[58] Simply being depressed can make your bones weaker: you are less likely to engage in exercise, eat correctly, and do other things that are essential for protecting bone health. It's not clear if antidepressants make you more fracture-prone because they disorient or impair good balance or because they actually hurt bone cells.[59]

Although many estrogens can help you build bone, some progestin-based birth control, such as Depo-Provera, can actually do damage. In her book *The Menopause Industry*, Sandra Coney writes that "after measuring the bones of young women who had been using Depo-Provera for over five years, if was found that they had 7.5% less bone in the spine and 6.5% less bone in the hip than women who had never used the drug."[60] The bone loss seems to result from the drug's blocking estrogen and causing periods not to come.

Partners in Crime: Illnesses That Might Make Your Bones Worse

A link between the thyroid and bone loss has also been suggested; for many years doctors have observed a connection between hyperthyroidism and osteoporotic fractures. The April 3, 2001, *Annals of Internal Medicine* reported that in a four-year study of 9,704 older women over sixty-five, those with hyperthyroidism faced a higher risk of new hip and spine fractures.[61]

Hypertension is another risk factor: a study published in the *Lancet* followed 3,676 women over the age of seventy-three. Study authors found that women with high blood pressure lost bone mass at almost twice the rate of those with low blood pressure. This may be because high blood pressure makes you lose calcium through your kidneys, although no one knows for sure why these two seem to have a connection.[62] One Danish study has gone so far as to suggest that the severity of cardiac events can be gauged by the severity of osteoporosis at the time of an attack.[63]

Women who survive breast cancer may be at risk for low bone density.[64] Some doctors theorize that this is in part because of lower hormone use among breast cancer patients. This seems unlikely to us, but if it's true, we should start to see similar weaknesses in the general female population as more women get off and stay off HT.

Having type 2 diabetes makes it more likely that you will sustain fractures. A study published in the *Journal of Clinical Endocrinology and Metabolism* found that over seven years, women with the metabolic disorder were much more likely to break bones at multiple sites than their healthy counterparts.[65] Add bone troubles to the long list of health complications inherent in this increasingly common disease.

We feel like a broken record saying it again, but having an oophorectomy is a major risk factor for osteoporosis and bone thinning.

What Can Help

It turns out that so much of preventing serious fractures comes down to, well, not falling. This is easier said than done.

Genetics play a huge role in bone health. Scientists estimate that as much as 70 percent of bone health is determined by what you were born with.[66] But it's far from the whole story.

Studies have found, for example, that African-American women have denser bones than white women: "The average rate of hip BMD loss is approximately twice as great in Caucasian as African-American women and increased with age in both groups."[67] Sounds like good news for black women, right? Well, not really. It turns out that even though their bones may be thicker, their rates of death from fracture are higher.[68] One explanation for this could be different bone alignments that would have a genetic base. Another would be to do with the way genetics and environment interact with each other. We know that in general low-income women of all races have less access to preventive care, receive less health education, and are less able to recognize risk factors for disease or make healthy lifestyle changes that would go a long way to keeping them well.

What are some lifestyle changes we can make to counterbalance genetic disadvantages?

Exercise

If there is one thing we would urge you to do to protect your bone health, it is exercise. It really will make all the difference.

Bone, like so many parts of the body, functions best through use; never was the old adage "use it or lose it" truer than in relation to your bones. New bone is built in response to stress. In addition, being steady on your feet makes a huge difference. Pat Crawshaw, a Canadian osteoporosis specialist, writes of a growing awareness that "much of the age-induced increased risk of fracture is an artifact of diminished muscle strength and balance."

A British study from the University of Cambridge found that "several popular forms of exercise," including "cycling, sculling, gymnastics, weights" could help to decrease the risk of serious fractures with aging.[69]

There are three major types of exercise that help prevent fracture: balance training (which prevents falls), strength training (which builds bone), and aerobic training (which builds muscle). Dr. Laura Toshi, an orthopedic surgeon who consults for the federal government's Office of Research on Women's Health, recommends balance training as the number one strategy against fractures.

You don't have to be running miles on the treadmill each day either. One of the safest and most effective methods of balance training is tai chi, a traditional Chinese exercise. It is particularly effective because it meets two of the three criteria for preventing fractures: it has been evaluated scientifically for benefits in balance and in cardiovascular health. Yoga is another option, which builds both balance and strength.

The importance of building muscle as well as bone through weight training and cardiovascular activity is illustrated in a 1996 Mayo Clinic study that found that strong back muscles played a role in preventing fracture in women with osteoporosis.[70]

Getting injured can be bad news for your skeleton because being inactive, even for a week or two, can reduce your bone mass. This kind of rapid change in bone density after being laid up dramatically underscores the importance of stress bearing and activity on maintaining skeletal health. If you are stuck in bed because of illness or being hurt, be sure to talk to your doctor about what you can do to protect your bones until you recover.

Home Safety

We all think of home as a place of safety and comfort. It's where we rest and relax, and we take measures to keep burglars or people who would hurt us out. As we age, though, we need to start to see the potential dangers *inside* our homes. Things that don't pose threats when we are young become much more dangerous as we age. Check your home for loose rugs and anything that might make you slip or trip. Move furniture that obstructs your path. Look at your lighting: Is it so dim that it makes it tough to see? This is also a hazard.

Check your shoe rack. High heels may make your legs look great, but there is no denying that they make taking a nasty spill a lot more likely. Be honest about which shoes help you walk better and which ones make you wobbly.

What's in your closet? As well as keeping you warm and toasty in the chill, a big down jacket in the winter can be a great safety precaution if it provides padding in case of a fall. There is also specially made padded underwear to help those at high risk of falling.

In general it is good to have a little extra something between you and the ground in case you do fall. Studies have found that thin people are more likely than heavier ones to fracture when they fall, so carrying a little (emphasis on *a little*) extra weight can be a good thing. Just to be clear, we're not suggesting you should gain weight to save your bones, but women with eating disorders like anorexia nervosa and those who diet to keep themselves in states of extreme thinness are doing serious damage.

A clinical study from June 2001 on the complications associated with eating disorders revealed that women suffering from anorexia and bulimia were two to three times more likely to suffer a fracture than women who were normal eaters. The study further revealed that anorexic young women can fail to achieve peak bone mass, which may increase risk of fracture "even more dramatically as they enter menopause."[71]

20

the golden bowl
incontinence and menopause

It is estimated that somewhere around 13 million Americans—between 10 and 30 percent of all U.S. women—experience some kind of incontinence.[1] The National Association for Continence puts the estimate at 25 million, although the majority of incontinent people will never seek appropriate treatment, so the real figure is possibly much higher—and those who do seek help wait an average of *nine years* to do so. This situation is changing: Dr. William H. Parker, a gynecologist and the author of the book *A Gynecologist's Second Opinion*, told Barbara recently that commercials for incontinence drugs have raised awareness among his female patients that urination control is not something to keep from your doctor: "Although I rarely treat incontinence with drugs—muscle rehabilitation works better—it has made women more comfortable with raising and discussing the issue."

Why do so many people fail to mention such a disruptive problem to their doctors? They may be embarrassed, or they may assume (wrongly!) that it is a natural part of aging. Regardless of the reason, countless Americans choose to suffer in silence, denying themselves access to treatments that can improve or cure the problem in nearly 90 percent of patients.[2]

Incontinence is a particularly important issue for midlife women because they are more than twice as likely to have the problem as men. Harvard Medical School describes the average person with the problem as "a 48-year-old woman who leaks when she coughs."[3] But is incontinence a menopause issue? What can be done to address this common but curable problem?

Like a water balloon, the kidneys expand as they fill. When the amount of urine in the bladder is around one and a half to two cups, nerves in the spine tell the brain that it is time to pee.[4] The urine travels through a sphincter muscle—a muscle that expands and contracts like the lips or the anus—into the urethra, a small tube through which liquid waste exits the body.

In healthy urinary tracts, urination is controlled through a series of muscle contractions and relaxation. The urine is held inside the body by the bladder muscle remaining relaxed while the sphincter muscle remains tightly contracted. When you urinate this reverses and the bladder contracts, forcing urine through the relaxed sphincter.

The Nature of the Beast: Identifying Incontinence

There are several different types of incontinence. The most common is called *stress incontinence* and is the type from which women under the age of sixty are most likely to suffer. It is often the result of damage caused by childbirth to the nerves of the urinary sphincter, but it can also happen after pelvic surgery or because of uterine prolapse or a number of other, less common causes. Stress incontinence occurs when the sphincter muscle is weakened and isn't able to stop urine from flowing out of the bladder. Also contributing are weakened pelvic floor muscles that offer support to the bladder.[5] If they aren't strong enough or are damaged, the bladder can push outward and prevent the muscles that shut the urethra from working.[6] One thing that weakens these muscles is pressure from a sagging bladder.

As the body ages, the bladder gradually loses sensitivity. This can have several consequences. One is that the connection between the bladder and the brain isn't as precise. Like an overflowing bathtub, the bladder is allowed to collect too much urine, which makes it more likely that something as simple as coughing will cause a spill.[7] It's worth mentioning, too, that as we age, the bladder can shrink, which means that it holds a little less urine to begin with.

According to the National Kidney and Urological Diseases Information Clearinghouse, stress incontinence "can worsen during the week before your menstrual period." Although this isn't entirely understood, it is theorized that lower estrogen levels might lessen muscle pressure around the urethra, again making leaks more likely.[8] Although the relationship between estrogen and incontinence is ill-understood, it doesn't stop doctors from extending this theory into menopause and assuming that lowered estrogen levels during menopause are the reason that more women experience incontinence with age.

Urge incontinence is the most common type of incontinence after the age of sixty. It happens when the bladder contracts sharply, often without much warning. A woman who experiences urge incontinence will, out of nowhere, realize that she needs to get to the bathroom urgently.

If stress incontinence is characterized by weakening of the muscles of the urinary tract, urge incontinence happens when the nerves that cue these muscles become unstable or overly sensitive.[9] It is also sometimes called *reflex incontinence*; it may be helpful to think about the way the leg moves after the doctor taps it with a rubber hammer: quickly and strongly. These contractions can be triggered by many different things. Sometimes the "rubber hammer" is sound—the rain or the flowing of tap water; other people find that they may want to urinate after similarly unlikely cues: after drinking a small glass of water or during sleep.[10]

Overflow incontinence happens when the nerves that tell the body to urinate become damaged. It can involve either an overflowing bladder or a blocked urethra. In the second cause, leaking occurs in part because the sufferer isn't able to empty his bladder completely when voiding. Because of this, urine dribbles slowly and constantly out of the body, sort of like a leaking faucet. This type of incontinence isn't seen in women often: its most common sufferer is a man who has been struggling with prostate problems.[11]

If you have trouble controlling urine because of a temporary external factor, such as a medicine you are taking in the short term or an infection, you are said to be experiencing *transient incontinence*.

Some people experience symptoms of more than one type of incontinence; these people are said to experience *mixed incontinence*.

The most common combination is symptoms of both stress and urge.

Urinary tract infections (UTIs) are a major cause of incontinence. *Interstitial cystitis* is a type of bladder infection that causes chronic inflammation of the bladder lining without the external symptoms of a UTI. It causes intense bladder pressure, and sufferers feel the frequent urge to urinate with only small amounts of urine resulting (very similar to urge incontinence). *Diverticulitis* is an intestinal disease in which stool becomes trapped in the intestine and breeds infection-causing bacteria. It causes swelling and bloating that can prevent proper urination. Likewise, constipation can prevent proper urination.

Some drugs known to cause leakage include certain sedatives, alpha-blockers, tricyclic antidepressants, and cold and sleep aids.

Two more terms you might hear are *functional* and *dysfunctional* incontinence. The first means urination problems cause by a disability, a problem communicating the need to use the bathroom, or other non-urinary-tract problems.[12] One cause of incontinence that has nothing to do with a malfunctioning urinary tract is depression. Doctors at Harvard Medical School note that "seriously depressed people may become incontinent because they no longer care about wetting themselves."[13] This is most likely in a seriously disabled or elderly population; however, antidepressants can also aggravate the problem.

Dysfunctional incontinence can involve symptoms of any of the three major types: stress, urge, or overflow. It happens when the brain and the bladder aren't communicating properly.[14]

Seeking Treatment: The Doctor's Visit

The prospect of talking about incontinence with a doctor is daunting for a lot of people. Some are embarrassed; they shouldn't be! Incontinence isn't a failure of will, it's a physical problem. Others just see the problem as one they can handle alone. There are many good reasons not to suffer in silence on this one, but one of the most compelling is that incontinence is rarely—but can be—an indicator of a more serious problem, such as a spinal cord injury, bladder cancer, or diabetes.[15] It is important to know why you are experiencing the problem as well as what you can do about it.

Unfortunately, many doctors aren't as prepared as they should be to deal with incontinence issues. The Public Citizen Health Research Group newsletter notes, "Most physicians are not trained to deal with incontinence, which was aptly described by an English physician more than 100 years ago as 'a symptom and not a disease.' Many doctors are unfamiliar with appropriate diagnostic tests and treatments, and, like their patients, erroneously believe that incontinence is a normal consequence of aging."[16]

Because of this, you may want to make sure that the doctor you are seeing has experience in treating bladder problems. Call the office and speak with the doctor. Ask her if she has treated incontinence before and what sort of treatment options are available—make sure the reply isn't just drugs and surgery.

Getting ready for your visit ahead of time can go a long way to making it easier for both you and your doctor to deal satisfactorily with your symptoms. A good thing to do before you go to the doctor is to keep a record of your urination habits. Most medical publications call this a voiding diary, but all it means is that for about a week, you should write down every day how often you urinate, what time of day you do it, and any episodes of leaking. Also note if anything seems to make the problem worse or better; this could be a medication, a food, an activity—anything that seems to correlate with experiences of incontinence. Write down if anything seems unusual: Is your urine a strange color? Does it have an unusual smell? Is there blood in it? You might also want to use a container and measure the amount of urine for a few days. Do you find that you urinate frequently but don't produce that much liquid?

In the Doctor's Office

The first thing a good doctor should do when you go in complaining of incontinence is to ask questions that would help identify any obvious problems such as UTIs.

UTIs cause burning with urination, the frequent desire to void with little output, pelvic pain, and, in bad cases, blood in the urine.

A woman with a UTI may feel the desire to pee to alleviate pain rather than to empty the bladder. A common instigator of incontinence, an infection is most often caused by the movement of bacteria during sexual intercourse (75 percent of UTIs begin within a day of having sex).

Doctors will treat UTIs with antibiotics, and they can often be prevented by drinking a glass of water before and after sex and being sure to urinate soon after intercourse. If you have recurrent UTIs, your doctor may want to perform a more extensive analysis of the urine to make sure that the correct antibiotic is being used, and that a more serious condition such as diabetes, multiple sclerosis, or cystocele (a condition where the bladder drops into the vagina) isn't the real problem.

Interstitial cystitis is a condition in which the lining of the bladder becomes chronically inflamed. Unlike a UTI, there aren't many outward symptoms of the infection such as blood or excessive bacteria in the urine. Dr. William H. Parker notes that it does, however, cause an "almost constant bladder or pelvic pain or pressure" and explains that sufferers "feel the urge to urinate when there are even small quantities of urine in their bladders."[17]

The cause of this condition is unknown, but doctors suspect that a layer of the bladder that is meant to protect the rest of the muscle from irritation may be either damaged or even absent. If the doctor suspects that this is the problem, a urologist can perform several tests to find out conclusively. Unfortunately, unlike UTI, this problem can't yet be permanently treated because the bladder lining can't be replaced. Dr. Parker explains that "there are a number of treatments presently available," but notes that "each of them is helpful to some women and not others."[18]

Once the doctor has eliminated certain possibilities and performed some routine physical exams, he may want to perform more specific tests to help determine what sort of incontinence you are experiencing and what the root causes might be.

Certain basic chemical tests can be very helpful in eliminating or confirming common causes of incontinence. Your doctor will almost certainly perform a urinalysis, testing a urine sample for the presence of a UTI, urinary stones, and other conditions that might contribute to loss of bladder control.[19] A blood test can check for certain sub-stances that could cause bladder problems.

Many women have ultrasounds as a part of their prenatal care. This procedure can also allow your doctor to see images of your blad-der, kidneys, ureters, or urethra. Another imaging technique is called cystoscopy, in which a small tube with a miniature camera is inserted into the urethra. It allows the doctor to see the urethra and bladder lining. This technology is used to evaluate a number of different uri-nary tract problems, including UTI, and can be used to perform bi-opsy or remove small bladder stones or growths.

If you don't keep a voiding diary before coming to the doctor or if there are still lingering questions, you may be given a special pan to place over the toilet rim to help measure urine quantities and be asked to keep a record of when and how much you pee.

Treatments

We cannot say this strongly enough: if your doctor recommends sur-gery before other options to deal with urinary incontinence, you should probably find another doctor. Again and again incontinence has been shown to respond more efficiently to muscular training than to either pharmaceutical options or surgical intervention. This is not to say that surgery is never the right option—sometimes it is—but there are many things that should be explored first.

The first line of treatment (and still the most successful) is *muscle therapy*. Kegel exercises, which are performed by tightening urethra and pelvic floor muscles, are a very effective way to treat stress prob-lems. Although there is some controversy about the exercises (some doctors feel it is too difficult to perform them correctly) it is believed that Kegels can improve incontinence in nearly 50 percent of women who practice them. For a description of how (and how often) to per-form Kegel exercises, see page 87. Your doctor may recommend using a weighted cone. The cone is inserted into the vagina and held there as you perform muscle contractions. Over time, the weight is in-creased as the muscles strengthen. The extra weight helps work the muscles that keep the urethra closed.[20]

A *therapeutic pessary*, a small, stiff, circular device, can be inserted into the vagina by a doctor or nurse. Once in, it presses against the vaginal walls, exerting pressure that slowly begins to reposition the urethra. This is generally used to treat only stress problems. The disadvantage of pessaries is that the device can increase your chances of developing a vaginal or urinary infection, which, as we know, can actually cause incontinence. A device called a urethral insert, a small plug that the patient can insert when not in the bathroom and then remove when ready to void and replace when finished, has similar problems. Urine seals work on a similar principle; a small pad is placed over the urethra. When it is time to go to the bathroom, the pad is removed and thrown out. Because it is disposable, it is less prone to bacterial growth and so less likely to cause a UTI.

Biofeedback and *electrical stimulation* are two other options in which small electrodes are affixed to the vagina and rectum. The purpose of biofeedback is to stimulate the muscles and make a patient aware of which parts are involved in controlling urination. Electrical stimulation seeks to strengthen the muscles by using currents to imitate the process of exercise and also to regulate overactive muscles.

For urge incontinence, *retraining the bladder* may be the best solution. The goal of this therapy is threefold: first, to increase the amount of urine the bladder can hold; second, to lengthen the amount of time between urination; and third, to increase the patient's overall bladder control.[21]

In addition to Kegel exercises, you start slowly increasing the time between bathroom visits. At first, this may mean waiting five or ten extra minutes before heading for the toilet. It is hoped that visits will soon be limited to around once an hour or once every two hours. Eventually, the time between toilet breaks is increased to once every three or four hours. If you have trouble delaying your visits, the American Academy of Family Physicians recommends practicing relaxation techniques: "Breathe slowly and deeply. Concentrate on your breathing until the urge goes away."[22] You may also want to try scheduling bathroom trips: write down an exact time to visit the bathroom and try to stick to it.

A lot of articles on incontinence advise drinking less coffee, alcohol, tea, and other liquids. While this isn't bad advice—caffeine and alcohol are dehydrating and are also diuretics (substances that increase your desire to urinate)—be very careful not to interpret this advice as a directive to stop drinking fluids; staying well hydrated is important to your overall health.

If you are overweight, you simply have more weight pressing on the bladder. Losing even small amounts of weight can sometimes go a long way to alleviating leakage. Another recent intervention is collagen injection. In this procedure, also called *urethral bulking*, bovine (cow) collagen is injected into the urinary sphincter. According to doctors at Harvard, this collagen is broken down by the body and becomes scar tissue that strengthens the pelvic muscles, like sandbags on the edge of a dam. Because this is a fairly new way to treat the problem, there is a lot of safety information still to be collected and a lot we still don't know about the mechanism by which this therapy works. Why, for example, is it so successful in treating certain women and totally ineffective in others? This is a temporary solution, with two or three injections providing relief for about a year.[23]

A July 2005 report in *Obstetrics and Gynecology* found that *acupuncture* provided relief for women with urge incontinence.[24] In a small trial performed through the department of obstetrics and gynecology at Oregon Health and Science University in Portland, Drs. Sandra Emmons and Lesley Otto found that women in their early fifties found comparable symptom relief from acupuncture as they did from drug or behavioral therapy. Since the trial didn't test for long-term efficacy, it would be interesting to see more work done in this area.

As we said at the beginning of the chapter, *incontinence drugs* are so much less effective in treating the problem than nonpharmaceutical options that most good doctors will recommend turning to pills only as a last resort. As one doctor explains bluntly, "Drug therapy is . . . only marginally helpful, partly because side effects may be nearly as troublesome as the incontinence itself." And we know that some drugs can also *cause* incontinence. The health advocate Maryann Napoli notes that diuretics, hypertension drugs such as Serpasil, ACE inhibitors, and tricyclic antidepressants can aggravate the problem.[25]

For many years HT was prescribed off label for treating incontinence. Once the WHI results were in, we learned that incontinence is yet another condition that is actually made worse, not better, by estrogen.[26] This is true of estrogen alone and estrogen plus progestin.

Something many articles about incontinence drugs don't make clear is that different types of the disorder are treated with different classes of drugs. What works for stress incontinence can be ineffective or even damaging for urge incontinence, and vice versa.

For stress incontinence, some doctors prescribe stimulants such as phenylpropanolamine and pseudoephedrine. These are more commonly used as decongestants, and if you look at any package of Ny-Quil, Tylenol Cold and Flu, or Sudafed, you will see pseudoephedrine listed as the major active ingredient. These drugs are technically called "alpha-adrenergic agonists" and they work by strengthening the urethra and bladder neck and helping them to hold in urine.

Detrol (tolterodine), the most famous brand in a class of drugs called anticholinergics, is commonly used to treat urge incontinence. If you are considering these drugs, you should know that they have some pretty nasty side effects. These include dry mouth, constipation, blurred vision, and (take a deep breath here) *inability to urinate*. Talk about going from the frying pan into the fire! Like just about every other drug class in the world, anticholinergics are now also available in patch form. While this could mean fewer side effects, it is far too early to say.

Overflow incontinence can be treated with a class of medications called alpha-blockers. These are more commonly prescribed for high blood pressure but are thought to help overflow incontinence by affecting the nerves that control the bladder.

Notice how we've left *surgery* for last? Well that's because surgery should always be a last resort. In some circumstances, other treatments are tried without success and a patient still continues to suffer. At this point, surgical options can reasonably be pursued. These options include repositioning a bladder that has slipped, and using a sling made out of synthetic material or tissue from the body to prevent urine leakage by supporting the urethra.

So finally, after all this discussion, you may be thinking: But what about menopause? *Is* there a relationship between incontinence and menopause? Again the truth is, we don't know.

As we discussed in chapter 6, on sexuality, there is good evidence that the urogenital tissues thin after menopause. This means that the vagina and bladder lose elasticity. That is why some women experience vaginal tearing with sex at midlife. It is possible that this can account for some of the failure to function on the part of the urethra and urinary sphincter. This thinning may be due to estrogen decline. It is worth remembering, though, that *all* the tissues in the body tend to thin or shrink with age.

Most likely, although there is probably some relationship between incontinence and hormone fluctuation, the problem itself is the result of multiple factors, including aging, wear and tear on the body, genetic predisposition, and luck. It is easy to simplify and say, "It's menopause," but this is taking the easy way out. Ignoring the complexity of women's medical experiences doesn't help us get any closer to improving our quality of life at menopause and beyond.

section four

meno-politics

21

male menopause
how the other half changes

Is there such a thing as male menopause?" a relative of Laura's
asked her in a hushed voice over a festive New Year's dinner.

"Sure there is, honey," Laura's cousin Gail retorted. "It's also
known as 'a sports car and a blonde.'"

While this answer is funny, the question is a serious one that men
and the women who love them ask us a lot. Gail's quick response
gives humorous treatment to a very serious divide in the way we talk
about men's and women's life transitions. For years now, we have assumed that men have a "midlife crisis"—a psychological transition—
and women have a "menopause"—a biological one.[1] Increasingly, we
are starting to acknowledge that much of what women define as
menopause is really a matter of dealing with various psychological
turning points at midlife, and likewise that men also experience a
profound physical transition as they enter their middle and later
years.[2]

But how do we define this male transition? When people ask us
if men go through menopause, we assume they are wondering if men
go through a comparable hormonal transition to the decline in female estrogen. While men don't undergo a dramatic, quick drop in
hormones, they do experience gradual declines in their natural hormone production. When doctors or scientists approach this question, the answer is confused, because some focus on this decline in
testosterone and sex drive, while others believe a more complicated
physical process is taking place.

In the past two decades, the language surrounding the idea of male menopause has ranged from humorous to unwittingly revealing of medical double standards. While doctors have been consistently willing to attribute physical symptoms to female menopause without adequate evidence, they balk at the notion of doing the same with andropause, the natural decline in testosterone that accompanies aging in men.

"Male menopause? Forget it! It's a myth," exclaimed the University of Chicago's *Better Health* newsletter dismissively. "The changes men go through have more to do with natural aging than the serious physical . . . upheaval women experience." This article was written in the mid-'90s, at a time when doctors were eagerly pushing HT on female patients for the yet-unproven purpose of preventing heart disease and were ignoring the well-known reproductive cancer risks. Yet the same doctors backed away from the possibility of hormone drugs—testosterone therapy in particular—for men because it "may lead to prostate hypertrophy or cancer and increased risk of heart disease"![3] (The exclamation point is ours.)

The same article explains that far from being the result of declining hormones, the symptoms experienced by many male patients are things that "many men experience in middle age, including an increase in body fat, increased cholesterol levels, a decrease in bone and muscle mass, and the loss of energy, virility and fertility."[4] It is fascinating that in women, the same problems are readily accepted as the result of hormone fluctuation, but when they occur in men, we are urged to understand each change as a discrete biological event.

Josh Fischman, in writing an article on the mood swings, sexual changes, and other physical symptoms encountered by men at midlife, found strong resistance to connecting these problems with hormone changes. He writes, "My own reviewers didn't want me to put 'male menopause' in the title because it's so controversial."[5] He ended up writing about "age-associated testosterone decline" in men, noting, "Low testosterone can be tied to a sense of figurative and literal impotence. . . . That doesn't mean that any man with midlife malaise should go on testosterone replacement therapy."

Couldn't we make the same argument about women? Aren't we,

like the men around us, hitting major psychological transitions in our forties and fifties?

The reality is that both male and female hormones are constantly changing throughout our lives. Estrogen decline begins years before it becomes evident to us that it's happening. Men begin to lose testosterone in midlife, but at a comparably slow rate. The confusion comes, in both cases, from a failure to identify clearly the points of intersection between hormonal shifts and multiple other biological processes.

Trying to grapple with what exactly is going on with men at midlife, Alvaro Morales, Jeremy P. W. Heaton, and Culley C. Carson III explain that while "a progressive decrease in androgen production is common in males after middle age," and the term *male menopause,* or *andropause,* "adequately conveys the concept of emotional and physical changes that, although related to aging in general, are associated with significant hormonal alterations,"[6] "menopause" is still inaccurate for a few reasons.

First, even though testosterone declines in most men, they don't lose fertility. Second, not all men experience testosterone decline, whereas all women who live long enough experience estrogen decline.

While it is true that all women eventually lose fertility, a failure to acknowledge the gradual nature of estrogen loss in women and a mistaken notion that it suddenly ceases has led to the cavalier overprescription of total hysterectomy in women.

It's not the idea that men change both biologically and mentally at this point in their lives that bothers Morales and his colleagues, it's the application to men of words that originally applied to women. The study authors suggest instead the more macho term "androgen decline in the aging male," or "ADAM." Take that, Eve!

Perhaps a conversation about the commonalities of men and women at midlife and beyond is as useful as cataloguing our differences. We know, for example, that many men, in addition to declining testosterone, experience "poor sex drive, tiredness and fatigue, acknowledgement of aging, hair loss and changes in body shape as they become less muscular and more rounded."[7] According to BBC

News, some men also have "irritability, sweating, flushing, general-ized aches and pains and low mood, sometimes depression." They conclude, "Many doctors acknowledge that a genuine change for men occurs, but believe it has a psychological basis rather than a hor-monal one. The realization that they've left youth behind is rein-forced by the signs of wrinkles, receding hairline and fat."

If hormone shifts in men aren't necessarily tied to mood, fatigue, and other symptoms, why do we assume they are in women?

We aren't suggesting that doctors are wrong about the limited nature of men's changes at midlife. Rather, we are saying that women should be a lot more skeptical about all of the things about our bod-ies or our minds that are quickly diagnosed and dismissed as results of "menopause." Midlife is a time of change, and the psychological impact on both men and women is broad and far-reaching.

Men are lucky in that so far a certain amount of sexism has led to skepticism in the medical community about unfounded claims of what is or isn't male menopause. However, dollars are without gen-der, and it seems just a matter of time before midlife pharmaceuti-cals—be they hormonal or of another kind—will be showered on men just as HT and so many other drugs have been on women.

Let's hope this doesn't happen. Let's hope we can learn from each other.

22

half the sky
menopause around the world

eventually, I had to stop asking." The anthropologist is talking about hot flashes. She is sitting in a rural Mayan village surrounded by smiling older women with weatherworn faces. The interview, recorded for the 1998 Canadian television documentary *Hot Flash on Menopause*, raises some important but hard-to-answer questions about how much of any of our menopause experiences are products of the time and place in which we live. How does our culture, which has so much to do with our understanding of the world around us, also shape the ways we view our own bodies and medical issues?

When the anthropologist first began working with Mayan women, she prodded them about hot flashes. When none of her subjects responded, she began to frame the questions in different ways, thinking that perhaps her meaning was lost in translation. At some point it became clear to her that in fact none of the women had ever experienced the thing we, living in North America, take for granted to be the calling card of the menopause transition. We can learn a lot both about culture and biology when we look at menopause around the world and ask some provocative questions about our own attitudes about aging.

In many ways, we're very lucky; we live in a culture that treats women pretty well. Both the first- and second-wave feminist movements helped to change forever the way that women live their lives and brought menopause into public life as a topic for discussion. Unfortunately, we don't live in a world that deals as well with aging. We believe in youth and don't have much time for anyone over forty, particularly older women.

Margaret Morganroth Gullette, a scholar at Brandeis University's Women's Studies Research Center, has written a lot about how we construct our midlife experiences. She writes, "Ageism is an ancient prejudice, but middle-ageism is our own local twentieth-century toxin."[1] Her belief is that we are taught to think so negatively about what might happen as we age that we turn decades of our lives into a "disease state." In the same way that we talk about menopause being medicalized, middle age is also turned into a time when we expect that the body will slowly break down along with the life we have built around it.

Getting older in American society has become something of a cautionary tale about who you don't want to become: the powerless, sick, unattractive person who spends all her time lamenting her youth. We tell this story to our young people and perpetuate the equally ludicrous notion that if you buy the right products and do the right things, you can somehow stay young forever.

The quest for the fountain of youth is as old as humanity. But for centuries, finding it had to do with avoiding death. Today, we fear age much more than death. Because of this, our middle years become an increasingly charged border between who we are told we should be—young people—and who we all, if we are lucky, become—old people.

Gullette writes that by middle age, we have come to understand that age means certain things and to associate negative qualities and experiences with it.[2] The story we have come to understand about the progressive decline of aging isn't true. It is created by a society that loves youth and hasn't tried to understand or appreciate age. While we have been busy thinking and obsessing over all the bad parts of getting older, we didn't notice that there are a lot of really wonderful qualities that come with the years, including maturity, experience, a sense of self, and compassion.

This is because we have let the idea of being "normal" become synonymous with being "youthful." This creates a situation where everyone who isn't young is necessarily abnormal and therefore sick.

It is a good way to create insecurities and sell lots of products, but it is ultimately a bad way to look at the world if you are a person getting older in it (as we all are).

What are some of the lessons we have learned from studying menopause around the world?

Most important, we find that women in countries where the end of menstrual periods constitutes a positive change in status have fewer physical symptoms—or mind them less—than those of us in places where the opposite is true. It was, after all, based on such an understanding of menopause around the world that led the legendary anthropologist Margaret Mead to coin her famous phrase, "postmenopausal zest."

One of the first recent anthropologists to do work in the field was a woman named Marcia Flint, who studied Rajput women in India in the 1970s. Before menopause, Rajput women were forced to live apart from men and wear veiled garments. After the end of menstruation, the women could "come downstairs from their women's quarters to where the men talked and drank their home brew. . . . The Rajput women could publicly visit and joke with men after attaining menopause."[3] Flint was struck by the women's lack of symptoms and concluded, "what we call 'menopausal symptomatology' may well be culturally defined."

Likewise, Yewoubdar Beyene famously found no hot flashes among rural Mayan women in the Yucatan. As part of her doctoral thesis, Bene compared the women with others from a Greek fishing village and found that while the Mayan women had no menopause symptoms, the Greek women had problems similar to those in North America.[4] The Mayan women understood menopause in these terms: you had a certain amount of menstrual blood, and when it was gone, you were done having babies. For others it simply meant never getting another period after your last baby.

The language we use to talk about menopause has a huge impact on how we experience it. A woman named Donna Lee Davis studied the transition in a Newfoundland fishing village and found that the women used culturally unique ways of talking about their experiences. For example, they felt that when you stopped menstruating, the remaining blood had nowhere to go. Believing this to be bad for the health, the women were more likely to experience certain problems and generally to be unwell.[5]

The anthropologist Margaret Lock found that rural Japanese women had no specific word for "hot flash." Perhaps partly because of biology and partly because of sociology, hot flashes are significantly less frequent in Japan.[6] There are certainly biological and environmental components to symptoms; the Mayan women's dearth of flashing may also be due in part to diet or genetics or environment. But there is more to it than that.

If you expect to experience a problem, it is more likely to happen. Lynnette Leidy Sievert, in gathering available international data on menopause, found joint pain—*not* hot flashes or bleeding—to be the most frequently mentioned and complained-about symptom.[7] In other places it is culturally understood as a common menopause problem and is a bonding point for women in the way that we deal with flashing. Thinking about menopause around the world—our differences and our similarities—helps us to imagine new possibilities for the transition. We can see that the lines between the medical and the social and psychological are more fluid than we may have imagined, and the positive aspects more numerous that we have been led to believe.

We can also understand that the line between pre-, peri-, and postmenopause is similarly fluid. In the end, our lives as women are at once continuous and the collection of so many discrete events. They are not the arbitrary transitions of the doctor's office but rather our own collection of moments and continuous biological changes that weave together in ways that are as unique as our fingerprints.

For decades, "menopause" was code for "middle age" as well as an illness. We have managed to gain at least some level of public acknowledgment that this last association of illness was erroneous and hurtful to women. Now let us work to a fight ageism and middle-ageism. It's more important that ever because, among other things, it will help us to connect effectively with our daughters and younger women on important health issues.

We believe that one of the reasons menopause has the potential to be so difficult is that young women don't prepare enough for the second half of their lives. It's easy to laugh about teenagers and twenty-somethings believing themselves to be invincible, but the truth is that in our culture, thinking about your health in later decades means admitting you are going to get old. We are unwilling to do that at forty and fifty, so why are we surprised when women in their teens and twenties and even thirties aren't interested? This is a shame, because crucial health interventions that could take place at younger ages don't. By the time your periods get irregular, you have already missed decades of lifestyle changes that could have made huge differences in how your menopause—and the decades beyond it—will be.

Menopause is a young women's issue in the way that aging health has so effectively become a menopausal women's issue. You can't compartmentalize your life and put off health decisions for another day.

Together we can change all of this. We can work toward a future that acknowledges both the good and the bad parts of aging and embraces its strengths as well as fearing its problems. We can better understand the big psychological and social changes going on in our middle years so that we don't act their stresses out on our bodies. We can come to see our lives as what they are: fluid, cohesive, challenging, and—if we are lucky—long enough to look back on menopause from some distance.

afterword
becoming a
no-nonsense patient
a crash course in the
basics of health literacy

Y ou start to become a "no-nonsense" patient when you realize that the healthiest thing you can do for yourself is to increase your health literacy. What exactly does this mean? Well, first, it means getting comfortable and confident enough to read medical information and learn for yourself what has been *proven* to be safe or helpful and what hasn't. It means becoming well-versed in your options, including the possibility of doing or taking nothing at all. It means learning to be assertive in doctors' visits, asking good questions, and making the most of your time with medical professionals. Most of all, it means when you know that you are healthy, having confidence and the wisdom to reach out for solid resources on the Internet or in the print media, as well as knowing when to go to the doctor's office when you aren't.

It is a very exciting, liberating thing to say, "I am in charge of my body and I am capable of deciding what is good for it." If you were never very good in biology, or if, like Laura, you find leafing through the *Journal of the American Medical Association* to be about as much fun as going to the dentist, this can also be a very scary process. Scientific and technical lingo can be intimidating or frustrating, and sometimes just the large amount of available information (half of which conflicts with the other half) can overwhelm even the most dedicated health connoisseur. But if we can do it, so can you, and this section is designed to help you cut your way through the jungle of health misinformation, to tell the real studies from the ersatz ones, and to understand some of the more complicated issues at stake in menopause medicine. It is no-nonsense boot camp.

Medical knowledge has always been understood to be a powerful tool, and possessing this knowledge gives doctors and scientists an authority unequaled in many other professions. This power is not maintained by making medical information easy to understand. After all, if we could do it ourselves, then we wouldn't need them as much. As far back as 1555, the Royal College of Physicians advised, "let no physicians teach the people about medicines or even tell them the names," and as recently as the 1930s there were laws mandating that the *Physicians Desk Reference* be "in language not understandable by the average person." For too long the right to understand medical information has been regulated through language. When information is presented in complicated, inaccessible words, it limits who can use or evaluate it.

At a January 2005 conference on Health Advocacy at Sarah Lawrence College, women, most of whom were nondoctors working in the health professions, puzzled over the question of how to help increase health literacy among the public. Laura was troubled by an assumption in some of the group that an average person *couldn't possibly* understand medical literature. We believe that with just a little extra knowledge, you can. The idea, of course, isn't to do without doctors; both of us love our doctors, and when we think something is wrong, we don't hesitate to consult with them. Rather it's that, in the words of Cy and Marcie Syms's clothing store commercials, "an educated consumer is the best customer." The best patient is someone who can interact confidently with her doctor and can fully understand the choices they are making.

What's Up, Doc? How to Have the Best Doctor's Visit Possible

A simple doctor's visit can be an incredibly complicated process; there's no guidebook that tells you which questions to ask, what drugs or treatments to avoid, and how to tell if your doctor is the right woman for the job. Moreover, while having a good visit can be a tough thing for anyone, for menopausal women there are unique challenges. Consider two different stories that both raise key issues women face when they go to discuss "the change" with their health care professional.

Several years ago, a friend of Barbara's complained that she was having a terrible time on hormone replacement therapy (HRT). When Barbara asked her why she continued taking the drug, her friend replied, "for heart disease prevention." Barbara assured her that there was no solid evidence that HRT was cardioprotective and reminded her that the FDA had never approved the drug for this purpose. "I asked my doctor how long I would have to be on it," her friend said, "and he said, 'Well, that depends; when do you want your first heart attack?'"

Several months ago, Laura was having a conversation with a friend who was experiencing common menopause symptoms like night sweats, hot flashes, and mood swings. Her friend was distraught and ready to try anything to alleviate her symptoms. Laura was about to launch into a standard speech she gives about how everything the woman was feeling was normal, and how she should just hold tight—yada yada yada—when her friend interrupted: "The worst part is, I went to my doctor last week. He told me I'm totally fine—everything is normal. I don't feel normal. And I feel like he was ignoring me."

What is a menopausal gal to do? How do you strike a balance between feeling that your doctor is ignoring you and avoiding physicians who unnecessarily advocate potentially dangerous long-term "preventive medicines"? On an even more basic level, how do you know which questions to ask and how to make sure that you are an active, informed, assertive health consumer?

Doing Your Homework: How to Find a Good Doctor

How do you find a good doctor? This can be a hard question and is one we are frequently asked by friends. You may not actually have a choice about who you see, as many managed care and insurance plans make it hard to be choosy. One way to find a good doctor is to ask friends; you can also ask other doctors you know for the names of colleagues whom they would recommend within a specific specialty. Either way, referrals are a good place to start.

Unfortunately, while your friends may know doctors they have a good rapport with, they may not be able to assess other important qualities. As one expert says, "While all good doctors may be kind, not all kind doctors are good." As a health consumer, you should be double-checking your doctor's credentials; *Consumer Reports* estimates that "5% of physicians applying to managed-care plans had made up phony credentials—including false residency training, board certification and clinical experience."[1] In a study performed in Connecticut in which doctors were investigated at random using the Yellow Pages, 12 percent of "specialists" lacked standard board certification for their specialty.

Obviously, a doctor has gone to medical school. In the United States, most med schools are roughly the same in quality; don't be overly concerned with finding a doctor who attended a certain school. You might want to watch out for doctors who attended medical school out of the country; while some non-U.S. medical schools are as fine— or finer—than many American ones, there are many offshore medical schools that have vastly lower standards. As one writer says, they can be "outright diploma mills." So if your doctor received her training outside the United States, you might want to look up her medical school to see how it's assessed by an objective third party.

Once doctors complete their first several years of school, they are asked in most states to perform a residency, which is a two-to-three-year training period, before they get a medical license. While most med schools are created equal, where a doctor performed her residency can make a big difference, particularly if you are trying to find a specialist. Two ways to check where a doctor did a residency are looking in the American Medical Association's (AMA) Medical Directory (which you can find at the library or online at the AMA's Web site) or simply calling and asking the doctor's staff.[2]

Another litmus test of a doctor's dedication and skill level vis-à-vis her particular specialty is whether or not she is board certified. While acquiring certification is a voluntary process, most studies suggest that board-certified doctors provide better care. *Consumer Reports* cautions, though, "Ignore the claim 'board-eligible.' It doesn't mean anything, and can simply mean that they failed the test."[3] You can find out if a doctor is board certified by calling the American Board of Medical Specialties, a seventy-year-old not-for-profit organization that monitors twenty-four major medical boards (www .abms.org or 1-866-ASK-ABMS).

Although certain types of continuing medical education (CME) can be a sign that a doctor is interested in keeping up on recent developments in a field, CME can have serious problems as it is often written or underwritten—paid for—by drug companies and therefore more often than not recommends pills and pharmaceutical approaches to problems. So while doctors may be reading "the latest" information on a certain subject, that knowledge may be biased. Another way doctors do CME is through membership in a medical specialty society. To confirm that a doctor is a member of such a society, contact the society by e-mail or phone.

Some other things to look for include hospital affiliation. Hospitals have access to databases and other information sources that health consumers don't have; in other words, they have more ways to double-check that a doctor's qualifications are legit. The National Practitioner Data Bank, for example, keeps records of all malpractice payments made by and disciplinary actions taken against a certain doctor.[4] It is unlikely that a respectable hospital, knowing of any seriously questionable behavior in a doctor's background, would want the responsibility of having that doctor on staff. (As a side note, consumer advocacy groups have been fighting for years to get the public and consumers the right to use this list.[5] Why it still isn't available is a mystery, and as far as we are concerned, patients have the right to full disclosure on such serious subjects.[6])

Before You Go: Making and Getting Ready for an Appointment

So you've chosen a doctor, you've looked into her qualifications, and you are ready to make an appointment. When you call, make sure you explain to the receptionist or the doctor herself the reasons you are coming in. One result of managed care has been that doctors are required to fit more patients into each day, so visits are generally shorter, and it is up to the patient to see that they aren't getting short-changed. Letting the staff know all of the medical issues you are coming in for is the first step in helping the doctor make sure you get the time you deserve.

If you don't like waiting, one thing you can do is to ask the receptionist to schedule you for either the first appointment of the day or for the first appointment after lunch. The doctor will usually be on time for these time slots, as there is no chance of the previous appointment running over.[7]

Don't be afraid to ask up front how much the visit will cost you. Remember that you are a consumer: you wouldn't buy a pair of pants without a price tag or without asking a salesperson how much they were, and a trip to the doctor's should be no different. As a consumer of health care, you have the right to know how much you will be paying and to shop comparatively if you want.

The week before a first trip to a new doctor, visit the doctor's office casually to get a feel for the place. If you find that you are already uncomfortable or see anything that concerns you, cancel your appointment. It's also a good idea to sit down at some point before the visit and write up a list of relevant information, including family histories, health problems you've had throughout your life, drugs you've taken (both prescription and over-the-counter as well as vitamins and herbal preparations), drugs that you are allergic to or have had bad experiences with, major illnesses, the dates of surgeries performed, and anything else that you might forget in the more rushed environment of the doctor's office. While you're at it, compose a list of all the health concerns that you want to discuss with the doctor, including information about when your symptoms occur, what seems to make them better, what seems to make them worse, and how long you've been having the problem. Once you've written down all your health concerns, rank them in order of importance. If you have pertinent medical records, copies of X-rays, or lab results, collect them to bring with you. If you are having these sent to the doctor, call ahead of time to make sure they have arrived.

Your doctor can't read your mind; *you* have to tell him what is going on. As women, we are not always as confident as we should be in speaking up and talking about personal health concerns. Many women need to work their way around to discussing certain menopausal topics such as vaginal dryness, sexual problems, or incontinence; these seem like such personal things, and we may be embarrassed that we are going through them. To prepare for the possibility that you might find yourself tongue-tied when it comes to discussing tough subjects, prepare a list of questions you want to ask. Underline the ones that you think might be harder to ask and make a promise to yourself not to let them go. Remember, your doctor has heard it all and is there to help, not to judge you.

You may want to do some research on your symptoms or health problems before you talk to the doctor, and there are many places to do this. The Internet has become a major destination for health information and can be very useful for just that purpose, but it can also be hard to tell the wheat from the chaff. A good general rule of thumb is that information from universities and federal government organizations tends to be more reliable (although they are certainly not without biases). That is, of course, insofar as it can be trusted that you are seeing real research, if not necessarily good research. Never forget that studies conducted by respected institutions and published in renowned journals can have serious flaws, provide you with spotty information, and come to unwarranted or even dangerous conclusions. A basic Web site like the Mayo Clinic (www.mayoclinic.com) or the government-run MedlinePlus (www.medlineplus.gov) is a good place to start because these sites are geared to helping you assess symptoms, not telling you how to treat them. They also have the advantage of being in simple English, not medical jargon. After reading our sections below on how to read and assess a study, we are sure you will also feel confident going to a more technical source such as medical journals or a health database like the National Library of Medicine's PubMed (pubmed.org will get you to the registration page).[8] These can be overwhelming in terms of both the sheer volume of information presented and the technical language that is used to present it. However, when it comes to your health, it always pays to act like the smartest kid in the class and do the extra work.

If you find information you want to discuss with your doctor, either print it out or take notes on it, including the Web site address. The same is true if you read something in a magazine or newspaper that piques your interest. Between doctor's visits, think about keeping a file with clippings of articles or printed information from the Web that you want to address on your next doctor's visit.

Doc Talk: Once You're in the Office

You have your lists, records, and questions to discuss and you are sitting in the doctor's office, waiting for the nurse in the white jacket holding the clipboard to call your name. Now what? Setting the right tone and creating open and equal lines of communication can be a major challenge. Lots of women have wonderful doctors who listen and encourage them to speak, but many women have a different experience; we want to make sure that they are equally prepared to take charge of office visits.

First things first: you might want to bring along a small tape recorder and ask if it is all right for you to record the appointment. If your doctor says no, or if you would prefer it, take notes. Make sure your doctor has all the information you have collected and either presented to her or sent in advance. In addition to the list of medications you're taking, you may also want to bring in the pill bottles themselves.

A study published in the *Journal of the American Medical Association (JAMA)* found that the majority of doctors interrupt their patients' opening statements, as well as the concerns and words that follow.[9] Doctors don't do this to be inconsiderate; they are usually just overeager to help. Since you want to set the right tone, however, don't be afraid to interrupt back if this happens to you. Say, "I'm sorry, I wasn't finished yet," and continue with what you were saying. If it happens again, just add, "I'd really appreciate it if you wouldn't speak until I'm done."

Kansas poet and wise women's health writer Barbara Seaman (yes, oddly enough, there is another) writes that part of the problem patients face in having a good doctor's visit has to do with lacking a common communication style and concept of what the doctor and patient roles are: "If you are wondering why so many office visits turn into a tug of war, it's partly because doctors and patients are on different ends of the rope. To the doctor, illness is a disease process that can be measured and understood through laboratory tests and clinical observation, but to the patient, illness is a disrupted life."[10] Many doctors still see themselves as authority figures imparting wisdom. While this certainly isn't always a problem, the *JAMA* report found that on the whole, doctors do much more talking at patients than listening to them.[11]

If you feel your doctor is talking over you or not addressing your concerns, be honest. Say, "I feel you aren't hearing what I'm saying. Please listen. It is extremely important for me to tell you that . . ." If your doctor responds that he is listening, just politely say, "Thank you. I'd feel better if I said it again, just for my own peace of mind." Remember, you can reiterate your concerns as many times as you would like until you are confident and comfortable that you have been heard. When your doctor is speaking, particularly when you are being offered advice, don't be afraid to ask for more information. Seaman notes that "doctors underestimate the amount of information patients want and overestimate how much they actually give."[12] If your doctor tells you that you are suffering from a specific condition or recommends a certain drug, it is absolutely in your best interest to ask *a lot* of questions.

Your doctor may want to prescribe medication for one or more of your symptoms or conditions. It is important that you understand why she is prescribing the drug and exactly how it should be taken. Dr. Alan N. Schwartz notes that while doctors are often good at discussing the common risks of taking a drug, they often "neglect to mention uncommon ones. Ask the doctor to explain all the risks of taking a drug, as well as the risks of forgoing treatment."[13] If you are

what to ask before you start popping: key questions about prescription drugs

1. Is this drug FDA-approved to treat my symptoms/health problem? (It's not illegal to prescribe a drug for off-label use, but it can be unwise.)
2. Why do you think a drug approach is the best way to go?
3. What might be some nonmedical things we could do that might also work?
4. What will happen if I decide not to treat this problem?
5. What kind of studies have been performed on this drug (including size, nature, and duration of the study)?
6. What are some of the known side effects of this drug? Which ones are either serious or potentially life-threatening?
7. How long do you think I should take this drug? Is it a long-term prescription?
8. How much does this drug cost? Will it add a financial burden to my life?

uncomfortable with taking a certain drug, then say so. Don't be afraid: it's your body, and you have the right to make decisions about what to do with it.

If your doctor is speaking in language that is too technical for you, speak up. Say, "I don't really understand what you mean. Can you say that in a different, more simple way?" or "Can you go over that in plain English [or Spanish, or whatever language you are conversing in]?" Say it again and again and again, until you feel confident that you have understood what is being said. If it would help you understand, don't hesitate to ask your doctor to show you photos or illustrations of what she is talking about. Some people learn better visually, and your doctor should be able to accommodate this.

Remember, the best doctor in the world can't help you if you aren't honest. Speak up about your concerns and symptoms. Don't say what you think the doctor wants to hear: don't tell your doctor you are exercising if you aren't or that you aren't smoking if you are. By withholding such information, you are potentially denying yourself crucial health knowledge. For example, if a young woman is a smoker and tells her doctor that she doesn't smoke, she may not be told that smoking and taking birth control pills can seriously compound risks of developing or aggravating chronic health problems.

When both you and your doctor feel that the appointment is over, ask your doctor to summarize some of the major points of the meeting. If you haven't taken notes or recorded the meeting, you could ask to have a written summary of the visit sent to you after you leave. After you finish, ask the receptionist for copies of lab test results and other information to keep in a personal medical file at home. Finally, make a plan to get in touch with the doctor and update her on any side effects with drugs or changes in your health that have occurred since your visit.

If You Decide to Go the Pharmaceutical Route

Should you opt to start taking a drug, you have to be very careful to educate yourself about some basic points, such as the generic name of the drug and its different prescribed doses. One reason is that prescription errors are a major source of serious health problems in America, particularly among older adults. In 1996, the FDA estimated that around 17 percent of all hospitalizations among elderly Americans were caused by the side effects of prescription drugs. According to Johns Hopkins Medical School, "these side effects often occur because errors are made when a prescription is written, filled, or taken home."[14]

It is also estimated that of the average five prescription drugs that the older American is asked to take, many are either unnecessary or inappropriate. According to a report issued by the Government Accounting Office, nearly 6 million of the nation's 30 million non-hospitalized Medicare patients take prescription drugs that either duplicate another drug or are considered unsafe for the patient's age group.[15]

As we age, getting the wrong medicine or the wrong amount of a necessary medicine is much more dangerous than when we were younger. Our kidney and liver functions slow down, which means our bodies break down chemicals at a slower rate. Also, our ratio of fat to muscle increases and the amount of water in our body tissues decreases, which has the effect of concentrating the amount of medication in our bodies. These changes can substantially, idiosyncratically affect the way a pill works for you, so don't be afraid to ask your doctor about the drugs she prescribes for you.

Always know both the brand names and generic names of your medications; this will help protect you if your doctor has messy handwriting. Tell the pharmacists the name of the drug you've been prescribed and make sure that it matches what they think is written on the prescription; if there are any problems, have them contact your physician. We all know the old jokes about doctors and how bad their handwriting is, but the consequences of this are far from humorous.

One way to tell a good pharmacy: it hands out printed information about your medications written in plain language. This should explain how to use the drug, what serious side effects to watch out for, and any other important information you should know. If the dosage on the package is different from the one on your prescription slip, check it with your doctor. Don't use the medicine if the dosage is not what you discussed with your doctor, even if it is the same drug. Check your refills; if the pills appear to be different from the original you might want to speak to your doctor about it.

There are more than fifteen thousand names of drugs on the market, each with one or more generic or brand names; Cornell University Medical School estimates that "overall, nearly 650 pairs of drugs have names that look or sound similar."[16] So you get drugs with names like Prozac and Prilosec, Lamisil and Lamictal, Zyrtec and Zyprexa, and Fosamax and Flomax. It is not uncommon for a pharmacist unintentionally (and again, perhaps because of the doctor's poor writing) to mix up the two.

Then there is always the controversial subject of pill splitting. Many older people don't need the amount of medicine contained in a standard dose. If you fall into this group, splitting pills can be safe as long as you do so in consultation with your doctor. But beware: not all drugs should be split, as some medications act by a time-release method built into the pill, and cutting them can cause the medicine to be distributed erratically in your body. Cutting the coatings on pills can also limit their ability to protect your stomach from irritation. If you are a candidate for pill splitting, don't try to cut pills by hand. Go to the pharmacy and get a pill cutter; they are much more accurate and easy to use.[17]

How to Read a Study: The Good, the Bad, and the Ugly

In October 2006, the *New York Times* published two separate articles about weight loss. The first announced that extreme calorie restriction, or eating an ultra-low-calorie vegan diet, could help prevent aging and extend life.[18] Later on the very same day, photos of some happy-looking mice graced the front page of the *Times* Web site, which announced that "researchers at the Harvard Medical School and the National Institute on Aging report that a natural substance found in red wine, known as resveratrol, offsets the bad effects of a high-calorie diet in mice and significantly extends their lifespan."[19] Guess which article—the one that suggested cutting calories and eating fermented soy paste or the one that encouraged a glass or two of wine with dinner—made the frequently e-mailed list?

But how do you figure out what information is important to you? How can you tell a good study from a bad one, or understand the difference between a clinical trial and an observational one? Does it make a difference if a study was performed by Pfizer, or the National Institutes of Health (NIH), or by an academic institution? These aren't always easy questions to answer, as even the professionals— doctors and journal editors—have trouble distinguishing between good and bad scientific work from time to time. But a little basic terminology can go a long way toward helping you become a more "no-nonsense" health consumer.

Where Did the Information Come From?

If you heard about an amazing new treatment option on a commercial or on a drug company's Web site, chances are you should take that "breakthrough" with a grain of salt. In general, if someone is trying to sell something—a pill, a product, a procedure (even a book!), the information may be skewed to support the product. A drugmaker who has an HT pill is probably not going to suggest treating hot flashes with patience, time, and a little yoga. This is not to suggest that many drugs aren't wonderful and life-changing but rather to say that the best sources of information are those who don't have a financial stake in the breakthrough product or research.

This can get complicated: for example, what if you are looking at the Web site of an organization that receives money from a drug company? How about a television news report where the majority of commercials are paid for by pharmaceutical manufacturers? We've all had this experience: you're watching your favorite evening news show and you see a peppy young reporter waxing on about the possibilities of a new drug treatment. Break to commercial, and suddenly there is that pill again, this time in a commercial. This is not a coincidence or an accident. Drug companies pay good money to support television and magazines for a reason: they are betting that the outlet won't want to lose valuable accounts by saying unfavorable things about their products.

We certainly aren't arguing that all TV health news is bad or biased or that you should never ask your doctor about a "new finding" you saw in your favorite women's magazine. We *are* saying that it is important to be aware of these financial relationships and be careful about being too readily convinced of a "breakthrough." If you receive information either directly or indirectly from a drug company, you may need to go a little further to find out what the original research said and if it applies to you.

Science Is about Conversations, Not Conclusions

Every scientific finding is based on research, usually a study of some sort published in a scientific or medical journal. That information is received and analyzed by doctors and journalists, and the journalists turn the study into the more basic news, magazine, and radio stories that bring most nonscientists their first flash of new medical news.

Studies rely on statistics; they use numbers to look at large groups of people and try to figure out things about individuals. But as the statistician Klaus Hinklemann notes, "With statistics one cannot prove anything, but that statistics, if used properly, can indeed demonstrate certain degrees of relationship among factors or variables."[20]

A study doesn't prove, for example, that eating cumin prevents Alzheimer's disease. Rather, it shows that women who ate food with high cumin content experienced fewer cases of Alzheimer's than those who ate no cumin. It's a small but crucial distinction.

The language in any report can tell you a number of things. First, if a reporter is using definite language—implying that something will certainly cure something or is absolutely a silver bullet—be wary. This is probably either a misunderstanding of the findings or a deliberate overstatement. Second, what are the writers actually saying? Often a headline will ask a big, open-ended question: "Does Coffee Prevent Parkinson's Disease?" The answer may be "no," it may be "possibly," but it will almost never be "yes." These headlines are designed to suck you in to the story. Once you are reading, more likely than not you will be presented with a small study that posits a possible relationship between two things. That will sound more like this:[21] "In a trial of fifty men between ages fifty-five and seventy, patients who drank two or more cups of coffee a day were 20 percent less likely to develop Parkinson's disease." And it will probably be followed by a statement like "More research on this topic is needed" or "Doctors are optimistic that this will lead to greater knowledge on this subject."

This is far from a firm answer to the very concrete question posed by the headline. Would there have been a difference if all the men had been in their late sixties? What other dietary factors did these men have in common? (For example, perhaps they all eat carrots or ice cream.) Were all the men being studied insured (meaning they've been receiving good health care)? And one of our favorites: How would these findings have been different if they had tested men *and* women? There are so many factors that can affect the results of scientific work that you always need to question the conclusive tone taken in many mainstream and nonscientific health resources.

Science Moves Slowly

Medical developments are in general the least dramatic things out there. It's not that the end product can't be breathtaking, it's just that the process of good research is so slow. Unfortunately, small, poorly conducted trials can sound very exciting, and journalists may or may not have the tools to realize that they aren't really looking at a good piece of science.

This has encouraged bad habits in both the press and the scientific community. If you are a researcher who wants to get your studies covered with the hopes of increasing your funding, you have an incentive to find positive or dramatic results. As a journalist, on the other hand, you may not scrutinize a study closely or reject a scientifically flawed but dramatically presented piece of work. If a reporter makes it sound as though the world has been turned on its head by new findings, it is likely that this isn't true. There is a handful of really revolutionary breakthrough drugs and procedures and findings out there, but certainly not enough to satisfy the insatiable appetite of health consumers for answers and cures.

Expert Reading: A Brief Primer in How Patients Can Get More from Medical Literature

An important thing to realize is that not all evidence—and the studies that present it—is created equal. The U.S. Preventive Services Task Force rates the quality of evidence on a scale that ranges from the least convincing evidence—"opinions of respected authorities based on clinical experience, descriptive studies or reports of expert committees"—to more convincing—uncontrolled trials and observational and cohort studies—to most convincing—randomized controlled clinical trials.

What are these different types of trials and studies, and how do you tell them apart?

An *observational study* involves human subjects. To perform such a study, researchers watch a certain group of people over a number of years. The NIH notes that the idea is to "help scientists find out who develops a disease, what those people have in common, and how they differ from the group that did not get sick. . . . What they learn can suggest a path for more research." For example, you could look at a group of three hundred women between the ages of forty and sixty.

You might keep records of numerous lifestyle factors, and if certain women develop breast cancer, you could check the records to see what things they had in common. Did they smoke? Take hormones? Did they eat a diet that wasn't high enough in certain chemicals? If you noticed, for example, that the women who developed breast cancer tended to exercise less than those who did not, you could create a new study specifically to test the relationship between exercise and breast cancer.

There are many different types of observational studies, including cohort, case-control, and cross-sectional studies. In a cohort study, a group of people—let's say a group of women—are recruited and observed for several years. Doctors will study the histories of those who develop a certain problem, such as a type of cancer, and will look for possible commonalities that might suggest a potential cause or factor in disease development.

Observational research has some big problems. Because you aren't testing and controlling for a specific factor, its tough to determine any specific relationships, and doctors may not always know why a certain group of people do or don't experience a disease. You might think a lack of exercise was causing women to develop breast cancer, but it might turn out to be chemicals in the water in the part of the country where you were conducting your study. In observational research it is common to theorize that one groups stays healthy for a certain reason, but the actual cause may turn out to be something very different.

Menopausal women in the late 1990s got a startling example of this problem. For years, observational trials gave us good news about hormones and heart disease. Women who took HT, researchers suggested, had healthier hearts. This belief was so prevalent that it was taken as earth-shattering news when the Heart and Estrogen-Progestin Replacement Study (HERS) Trial, a four-year study (and not an observational one) of estrogen plus progestin, and the heart, found that estrogen "didn't help lower heart disease."[22] In an accompanying editorial, Dr. Drana Pettiti wrote that HERS was "a sobering reminder of the limitations of observational research, the incompleteness of current understanding of the mechanisms of vascular disease and the dangers of extrapolation." In other words, an observational trial can be the first step in knowledge about disease prevention, but it is far from the final word.

A case-control study, a type of epidemiological research, works in the opposite way from cohort trials: rather than looking for similarities, it tries to hash out differences. In this instance, the group of people being studied are recruited because they already have a specific commonality, such as a group of women who all have breast cancer. Researchers will then look for differences in their histories and lifestyle factors. This second type of observational research is faster and cheaper than the first, but it can be less reliable.

A cross-section study is cheaper still but even less reliable. These studies look at a group at a certain moment in time: it is a sort of scientific snapshot. For example, you could look at a group of women, noting who takes HT and who has developed breast cancer to see if the numbers of women with breast cancer are higher among those taking hormones. The problem with this research is that it has no context: diseases and health conditions develop over time, so while HT might cause breast cancer, many of the women taking HT might not develop cancer for many years to come. It is very difficult to demonstrate any kind of causality reliably with this sort of study.

The next step after an observational trial should be a *clinical trial*. Randomized controlled clinical trials are considered the gold standard in medical research. Such a trial would involve a number of human volunteers. The NIH explains that they "are assigned to two or more study groups by chance" (that "chance" is the randomization part.) Let's say we're testing a new antidepressant. We break our total group of six hundred people into a group of two hundred who take a 100 mg dose of the new drug, a group of two hundred who take a 150 mg dose of the new drug, and a group of two hundred who take a pill filled with artificial sweetener. This last group is called the placebo group and the sugar pill is the placebo. Having a placebo group insures that any positive benefits we might see in the other two groups are really the result of the drug and not of another factor. If a trial is a good one, it may be "double-blinded," or "masked," meaning that even the doctors conducting the trial don't know ahead of time which patients are receiving a medication and which are getting the placebo.

Dr. Marcia Angell, the former editor of the *New England Journal of Medicine*, observes that for drugs, the *real* gold standard would be a trial that compared new drugs head-on with older prescriptions for the same problem as well as with placebos. New drugs are rarely tested against existing prescriptions, yet they are rarely better than

Other Types of Studies You Might Encounter

NAME	DESCRIPTION	PROBLEMS AND BENEFITS
Pilot study	A smaller, quicker version of a bigger study. Often performed to see if a study design will work and to identify problems that could confound the bigger trial.	Too small to yield any conclusive information about disease prevention or health benefits of a given procedure, drug, etc. A test of the trial itself.
Prevention trial	Designed to see if a drug or lifestyle intervention can prevent a certain health problem.	While they can help doctors identify individuals who might be at risk for a serious health problem early, these studies may identify individuals who will not have a certain health problem, and people may be prematurely urged to take aggressive action to prevent or treat an illness they might not have.

(continued)

NAME	DESCRIPTION	PROBLEMS AND BENEFITS
Descriptive study (a category of epidemiological research)	Done to create a picture of an individual or a group, not to test a hypothesis or determine causality. This can be incredibly small—an individual case study—or can involve larger groups who are profiled orsurveyed.	These studies are more anecdotal than scientific.
Analytical study (a category of epidemiological research)	Scientists observe a certain behavior and record health results.	
Screening trial	Done on an individual or a group of people to test for a certain illness—for example, testing for a gene that is associated with higher rates of breast cancer.	
Epidemiology trial	A general term used for many types of obser-vational research. Usually an observational study tests whether a certain drug, life-style factor, or other variable is associated with a certain disease.	

the old drugs and nearly always more expensive. When they are tested against older drugs—say, a new SSRI against an older tricylic—the dosages are usually not equivalent. A lower dose of the older drug will be used purposely to skew the results.

Understanding Risk Factors

You don't have to be very good at math to understand that numbers can be presented in different ways to dissimilar effects. Small results can be made to look dramatic, and huge and world-changing findings can be explained in a way that makes them boring.

With trial results, numbers are presented as showing an absolute risk or benefit, or a relative one. In scientific literature and in mainstream health articles, you will almost always hear about *relative risks* generally presented as a percentage—for example, there were 30 percent fewer heart attacks—or a ratio—heart attacks were cut by one third.

These numbers are used for a lot of reasons, but in many cases they are good because they sound dramatic. For example, let's say we are conducting a study with two hundred women: one hundred taking a drug and one hundred taking a placebo. We're testing to see if our drug helps prevent stroke. Of the hundred women in the placebo group, let's say two women had a stroke. In the group taking the drug, imagine only one woman suffered a stroke. Laura writes up our report and announces breathlessly that women on the drug experienced 50 percent fewer strokes than women on the sugar pill. Or better yet, we say that our drug cuts stroke risk in half. Both of these things are true. But do they really tell us anything?

Probably not. The truth is that that extra stroke in the placebo group could have been the result of chance, not our wonder drug. By the time this information gets to you, the health consumer, you have no idea that the original numbers were so small and that the way the numbers are presented overstates the benefit of the pharmaceutical.

Of course we're presenting an extreme example here, but you would be amazed how often small studies are manipulated to make results look conclusive when data is weak.

The other number—the *absolute risk* or benefit—is something we find through simple arithmetic. It is the actual number of people in the trial compared with the real number of health problems that were experienced or avoided. For most of us who left math back in high school or college, this is a much easier number to understand. Like Waldo being spotted in his striped red shirt amidst thousands of other people, this number puts in perspective both the scope of the trial and the frequency of a given problem. In our stroke study, one fewer patient had a stroke while taking the drug when compared with the placebo group.

Because absolute numbers don't seem to make their way into most health reports, one way to find them out is to check the results in the original trial. Most articles in magazines or stories on television will mention the original journal in which a certain study was published or the school or organization that conducted it. You can Google the name of a scientist or a medical school, or go directly to a journal Web site to look for the real numbers. If you still have trouble understanding, call your doctor and ask her to explain the absolute benefits in a simple way.

Is Bigger Better?

Our fictional stroke study raises another issue to think about when scrutinizing a study. How big was the study? Our example was so small that one or two strokes could generate very shocking statistics that didn't mean very much. In addition, a small trial is less likely to reveal extensive side effects and problems that should be identified before drugs reach the general public. Although a large study isn't necessarily a good one, and a small one isn't always a bad one, in general, large studies are more reliable for identifying side effects and also giving confidence about really significant benefits.

The bigger a trial is, the more likely it is that sufficient numbers of individuals with different health concerns and predispositions will be included to demonstrate problems. But such big trials are expensive. Dr. Romano Deghenghi, a brilliant Italian endocrinologist with a knack for getting to the heart of issues with drugs, explains, "It takes tens of thousands of patients to show a side effect. Who has that kind of time or money?" [23] He adds that drugmakers with successful blockbuster drugs have less interest than anyone in performing such tests: "If you have, say, the best-selling statin on the market, why do you want to spend lots of your own money to show that your best-selling product does bad things?"

In the end, a trial's construction is the most important factor in its ability to give accurate results.

Because conducting huge trials is so expensive, a popular alternative has been to perform a *meta-analysis*. In this kind of study, a scientist plugs the data from lots of other trials into a computer and compares their findings. For example, you might look at fifteen different trials of the herb black cohosh for curbing hot flashes. It's a great way of reconciling different results and determining the best consensus we have on a given drug or treatment. Since all the clinical work has already been performed, meta-analyses are extremely economical.

There are also a lot of potential problems with this type of study. First of all, the studies analyzed may all track the relationship between black cohosh and hot flashes, but this doesn't mean they are similar enough in design to compare in a way that will be meaningful. Imagine for a minute that five of the studies used black cohosh supplements, six used creams, and the rest tested the effects of the fresh herb. These studies are different in such substantial ways that just plugging their results into a computer together won't be helpful.

Another problem is the prejudice of the scientists or statisticians conducting the trial. A *New England Journal of Medicine* editorial says that "problems were so frequent and so serious, including bias on the part of the meta-analyst, that it was difficult to trust" some current methods of conducting meta-analysis.[24] There are very different methods of conducting this type of science, and part of the challenge may be finding ways to do it that are more resistant to researchers' personal partialities.

Another money-saving strategy has been to perform data analysis on existing large clinical trials, for example, using information from a study like the WHI or HERS. In this case, you are looking at data from only one study, but analyzing it to look at a factor the study wasn't originally designed to test. This can be problematic because it doesn't necessarily ask questions that the study was created to answer. A dramatic example came from Wayne State University, where a group of doctors headed by Rahi Victory and Michael Diamond announced the news that birth control pills might reduce the risk of heart disease.[25] The problem was that this conclusion was drawn from reexamining records from the WHI. The WHI was not designed to test the effects of oral contraceptives, and therefore its data on their use among its participants were based on self-reporting by women in the study. This would be different from, say, its data on Prempro use, one of the things the trials *was* designed to test. By the time the Victory study hit newsstands, it was very hard to tell anything about its methodology. What came through loud and clear was that the pill was good for the heart. That this claim was based on spurious evidence was less apparent.

how to read a medical journal article

1. Look at the methods and results, not the conclusion. The conclusion may just be the opinion of the study authors; the results will tell you what happened.
2. Who was studied? Were they similar to you in age, sex, race, other ways? Be careful of trusting studies where the people being studied had little in common with you.
3. How many people were included in the trial group? In general, bigger is better, although not always. Study design is more important but harder to pick up on and discern from a brief news story.
4. What was being tested?
5. What did the trial actually find?
6. If there was a placebo group, how did the subject of the test stack up against the placebo?
7. Did the placebo group experience benefits similar to the test group?
8. If it was a drug, a procedure, or surgery, was it tested against another similar drug, procedure, or surgery? If so, was it shown to be any better than an existing, older pill or procedure?
9. Were risks and benefits stated absolutely or relatively? If they are relative risks, what were the actual numbers (for example, how many fewer heart attacks or hot flashes). If this is confusing to you, ask your doctor about it.

notes

Introduction

1. Women's Health Initiative, Department of Health and Human Services, National Institutes of Health: http//www.nhibi.nihi.gov/whi/, updated 10/10/07.

2. Margaret Lock, "Deconstructing the Change: Female Maturation in Japan and North America," in *Welcome to Middle Age! And Other Cultural Fictions*, ed. Richard A. Shweder (Chicago and London: University of Chicago Press, 1998), 45–75.

3. Ibid.

4. World Health Organization, "Research on the Menopause in the 1990's" (proceedings of a meeting in Geneva, Switzerland), *Maturitas* 23 (2) (March 1996): 109–259.

5. Sherry S. Sherman, "Defining the Menopause Transition," NIH State-of-the-Science Conference on Management of Menopause-Related Symptoms, Mar. 21–23, 2005, conference abstracts, 25–28, http://consensus.nih.gov/2005/2005MenopausalSymptomsSOS025Program.pdf.

1. Flashing Back: A Brief History of Menopause

1. Amber Coverdale Sumrall, "Off the Edge," in *Women of the 14th Moon: Writings on Menopause*, ed. Dena Taylor and Amber Coverdale Sumrall (Freedom, CA: The Crossing Press, 1991).

2. Lynnette Leidy Sievert, *Menopause: A Biocultural Perspective* (New Brunswick, NJ: Rutgers University Press, 2006), 47.

3. Ibid., 48.

4. Jocelyn Scott Peccei, "A Critique of the Grandmother Hypothesis," *American Journal of Human Biology* 13 (2001): 434–452.

5. Barry Bogin and B. Holly Smith, "Evolution of the Human Life Cycle," *American Journal of Human Biology* 8 (1996): 703–716.

6. Jocelyn Scott Peccei, "A Hypothesis for the Origin of Evolution of Menopause," *Maturitas* 21 (1995): 83–89.

7. Ibid.

8. Grace Paley, Preface to Taylor and Sumrall, *Women of the 14th Moon*.

9. Deborah Sweeney, "Elder Women in Ancient Egypt," Tel Aviv University, http://www.tau.ac.il/humanities/archaeology/projects/proj_past_elder .html.

10. Ibid.

11. *Women's Lives in Medieval Europe: A Sourcebook*, ed. Emilie Amt (London: Routledge, 1992).

12. Michael Stolberg, "A Woman's Hell? Medical Perceptions of Menopause in Pre-Industrial Europe," *History of Medicine Bulletin* 73 (3) (1999): 404–428.

13. Ibid.

14. Margaret Lock and Patricia Kaufert, "Menopause Local Biologies and Cultures of Aging," *American Journal of Human Biology* 13 (2001): 494–504.

15. Ibid.

16. Janice Delaney, Mary Jane Lupton, and Emily Toth, *The Curse* (New York: E. P. Dutton, 1976), 182.

17. Ibid.

18. Ibid.

19. Introduction to Taylor and Sumrall, *Women of the 14th Moon*.

20. Paley, in Taylor and Sumrall, *Women of the 14th Moon*.

21. Nancy Fugate Woods, "Symptoms During the Perimenopause: Prevalence, Severity, Trajectory and Significance in Women's Lives," NIH State-of-the-Science Conference on Management of Menopause-Related Symptoms, Mar. 21–23, 2005, conference abstracts, 31–36, http://consensus.nih.gov/ 2005/2005MenopausalSymptomsSOS025Program.pdf.

22. Yewoubdar Beyene, *From Menarche to Menopause: Reproductive Lives of Peasant Women in Two Different Cultures* (Albany: State University of New York Press, 1989).

23. Marcia Flint, *Menarche and Menopause in Rajput Women* (PhD diss., City University of New York, 1974).

24. Ursula K. LeGuin, "The Space Crone," in *Meanings of Menopause: Historical, Medical, and Cultural Perspectives*, ed. Ruth Formank (London: Analytic Press, 1990).

2. At First Glance: Perimenopause, Beginnings and Ends

1. Madeline Gray, *The Changing Years* (Garden City, NY: Doubleday, 1953), 13.

2. Ibid., 16.

3. Alex Kuczynski, "Menopause Forever," *New York Times*, June 23, 2002.

4. Ibid.

5. Ibid.

6. Lori A. Bastian, Crystal M. Smith, and Kavita Nanda, "Is This Woman Perimenopausal?" *Journal of the American Medical Association* 289 (3) (2003): 895–902.

7. Matthew A. Cohen and Mark V. Sauer, "Fertility Problems in Perimenopausal Women," *Clinical Obstetrics and Gynecology* 41 (4) (1998): 958–965.

8. Ibid.

9. Barbara Seaman, "Is This Any Way to Have a Baby?" *O (The Oprah) Magazine* (February 2004), 190–191.

10. Boston Women's Health Collective and Vivian Pinn, *Our Bodies, Ourselves: Menopause* (New York: Touchstone, 2006), 57–73.

11. A. W. Bergen and N. Caporaso, "Cigarette Smoking," *Journal of the National Cancer Institute* 91 (1999): 1365–1375.

12. J. Bradbury, "Mechanism Found for Smoking-Induced Early Menopause," *Lancet* 358 (9277) (July 21, 2001): 2115.

13. Herschel Jick, "Cigarette Smoking and Early Menopause," *Western Journal of Medicine* 130 (3) (March 1979): 235.

14. Walter Willett, Meir J. Stamfer, Christopher Bain et al., "Cigarette Smoking, Relative Weight and Menopause," *American Journal of Epidemiology* 117 (6) (1983): 651–658; and A. S. Midgette and J. A. Baron, "Cigarette Smoking and the Risk of Natural Menopause," *Epidemiology* 1 (6) (November 1990): 474–480.

15. Bastian, Smith, and Nanda, "Is This Woman Perimenopausal?" 895–902.

16. Bradbury, "Mechanism," 2115.

17. B. W. Hartmann, S. Kirchengast, A. Albrecht et al., "Hysterectomy Increases the Symptomatology of Postmenopausal Syndrome," *Gynecological Endocrinology* 9 (1995): 247–252.

18. Evelyn M. Parke, "A Funny Thing Happened on My Way to Middle Age," in Dena Taylor and Amber Coverdale Sumrall, *Women of the 14th Moon* (Freedom, CA: The Crossing Press, 1991).

19. Lynette Leidy Sievert, *Menopause: A Biocultural Perspective* (New Brunswick, NJ: Rutgers University Press, 2006), 28–29.

20. Ibid.

21. Ibid.

22. H. Snieder, A. J. MacGregor, and T. D. Spector, "Genes Control the Cessation of a Woman's Reproductive Life: A Twin Study of Hysterectomy and Age at Menopause," *Journal of Clinical Endocrinology and Metabolism* 83 (6) (1998): 1875–1880.

23. D. W. Cramer, H. Xu, and B. L. Harlow, "Family History as a Predictor of Early Menopause," *Fertility and Sterility* 64 (4) (1995): 740–745.

24. M. R. Soules, S. Sherman, E. Parrott et al., "Executive Summary: Stages of Reproductive Aging Workshop (St. R. A. W.) Park City, UT, 2001," *Menopause* 8 (6) (2001): 402–407.

25. Jerilynn C. Prior, *Estrogen's Storm Season: Stories of the Perimenopause* (Vancouver, BC: Centre for Menstrual Cycle and Ovulation Research, 2005), ix.

26. Jerilynn C. Prior, "Perimenopause: The Complex Endocrinology of the Menopausal Transition," *Endocrine Reviews*, 19 (4) (1998): 397–428.

27. Prior, *Estrogen's Storm Season*, ix.

3. Seeing Red: Excessive Bleeding, Menorrhagia, and Perimenopause

1. National Institutes of Health, State-of-the-Science Conference Statement on Management of Menopause-Related Symptoms, Mar. 21–23, 2005, http://consensus.nih.gov/2005/2005MenopausalSymptomsSOS025html.htm.

2. Thomas J. Graham, *On the Diseases of Females* (London: Simpkin, Marshal & Co., 1837).

3. Mayo Clinic, "Menorrhagia," http://www.mayoclinic.com/health/menorrhagia/DS00394.

4. Jerilynn C. Prior, "Managing Menorrhagia Without Surgery," Center for Menstrual Cycle and Ovulation Research, Nov. 6, 2003: http://www.cemcor.ubc.ca/articles/misc/managing_menorrhagia.shtml.

5. Mayo Clinic, "Menorrhagia."

6. Prior, "Managing Menorrhagia."

7. "Menorrhagia aka 'Flooding' aka Abnormal Uterine Bleeding," Menopause and Beyond Archives, http://www.geocities.com/menobeyond/bleeding.html.

8. Susan Love and Karen Lindsey, *Dr. Susan Love's Menopause and Hormone Book* (New York: Three Rivers Press, 2003), 57.

9. Ibid.

10. Prior, "Managing Menorrhagia."

11. McGill University, Student Health Service: http://www.mcgill.ca/studenthealth/information/nutritionalhealth/ironrich.

12. R. F. Casper, S. Dodin, and R. L. Reid, "The Effect of 20 mg Ethinyl Estradiol/1 mg Norethindrone Acetate (Minestrin), a Low-Dose Oral Contraceptive, on Vaginal Bleeding Patterns, Hot Flashes, and Quality of Life in Symptomatic Perimenopausal Women," *Menopause* 4 (1997): 139–147.

13. G. A. Irvine, M. B. Campbell Brown, M. A. Lumsden et al., "Randomised Comparative Trial of the Levonorgestrel Intrauterine System and Norethisterone for Treatment of Idiopathic Menorrhagia," *British Journal of Obstetrics and Gynaecology* 105 (6) (1998): 592–598.

14. J. Majoribanks, A. Lethaby, and C. Farquar, "Surgery versus Medical Therapy for Heavy Menstrual Bleeding," *Cochrane Database of Systemic Reviews* 3 (2003): 1–65.

15. J. T. Preston, "Tranexamic Acid and Norethisterone in the Treatment of Ovulatory Menorrhagia," *British Journal of Obstetrics and Gynaecology* 102 (1995): 401.

16. Ruth Savage, "Thrombosis with Tranexamic Acid for Menorrhagia," *Prescriber Update* 24 (2) (2003): 26–27; Y. Endo et al, "Deep Vein Thrombosis Induced by Tranexamic Acid in Idiopathic Thrombocytopenic Purpura,"

Journal of the American Medical Association 259 (24) (1998): 3561–3562; and M. Taparia, F. T. Cordingley, and M. F. Leahy, "Pulmonary Embolism Associated with Tranexamic Acid in Severe Acquired Haemophilia," *European Journal of Haematology* 68 (2002): 307–309.

17. Prior, "Managing Menorrhagia."

18. Love and Lindsey, *Menopause and Hormone Book*, 57.

4. "Is It Hot in Here, or Is It Just You?": Hot Flashes, Night Sweats, and Other Things That Keep You Up at Night

1. N. E. Avis and S. M. McKinley, "The Massachusetts Women's Health Study: An Epidemiologic Investigation of the Menopause," *Journal of the American Medical Women's Association* 50 (1995): 45–49.

2. Nancy Fugate Woods, "Symptoms During the Perimenopause: Prevalence, Severity, Trajectory and Significance in Women's Lives," NIH State-of-the-Science Conference on Management of Menopause-Related Symptoms, Mar. 21–23, 2005, conference abstracts, 31–33, http://consensus.nih.gov/2005/2005MenopausalSymptomsSOS025Program.pdf.

3. Erica Weir, "Hot Flashes . . . In January," *Canadian Medical Journal* 170 (1) (Jan. 6, 2004): 39–40.

4. George Henry Napheys, "The Change of Life," *The Physical Life of Women: Advice to the Wife, Mother and Maiden* (Toronto: Musson Book Co., 1869).

5. Anna M. Longshore-Potts, *Discourses to Women on Medical Subjects* (London: privately printed 1887), http://www.geocities.com/menobeyond/menscess.html.

6. E. W. Freeman, M. D. Sammel et al., "Hot Flashes in the Late Reproductive Years: Risk Factors for African Women and Caucasian Women," *Journal of Women's Health and Gender-based Medicine* 10 (1) (2001): 67–76.

7. North American Menopause Society, *Early Menopause Guidebook*, 6th ed. (Cleveland: North American Menopause Society, 2003), 13–14.

8. Weir, "Hot Flashes . . . In January."

9. Medical University of South Carolina, http://www.musc.edu/.

10. Susan Love and Karen Lindsey, *Dr. Susan Love's Menopause and Hormone Book* (New York: Three Rivers Press, 2003), 52.

11. *Harvard Women's Health Watch*, February 1997.

12. R. R. Freedman, "Pathophysiology and Treatment of Menopausal Hot Flashes," *Seminars in Reproductive Medicine* 23(2) (May 2005): 117–125.

13. Ellen B. Gold, Barbara Sternfeld, Jennifer L. Kelsey et al., "Relation of Demographic and Lifestyle Factors to Symptoms in a Multi-Racial/Ethnic Population of Women 44–55 Years of Age," *American Journal of Epidemiology* 152 (5) (2000): 463–473.

14. Freeman, Sammel et al., "Hot Flashes," 67–76.

15. Gina Kolata, "Gauging Body Mass Index in a Changing Body," *New York Times*, Jun. 28, 2005.

16. Erin J. Aiello et al., "Effect of a Yearlong, Moderate Intensity Exercise Intervention on the Occurrence and Severity of Menopause Symptoms in Postmenopausal Women," *Menopause* 11(4) (July-August 2004): 382–388.

17. K. Smith-Dijulio, D. Percival, N. Woods et al., "Hot Flash Severity in Hormone Therapy Users/Nonusers Across the Menopausal Transition, *Maturitas* 58(2): 191–200.

18. E. A. Jakab, "Anatomy of a Hot Flash," *Seasons* 5 (1) (1995).

19. North American Menopause Society, *Early Menopause Guidebook*, 13–14.

20. Nima Sharifi et al., "Androgen Deprivation Therapy for Prostate Cancer," *Journal of the American Medical Association* 294 (2) (2005): 238–244.

21. Helena Rodbard, *Bottom Line/Health*, October 2000.

22. North American Menopause Society, *Early Menopause Guidebook*, 13–14.

23. R. R. Freedman and T. A. Roehrs, "Lack of Sleep Disturbance from Menopausal Hot Flashes," *Fertility and Sterility* 82 (1) (July 2004): 138–144.

24. K. M. Sharkey, H. M. Bearpark et al., "Effects of Menopausal Status on Sleep in Midlife Women," *Behavioral Sleep Medicine* 1(2) (2003): 69–80.

25. Rachel Lynn Palmer and Sarah K. Greenberg, *Facts and Frauds in Woman's Hygiene: A Medical Guide against Misleading Claims and Dangerous Products* (New York: Vanguard Press, 1936).

26. Heidi D. Nelson et al., "Nonhormonal Therapies for Menopausal Hot Flashes," *Journal of the American Medical Association* 295 (17) (2003): 2057–2071.

27. P. W. Whiting, A. Clouston, and P. Kerlin, "Black Cohosh and Other Herbal Remedies Associated with Acute Hepatitis," *Medical Journal of Australia* 177 (8) (2002): 440–443.

28. "Vasomotor Symptoms," *Obstetrics and Gynecology* 104 (4) (October 2004): 106S–117S.

29. P. A. Komesaroff, C. V. Black, V. Cable, and K. Sudhir, "Effects of Wild Yam Extract on Menopausal Symptoms, Lipids and Sex Hormones in Healthy Menopausal Women," *Climacteric* 4 (2) (2001): 144–150.

30. Gary Elkins, Joel Marcus, Lynne Palamara, and Vered Stearns, "Can Hypnosis Reduce Hot Flashes in Breast Cancer Survivors? A Literature Review," *American Journal of Clinical Hypnosis* 47 (1) (July 2004): 29–42.

31. Y. Wyon, R. Lindgren, T. Lundberg, and M. Hammar, "Effects of Acupuncture on Climacteric Vasomotor Symptoms, Quality of Life and Urinary Excretion of Neuropeptides among Postmenopausal Women," *Menopause* 2 (1) (1995): 3–12.

32. J. S. Carpenter, N. Wells, B. Lambert et al., "A Pilot Study of Magnetic Therapy for Hot Flashes after Breast Cancer," *Cancer Nurse* 25 (2002): 104–109.

33. A. MacLennan, S. Lester, and V. Moore, "Oral Estrogen Replace-

ment Therapy versus Placebo for Hot Flashes: A Systematic Review," *Climacteric* 4 (1) (2001): 58–74.

34. Bruce Ettinger et al., "Reduction of Vertebral Fracture Risk in Postmenopausal Women with Osteoporosis Treated with Raloxifene: Results from a 3-Year Randomized Clinical Trial; Multiple Outcomes of Raloxifene Evaluation (MORE) Investigators," *Journal of the American Medical Association* 282 (1999): 637–645.

35. "Vasomotor Symptoms," 106S–117S.

36. J. M. Foidart, J. Vervliet, and P. Buytaert, "Efficacy of Sustained-Release Vaginal Oestriol in Alleviating Urogenital and Systemic Climacteric Complaints," *Maturitas* 13 (1991): 99–107; and J. Vartiainen, T. Wahlstrom, and C. G. Nilsson, "Effects and Acceptability of a New 17 Beta-Oestradiol-Releasing Vaginal Ring in the Treatment of Postmenopausal Complaints," *Maturitas* 17 (1993): 129–137.

37. Morris Notelovitz, "Hot Flashes and Androgens: A Biological Rationale for Clinical Practice," *Mayo Clinic Proceedings* 79 (4) (April 2004): S8–S13.

38. Charles L. Loprinzi et al., "Venlafaxine in Management of Hot Flashes in Survivors of Breast Cancer: A Randomized Controlled Trial," *Lancet* 356 (9247) (2000): 2059–2064. This study, like so many others, was performed on women who had had breast cancer and often experienced early menopause due to chemotherapy.

39. Vered Stearns et al., "Paroxetine Controlled Release in the Treatment of Menopausal Hot Flashes," *Journal of the American Medical Association* 289 (21) (2003): 2827–2834.

40. "Glaxo Resumes Paxil CR Sales after Seizure," *Los Angeles Times*, Jun. 28, 2005.

41. Charles L. Loprinzi, "Centrally Active Non-Hormonal Hot Flash Therapies," NIH State-of-the-Science Conference on Management of Menopause-Related Symptoms, Mar. 21–23, 2005, conference abstracts, 109–112, http://consensus.nih.gov20052005MenopausalSymptomsSOS025Program.pdf.

42. K. J. Pandya, J. Roscoe, E. Pajon et al., "A Preliminary Report of a Double Blind Placebo Controlled Trial of Gabapentin for Control of Hot Flashes in Women with Breast Cancer: A University of Rochester Cancer Center CCOP Study," *Proc ASCO* 23 (2004): 801.

5. The Science of Sleep: Night Sweats, Wakefulness, and Getting Some Shut-Eye

1. R. Manni, "Rapid Eye Movement Sleep, Non-Rapid Eye Movement Sleep, Dreams and Hallucinations," *Current Psychiatry Reports* 7 (3) (June 2005): 196–200.

2. Marcos G. Frank, "The Role of Sleep in Memory Consolidation and Brain Plasticity: Dream or Reality," *Neuroscientist* 12 (6) (2006): 477–488.

3. Jie Zhang, "Memory Process and the Function of Sleep," *Journal of Theoretics* 6 (6) (December 2004).

4. Peter Stern, "Social Experience and the Need to Sleep," *Sci. STKE* 354 (September 2006): tw366.

5. H. P. Van Dongen, G. Maslin, J. M. Mullington, and D. F. Dinges, "The Cumulative Cost of Wakefulness: Dose-Response Effects on Neurobehavioural Functions and Sleep Physiology from Chronic Sleep Restriction and Total Sleep Deprivation," *Sleep* 26 (2) (Mar. 15, 2003): 117–126.

6. Christine Gorman, "Why We Sleep," *Time* Dec. 20, 2004, http://www.time.com/time/magazine/article/0,9171,1009765,00.html.

7. Eve VanCauter, Rachel Leproult, and Laurence Plat, "Age-Related Changes in Slow Wave Sleep and REM Sleep and Relationship with Growth Hormone and Cortisol Levels in Healthy Men," *Journal of the American Medical Association* 284 (7): (August 16, 2000): 861–868.

8. Cathryn Jakobson Ramin, *Carved in Sand: When Attention Fails and Memory Fades at Midlife* (New York: HarperCollins, 2007), 155.

9. "NSF's Latest Poll Shows that Sleep, Health and Aging Are Linked," National Sleep Foundation, 2003, http://www.sleepfoundation.org/site/c.hulXKjM0IxF/b.2417365/k.1460/2003_Sleep_in_America_Poll.htm.

10. Daniel F. Kripke, Lawrence Garfinkel et al., "Mortality Associated with Sleep Duration and Insomnia," *Archives of General Psychiatry* 59 (2002): 131–136.

11. Rhonda Rowland, "Experts Challenge Study Linking Sleep, Life Span," Feb. 15, 2002: http://archives.cnn.com/2002/HEALTH/02/14/sleep.study/index.html.

12. Carol M. Worthman and Melissa K. Melby, "Toward a Comparative Developmental Ecology of Human Sleep," in *Adolescent Sleep Patterns: Biological, Social, and Psychological Influences*, ed. M. A. Carskadon (New York: Cambridge University Press, 2002).

13. Ibid.

14. Ibid., 100.

15. Lynnette Leidy Sievert, *Menopause: A Biocultural Perspective* (New Brunswick, NJ: Rutgers University Press, 2006), 112–117.

16. National Sleep Foundation, *SleepMatters* 7 (3) (November 2005), www.sleepfoundation.org.

17. Sleep Apnea Information, American Sleep Apnea Association, 2007, http://www.sleepapnea.org/info/index.html.

18. National Sleep Foundation, *SleepMatters* 5 (4) (Fall 2003), www.sleepfoundation.org.

19. National Sleep Foundation, *SleepMatters* 7 (3) (Summer 2005), www.sleepfoundation.org.

20. "What Are the Possible Side Effects of Requip?," http://www.requip.com/requip.

21. Michael H. Silber, "What Causes Narcolepsy?" *SleepMatters* (Fall 2002), http://www.sleepfoundation.org/site/c.hulXKjM0IxF/b.2422635/k.4492/Ask_the_Sleep_Expert_Narcolepsy_and_Cataplexy.htm.

22. Carlin Flora, "Sleep Deprived in Menopause," *Psychology Today*, Nov. 13, 2003.

23. Helen Fields, "Losing Sleep," *U.S. News and World Report*, Oct. 10, 2005.

24. U.S. Food and Drug Administration, Aug. 29, 2005, http://www.fda.gov/cder/foi/label/2005/021774lbl.pdf, 4.

25. "New Data Support Long-Term Use of AMBIEN CRTM (zolpidem Tartrate Extended-Release) Tablets C(IV) for Up to 24 Weeks," Jul. 14, 2006, http://www.medicalnewstoday.com/articles/47098.php.

26. Sonia Ancoli-Israel, Gary S. Richardson, Richard M. Mangano et al., "Long-Term Use of Sedative Hypnotics for Older Patients with Insomnia," *Sleep Medicine* 6 (2) (March 2005): 107–113.

27. Martin F. Downs, "To Sleep, Perchance to . . . Walk," *Washington Post*, Mar. 14, 2006.

28. Ramin, *Carved in Sand*, 158–164.

6. Getting It On as You Get On: Menopause, Aging, and Sexuality

1. Marie Stopes, like Margaret Sanger, was an advocate for eugenics and even more outspoken than Sanger in her support. It is a sad fact that many pioneers of contraception and sexuality were supporters of this discriminatory pseudoscience.

2. "Historic Figures: Marie Carmichael Stopes: 1880–1958," http://www.bbc.co.uk/history/historic_figures/stopes_marie_carmichael.shtml.

3. Marie Carmichael Stopes, *Enduring Passion: Further New Contributions to the Solution of Sex Difficulties Being the Continuation of Married Love* (London: G. P. Putnam's Sons, 1929).

4. "Libido Change," Menopause and Beyond Archives, http://www.geocities.com/menobeyond.

5. Colette Bouchez, "Sex in the Menopause City," Nov. 19, 2004, www.webmd.com.

6. Stephen B. Levine, "The Sexual Consequences of Perimenopause and Menopause," *American Menopause Foundation* 3 (6) (Winter 1998).

7. "Sex After 50," Cornell University, *Women's Health Advisor*, September 1999.

8. Levine, "Sexual Consequences."

9. "Sex After 50."

10. Mount Sinai School of Medicine, "Enjoying Sex in the Second Half of Life," *Focus on Healthy Aging* 1 (2) (September 1998).

11. Pat Wingert and Barbara Kantrowitz, *Is It Hot in Here, or Is It Me? The Complete Guide to Menopause* (New York: Workman, 2006), 118–119.

12. "Enjoying Lifelong Sexual Vitality," *Johns Hopkins Medical Letter: Health After 50*, May 2000.

13. "Sex After 50."

14. Mary Duenwald, "Effort to Make Sex Drugs for Women Challenges Experts," *New York Times*, Mar. 25, 2003.

15. We do not use the term *sexual dysfunction* because it has not been determined if it is a real medical condition or merely the invention of a pharmaceutical company.

16. R. Basson, J. Berman, A. Burnett et al., "Report of the International Consensus Development Conference on Female Sexual Dysfunction: Definitions and Classifications," *Journal of Urology* 163 (2000): 888–893.

17. "Sexual Dysfunction and Hormone Therapy," *Obstetrics and Gynecology* 104 (4) (October 2004): s85–s91.

18. Jack Hitt, "The Second Sexual Revolution," *New York Times Magazine*, Feb. 20, 2000.

19. "Restoring Sexual Health," *Consumer Reports on Health*, March 2001.

20. Duenwald, "Sex Drugs."

21. Hitt, "Second Sexual Revolution."

22. Duenwald, "Sex Drugs."

23. New View of Women's Sexual Problems, http://www.fsd-alert.org/.

24. Duenwald, "Sex Drugs."

25. Ray Moynihan, "The Making of a Disease: Female Sexual Dysfunction," *British Medical Journal* 326 (Jan. 4, 2003): 45–47.

26. National Women's Health Network, "Female Sexual Dysfunction: For Women or For Sale?" *Network News*, January-February 2000.

27. Justin Clark, "Sex: The Big Turnoff," *Psychology Today*, January-February 2005.

28. Leonore Tiefer, "Historical, Scientific, Clinical and Feminist Criticisms of 'The Human Sexual Response Cycle' Model," *Annual Review of Sex Research* 2 (1991): 1–23.

29. E. J. Mundell, "FDA Panel Votes Against Testosterone Patch for Women," *HealthDay*, Dec. 2, 2004.

30. Ibid.

31. Ray Moynihan, "FDA Panel Rejects Testosterone Patch for Women on Safety Grounds," *British Medical Journal* 329 (Dec. 11, 2004): 1363.

32. Mundell, "FDA Panel Votes."

33. "Sexual Dysfunction and Hormone Therapy," s85–s91.

34. B. J. Messinger and H. L. Thacker, "Prevention for the Older Woman: A Practical Guide to Hormone Replacement Therapy and Urogynecologic Health," *Geriatrics* 56 (2001): 32–34, 37–38, 40–42.

35. W. H. Utian, D. Shoupe, G. Bachmann et al., "Relief of Vasomotor Symptoms and Vaginal Atrophy with Lower Doses of Conjugated Equine Estrogens and Medroxyprogesterone Acetate," *Fertility and Sterility* 75 (2001): 1065–1079.

36. "Sexual Dysfunction and Hormone Therapy," s85–s91.

37. Ibid.

38. North American Menopause Society, *Menopause Guidebook*, 6th ed.

(Cleveland: North American Menopause Society, 2007), 21: http://www
.menopause.org/edumaterials/guidebook/guidebook.htm.

39. Bouchez, "Sex in the Menopause City."

40. Duenwald, "Sex Drugs."

41. Bouchez, "Sex in the Menopause City."

42. Ibid.

43. Betty Dodson, *Orgasms for Two* (New York: Harmony, 2002), 202–214.

44. Hitt, "Second Sexual Revolution."

45. "Cupid's Arrows," *Harvard Health Letter*, February 2000.

46. Kristina Orth-Gomer, Sarah P. Wamala, Myriam Horsten et al., "Marital Stress Worsens Prognosis in Women with Coronary Heart Disease," *Journal of the American Medical Association* 284 (23) (December 2000): 3008–3014.

47. Mount Sinai School of Medicine, "Enjoying Sex in the Second Half of Life," *Focus on Healthy Aging* 1 (2) (September 1998).

48. Some women swear by them. Betty Dodson, for one, talks about the advantages of massage oil in her most recent book, *Orgasms for Two*.

49. "Sex After 50."

50. Dagmar O'Connor, ". . . How to Make Sex Exciting," *Bottom Line/ Health*, July 2001.

51. "Midlife Sexuality: A Time of Change, a Time of Opportunity," *Mayo Clinic Women's Health Source*, January 2006.

52. O'Connor, "How to Make Sex Exciting."

53. Dodson, *Orgasms*, 202–214.

54. "Sex After 50."

55. "Midlife Sexuality."

56. "How to Make Sex Fun and Fulfilling . . . Again," *Bottom Line/Health*, January 1999.

57. Eros Therapy, www.eros-therapy.com.

58. "Midlife Sexuality."

59. "How to Make Sex Fun and Fulfilling . . . Again."

60. Mount Sinai School of Medicine, "Enjoying Sex."

61. Ibid.

62. Arnold Lorand, *Old Age Deferred* (Philadelphia: F. A. Davis, 1925).

63. Bouchez, "Sex in the Menopause City."

64. Levine, "Sexual Consequences."

65. "Midlife Sexuality."

66. Stacy Tessler Landau et al., "A Study of Sexuality and Health among Older Adults in the United States," *New England Journal of Medicine* 357 (8) (2007): 762–774.

7. The Swing versus the Slump: Menopause, Mood, and Depression

1. "There is Help for PMDD Sufferers," Eli Lilly and Company, http://www.lilly.com/products/health_women/pmdd/index.html.

2. Although we will be exploring the subject further in this chapter, please keep in mind that it is difficult to secure statistics on depression that are *not* pharmaceutically biased.

3. Ray Moynihan and Alan Cassels, *Selling Sickness* (Vancouver, BC: Greystone Books, 2005), 23.

4. Jeffrey R. Lacasse and Jonathan Leo, "Serotonin and Depression: A Disconnect between the Advertisements and the Scientific Literature," *PLoS Med* 2(12) (2005): e392.

5. Ibid.

6. Jacky Law, *Big Pharma: How the World's Biggest Drug Companies Control Illness* (London: Constable and Robinson, Ltd., 2006), 104–120.

7. K. Schulz, "Did Antidepressants Depress Japan?" *New York Times*, Aug. 22, 2004.

8. Edward Shorter, *A History of Psychiatry* (New York: John Wiley, 1997).

9. Peter J. Schmidt, "Mood, Depression and Reproductive Hormones in the Menopause Transition," NIH State-of-the-Science Conference on Management of Menopause-Related Symptoms, Mar. 21–23, 2005, conference abstracts, 53–56, http://consensus.nih.gov/2005/2005MenopausalSymptoms Program.pdf.

10. R. C. Kessler, P. Berglund, O. Demler, R. Jin et al., "The Epidemiology of Major Depressive Disorder: Results from the National Comorbidity Survey Replication (NCS-R)," *Journal of the American Medical Association* 289 (2003): 3095–3105.

11. National Institutes of Health, *Depression: What Every Woman Should Know*, NIH Publication No. 00-3679 (Bethesda, MD: Department of Health and Human Services, August 2000): 5.

12. Joyce T. Bromberger, "A Psychosocial Understanding of Depression in Women: For the Primary Care Physician," *Journal of the American Medical Women's Association* 59 (3) (Summer 2004): 198–206.

13. J. M. Cyranowski, E. Frank, E. Young, and M. K. Shear, "Adolescent Onset of the Gender Difference in Lifetime Rates of Major Depression," *Archives of General Psychiatry* 57 (2000): 21–27.

14. Mayo Clinic, "Depression in Women: Understanding the Gender Gap," Sep. 20, 2006, http://mayoclinic.com/health/depression/MH00035.

15. B. Mc Ewan, "Ovarian Steroids Have Diverse Effects on Brain Structure," in *The Modern Management of the Menopause: A Perspective for the 21st Century*, ed. G. Berg and M. Hammer (New York: Parthenon, 1994), 269–278.

16. Bromberger, "Psychosocial Understanding."

17. Ibid.

18. Schmidt, "Mood, Depression, and Reproductive Hormones."

19. National Institutes of Health, *Depression: What Every Woman Should Know*, 9.

20. Joyce T. Bromberger, Peter M. Meyer, Howard M. Kravitz et al., "Psychological Distress and Natural Menopause: A Multiethnic Community Study," *American Journal of Public Health* 91 (9) (September 2001): 1435–1442.

21. H. Joffe and L. Cohen, "Estrogen, Serotonin and Mood Disturbance: Where Is the Therapeutic Bridge?" *Biological Psychiatry* 157 (1998): 924–930.

22. Schmidt, "Mood, Depression, and Reproductive Hormones."

23. Ellen W. Freeman, Mary D. Sammel, Hui Lin, and Deborah B. Nelson, "Associations of Hormones and Menopausal Status with Depressed Mood in Women with No History of Depression," *Archives of General Psychiatry* 63 (4) (2006): 375–382.

24. Lee S. Cohen, Claudio N. Soares, Allison F. Vitonis, Michael W. Otto et al., "Risk for New Onset of Depression During the Menopause Transition: The Harvard Study of Moods and Cycles," *Archives of General Psychiatry* 63 (4) (2006): 385–390.

25. Adel Aziz, Christer Bergquist, Mats Brannstrom, Lena Nordholm et al., "Differences in Aspects of Personality and Sexuality Between Perimenopausal Women Making Different Choices Regarding Prophylactic Oophorectomy at Elective Hysterectomy," *Acta Obstetricia et Gynecologica Scandinavica* 84 (9) (September 2005): 854.

26. M. Jawor, A. Dimter, K. Marek, D. Dudek et al., "Anxiety-Depressive Disorder in Women after Hysterectomy," *Psychiatria Polska* 35(5) (September-October 2001): 771–780.

27. S. B. Ewalds-Kvist, T. Hirvonen, M. Kvist, K. Lertola et al., "Depression, Anxiety, Hostility and Hysterectomy," *Journal of Psychosomatic Obstetrics and Gynaecology* 26 (3) (September 2005): 193–204.

28. S. Gulseren, L. Gulseren, Z. Hekimsoy, P. Cetinay, et al., "Depression, Anxiety, Health-Related Quality of Life and Disability in Patients with Overt and Subclinical Thyroid Dysfunction," *Archives of Medical Research* 37(1) (January-February 2006): 133–139.

29. Mayo Clinic, "Depression in Women: Understanding the Gender Gap."

30. National Institutes of Health, *Depression: What Every Woman Should Know*, 8.

31. "Increased Irritability and Rage, Mood Swings," Menopause & Beyond, http://www.geocities.com/menobeyond/.

32. J. E. Zweifel and W. H. O'Brien, "A Meta-Analysis of the Effect of Hormone Replacement Therapy upon Depressed Mood," *Psychoneuroendocrinology* 22 (1997): 189–212.

33. M. F. Morrison, M. J. Kallan, T. Ten Have, I. Katz et al., "Lack of Efficacy of Estradiol for Depression in Postmenopausal Women: A Randomized, Controlled Trial," *Biological Psychiatry* 55 (2004): 406–412.

34. Jerry M. Cott, "St. John's Wort (*Hypericum perforatum*)," in *The Ency-*

clopedia of Dietary Supplements, ed. Paul M. Coates, Marc C. Blackman, Gordon M. Bragg, Mark Levine et al. (New York: Marcel Dekker, 2005).

35. K. Linde, G. Ramirez, C. D. Mulrow, A. Pauls et al., "St. John's Wort for Depression: An Overview and Meta-Analysis of Randomised Clinical Trials," *British Medical Journal* 313 (7052) (1996): 253–258.

36. Richard C. Shelton, Martin B. Keller, Alan Gelenberg, David L. Dunner, et al., "Effectiveness of St. John's Wort in Major Depression: A Randomized Controlled Trial," *Journal of American Medical Association* 285 (15) (April 18, 2001): 1978–1986.

37. Hypericum Depression Trial Study Group, "Effect of *Hypericum Perforatum* (St. John's Wort) in Major Depressive Disorder: A Randomized Controlled Trial," *Journal of the American Medical Association* 287 (14) (2002): 1807–1814.

38. K. Linde, C. D. Mulrow, M. Berner and M. Egger, "St. John's Wort for Depression," *Cochrane Database of Systematic Reviews* (2) (2005).

39. Cott, "St. John's Wort."

40. E. J. Mundell, "Workouts Can Lighten Heavy Hearts," *HealthDay,* Nov. 6, 2005.

41. Andrea L. Dunn, Madhukar H. Trivedi, James B. Kampert et al., "Exercise Treatment for Depression," *American Journal of Preventive Medicine* 28 (1) (January 2005): 1–8.

8. The Secret Hystery: The Truth about Hysterectomy and Oophorectomy

1. Madeline Gray, *The Changing Years* (Garden City, NY: Doubleday 1951), 12.

2. William H. Parker, MD, with Rachel L. Parker, *A Gynecologist's Second Opinion* (New York: Plume, 2003).

3. Edith Sunley, "Sex After Hysterectomy: Another Look" (unpublished manuscript), 1974. It is amazing how much information Sunley gathered and how many of her conclusions were ahead of their time.

4. N. P. Roussis et al., "Sexual Response in the Patient After Hysterectomy: Total Abdominal versus Supercervical versus Vaginal Procedure," *American Journal of Obstetrics and Gynecology* 190 (2004): 1427–1428; and S. A. Farrell and K. Kaiser, "Sexuality After Hysterectomy," *Obstetrics and Gynecology* 95 (2000): 1045–1050.

5. K. McPherson et al., "Psychosexual Health 5 Years After Hysterectomy: Population-Based Comparison with Endometrial Ablation for Dysfunction Uterine Bleeding," *Health Expectations* 8 (2005): 234–243.

6. L. Lowenstein et al., "Does Hysterectomy Affect Genital Sensation?" *European Journal of Obstetrics, Gynecology and Reproductive Biology* 119 (2005): 242–245.

7. Maryann Napoli, "Sexual Response After Hysterectomy," *HealthFacts,* Dec. 1, 1990.

8. Beverly Whipple, Carlos Beyer-Flores, and Barry R. Komisaruk, *The Science of Orgasm* (Baltimore: John Hopkins University Press, 2006).

9. Beverly Whipple, "What's Going On Down There?" (lecture, New York, NY, Jun. 19, 2007).

10. Chris Sutton, "Hysterectomy: A Historical Perspective," *Bailliere's Clinical Obstetrics and Gynaecology* 11 (1) (1997): 1–22.

11. Ibid.

12. Jason Hall and Don J. Hall, "The Forgotten Hysterectomy: The First Successful Abdominal Hysterectomy and Bilateral Salpingo-Oophorectomy in the United States," *Obstetrics & Gynecology* 107 (2c) (February 2006): 541–543.

13. Sutton, "Hysterectomy: A Historical Perspective."

14. Barbara Seaman, "Keeping All Your Eggs in One Basket," *O (The Oprah) Magazine,* October 2006.

15. National Women's Health and Information Center, "Hysterectomy," US Department of Health and Human Services, May 2006.

16. Parker, *A Gynecologist's Second Opinion.*

17. Gray, *The Changing Years,* 229.

18. William Parker et al., "Ovarian Conservation at the Time of Hysterectomy for Benign Disease," *Obstetrics & Gynecology* 106 (2005): 219–226.

19. JoAnn E. Manson et al. for the WHI and WHI-CACS Investigators, "Estrogen and Coronary-Artery Calcification," *New England Journal of Medicine* 356 (25) (Jun. 21, 2007): 2591–2602.

20. A group of women with intact uteri were originally in the "Estrogen Only" arm of the Women's Health Initiative. However, in 1995, after concerns about endometrial cancer were raised, they were reassigned to the Prempro section.

21. Mayo Clinic, "Preventive Ovary Removal Linked to Early Death in Younger Women, Mayo Clinic Discovers," *Science Daily,* September 15, 2006.

22. W. A. Rocca, J. H. Maraganore et al., "Increased Risk of Parkinsonism in Women Who Underwent Oophorectomy Before Menopause," *Neurology* 70 (2008): 200–209.

23. "Too Many Hysterectomies?" *Time,* Feb. 7, 1969.

9. Down Under: Vaginal and Reproductive Health As You Age

1. "Treating Fibroids: Alternatives to Hysterectomy," *Cornell Women's Health Advisor,* October 1999.

2. "Fibroids," *Harvard Women's Health Watch,* August 1995.

3. William H. Parker with Rachel L. Parker, *A Gynecologist's Second Opinion* (New York: Plume, 2003), 105.

4. "Treating Fibroids: Alternatives to Hysterectomy," *Cornell Women's Health Advisor,* October 1999.

5. "Fibroids," *Harvard Women's Health Watch*.

6. Susan Love and Karen Lindsey, *Dr. Susan Love's Menopause and Hormone Book* (New York: Three Rivers Press, 2003), 195.

7. "Fibroids," *Harvard Women's Health Watch*.

8. Ibid.

9. Ibid.

10. Parker, *A Gynecologist's Second Opinion*, 120.

11. Ibid.

12. "Treating Fibroids: Alternatives to Hysterectomy."

13. Parker, *A Gynecologist's Second Opinion*, 121.

14. Ibid., 129.

15. "Treating Fibroids: Alternatives to Hysterectomy."

16. Ibid.

17. Ibid.

18. Parker, *A Gynecologist's Second Opinion*, 144–145.

19. Ibid., 146.

20. Stefano Palombo et al., "Transdermal Hormone Replacement Therapy in Postmenopausal Women with Uterine Leiomyomas," *Obstetrics and Gynecology* 98 (6) (2001): 1053–1058.

21. Ingrid A. Rodi, "Endometriosis," in Parker with Parker, *A Gynecologist's Second Opinion*, 203–229.

22. Mayo Clinic, "Adenomyosis," Feb. 21, 2006, http://www.mayoclinic.com/health/Adenomyosis/DS00636.

23. "Ovarian Cyst," American Academy of Family Physicians, October 2005, http://familydoctor.org/online/famdocen/home/women/reproductive/gynecologic/279.htm.

24. Mayo Clinic, "Ovarian Cysts," Jul. 20, 2007, http://www.mayoclinic.com/health/ovarian-cysts/DS00129.

25. Ibid.

26. Ibid.

27. "Women's Health: Uterine Prolapse: A Common Problem for Older Women," *University of Texas Lifetime Health Letter*, October 1995.

28. Ibid.

29. Ibid.

10. The World Is Flat: The New and Changing Role of Hormone Therapy in Menopause

1. Barbara and Gideon Seaman, *Women and the Crisis in Sex Hormones* (New York: Rawson Publishing, 1977).

2. Robert Wilson, *Feminine Forever* (New York: M. Evans, 1966).

3. Barbara Seaman, "History of Hormone Replacement Therapy," in *Controversies in Science and Technologies: From Maize to Menopause*, ed. Daniel Lee Kleinman et al. (Madison: University of Wisconsin, 2005), 220–221.

4. Elizabeth Siegel Watkins, "The Neutral Gender and the Problem of

Aging" (abstract, Annual Meeting of the American Association for the History of Medicine, 2004).

5. Barbara Seaman, *The Greatest Experiment Ever Performed on Women* (New York: Hyperion, 2003), 51.

6. Harry Genant et al., "Qualitative Computed Tomography of Vertebral Spongiosa: A Sensitive Method for Detecting Early Bone Loss After Oophorectomy," *Annals of Internal Medicine* 97 (1982): 699–705.

7. Stephen Hulley et al., "Randomized Trial of Estrogen Plus Progestin for Secondary Prevention of Coronary Heart Disease in Postmenopausal Women," *Journal of the American Medical Association* 280 (1998): 605–613.

8. Jennifer S. Haas et al., "Changes in Newspaper Coverage About Hormone Therapy with the Release of New Medical Evidence," *Journal of General Internal Medicine* 21 (2006): 304–309.

9. Margaret Morganroth Gullette, "Hormone Nostalgia: Estrogen, Not Menopause, Is the Public Health Issue," *American Prospect*, Jan. 22, 2007.

10. "Understanding the WHI Results," in *Our Bodies, Ourselves: Menopause*, ed. Boston Women's Health Book Collective (New York: Simon and Schuster, 2006), 101.

11. Tara Parker-Pope, *The Hormone Decision* (New York: Rodale, 2007), 9.

12. JoAnn E. Manson et al., "Estrogen Therapy and Coronary-Artery Calcification," *New England Journal of Medicine* 356 (25): 2591–2602.

13. Sylvia Wassertheil-Smoller et al., "Effect of Estrogen Plus Progestin on Stroke in Postmenopausal Women: The Women's Health Initiative: A Randomized Trial," *Journal of the American Medical Association* 289 (20) (May 28, 2003): 2673–2684.

14. Allison Gandey, "Sudden Decline in Breast Cancer Could Be Linked to HRT," *Medscape Medical News*, Dec. 14, 2006: www.medscape.com.

15. Christina A. Clarke et al., "Recent Declines in Hormone Therapy Utilization and Breast Cancer Incidence: Clinical and Population-Based Evidence," *Journal of Clinical Oncology* 24 (33) (Nov. 20, 2006): e49–e50.

16. Parker-Pope, *Hormone Decision*, 87.

17. L. H. Kuller, K. A. Mathews, E. N. Meilahn et al., "Recency and Duration of Postmenopausal Hormone Therapy: Effects on Bone Mineral Density and Fracture Risk in the National Osteoporosis Risk Assessment (NORA) Study," *Menopause* 10 (5) (September-October 2003): 412–419.

18. S. A. Shumaker, C. Legault, L. Kuller et al., "Conjugated Equine Estrogens and Incidence of Probable Dementia and Mild Cognitive Impairment in Postmenopausal Women: Women's Health Initiative Memory Study," *Journal of American Medical Association* 291 (2004); 2947–2958.

19. Barbara and Gideon Seaman, *Women and the Crisis in Sex Hormones*.

20. Joel A. Simon, Donald B. Hunninghake, Sanjay K. Agarwal et al., "Effect of Estrogen plus Progestin on Risk for Biliary Tract Surgery in Postmenopausal Women with Coronary Artery Disease: The Heart and Estrogen/Progestin Replacement Study," *Annals of Internal Medicine* 135 (7) (Oct. 2, 2001): 493–501.

21. Dominic J. Cirillo, Robert B. Wallace, Rebecca J. Rodabough et al., "Effect of Estrogen Therapy on Gallbladder Disease," *Journal of the American Medical Association* 293 (3) (Jan. 19, 2005): 330–339.

22. Susan L. Hendrix, Barbara B. Cochrane, Ingrid E. Nygaard et al., "Effects of Estrogen With and Without Progestin on Urinary Incontinence," *Journal of the American Medical Association* 293 (8) (Feb. 23, 2005): 935–948.

23. Vanessa Barnabei, Barbara Cochrane, Aaron K. Aragaki et al., "Menopausal Symptoms and Treatment-Related Effects of Estrogen and Progestin in the Women's Health Initiative," *Obstetrics and Gynecology* 105 (May 2005): 1063–1073.

24. Jennifer Hays, Judith K. Ockene, Robert L. Brunner et al., "Effects of Estrogen plus Progestin on Health Related Quality of Life," *New England Journal of Medicine* 348 (19) (May 8, 2003): 1839–1854.

25. D. E. Bonds, N. Nasser, L. Qi, R. Brzyski et al., "The Effect of Conjugated Equine Oestrogen on Diabetes Incidence: The Women's Health Initiative Randomized Trial," *Diabetologia* 49 (3) (Jan. 27, 2006): 459–468.

26. Natalie Angier, "New Respect for Estrogen's Influence," *New York Times*, Jun. 24, 1997.

27. Ibid.

28. Million Women Study Collaborators, "Breast Cancer and Hormone Replacement Therapy in the Million Women Study," *Lancet* 362 (2003): 419–427.

29. Parker-Pope, *Hormone Decision*, 149.

30. Camille Sweeney, "Not Tonight," *New York Times*, Jun. 5, 2005.

31. Parker-Pope, *Hormone Decision*, 98–99.

32. B. Fisher et al., "Tamoxifen for Prevention of Breast Cancer: Report of the National Surgical Adjunvant Breast and Bowel Project P-1 Study," *Journal of the National Cancer Institute* 90 (18) (1998): 1371–1389.

33. National Women's Health Network, *The Truth About Hormone Replacement Therapy* (Roseville, CA: Prima Publishing, 2002), 59.

34. Abby Ellin, "A Battle Over 'Juice of Youth,'" *New York Times*, Oct. 15, 2006.

35. Ibid.

36. "Pharmacy Compounding Is . . . ," The International Academy of Compounding Pharmacists, www.iacprx.org.

37. National Women's Health Network, *The Truth About Hormone Replacement Therapy*, 131.

38. Kathryn M. Rexrode and JoAnn E. Manson, "Are Some Types of Hormone Therapy Safer Than Others?" *Circulation* 115 (2007): 820–822.

39. Judith K. Ockene, David H. Barad, Barbara B. Cochrane, Joseph C. Larson et al., "Symptom Experience After Discontinuing Use of Estrogen plus Progestin," *Journal of the American Medical Association*, 294 (2)(Jul. 13, 2005): 183–193.

40. Deborah Grady and George F. Sawaya, "Discontinuation of Postmenopausal Hormone Therapy," *American Journal of Medicine* 118 (12b) (2005): 163S–165S.

41. Dr. Jacques Rossouw, e-mail message to author, Sept. 19, 2007.

42. Ibid.

43. T. S. Eliot, *Four Quartets*, ed. Bernard Bergonzi (New York: Macmillan, 1972).

11. Menopause, Naturally? What We Know about the Wild West of Natural, Alternative, and Bioidentical Menopause Medicine

1. Barbara Ehrenreich and Deirdre English, *Witches, Midwives and Nurses: A History of Women Healers* (New York: Feminist Press at the City University of New York, 1973), 1.

2. Wayne B. Jonas, "Alternative Medicine—Learning From the Past, Examining the Present, Advancing to the Future," *Journal of the American Medical Association* 280 (1998): 1616–1618.

3. Stella M. Yu, Reem M. Ghandour, and Zhihaun J. Huang, "Herbal Supplement Use among US Women, 2000," *Journal of the American Medical Women's Association* 59 (2004): 17–24.

4. Judith Garrard, Susan Harms, Lynn E. Eberly, and Amy Matiak, "Variations in Product Choices of Frequently Purchased Herbs," *Archives of Internal Medicine* 163 (2003): 2290–2295.

5. Yu, Ghandour, and Huang, "Herbal Supplement Use," 17–24.

6. G. B. Mahady, J. Parrot, and C. Lee, "Botanical Dietary Supplement Use in Peri and Postmenopausal Women," *Menopause* 10 (2003): 65–72.

7. Barbara Seaman, "Did You Know Labels Can Lie?" *Hadassah Magazine*, June-July 2003.

8. Jay Udani, "Integrating Alternative Medicine into Practice," *Journal of the American Medical Association* 280 (1998): 1620.

9. Ibid.

10. Phil B. Fontanarosa and George D. Lundberg, "Alternative Medicine Meets Science," *Journal of the American Medical Association* 280 (1998): 1618–1619.

11. Dan Hurley, *Natural Causes: Death, Lies and Politics in America's Herbal Supplement Industry* (New York: Broadway Books, 2006): 54–71.

12. Christine M. Gilroy, John F. Steiner, Tim Byers, Howard Shapiro, and William Georgian, "Echinacea and Truth in Labeling," *Archives of Internal Medicine* 163 (2003): 699–704.

13. "Natural Remedies for Menopause Gain in Popularity," *New York Times*, Jun. 20, 2000.

14. Garrard, Harms, Eberly, and Matiak, "Variations in Product Choices," 2290–2295.

15. Gilroy, Steiner, Byers, Shapiro, and Georgian, "Echinacea and Truth in Labeling," 699–704.

16. "Herbal Roulette," *Consumer Reports* (November 1995): 698–705.

17. Nancy L. Booth, Cassia R. Overk, Ping Yao, Joanna E. Burdette et al., "The Chemical and Biologic Profile of a Red Clover (*Trifolium pratense L*) Phase II Clinical Extract," *Journal of Alternative and Complementary Medicine* 12 (2) (2006): 133–139.

18. Peter Whitton, Julie Whitehouse, and Christine Evans, "Response to Reported Hepatotoxicity of High Lactone Extractions of Piper Methysticum Forst (Kava)," *Journal of Alternative and Complementary Medicine* 8 (3) (2002): 237–263.

19. Gilroy, Steiner, Byers, Shapiro, and Georgian, "Echinacea and Truth in Labeling," 699–704.

20. Robert S. DiPaola and Timothy Gower, *The Doctor's Guide to Herbs and Supplements* (New York: Henry Holt, 2001), 41.

21. Ibid.

22. Leslie Berger, "Herbs for Hot Flashes: New Attention, Mixed Results," *New York Times*, Aug. 12, 2003.

23. Fredi Kronenberg and Adriane Fugh-Berman, "Complementary and Alternative Medicine for Menopausal Symptoms: A Review of Randomized, Controlled Trials," *Annals of Internal Medicine* 137 (2002): 805–813.

24. Tieraona Low Dog, "Menopause: Review of Botanical Dietary Supplement Research," NIH State-of-the-Science Conference on Management of Menopause-Related Symptoms, Mar. 21–23, 2005, conference abstracts, 95–102, http://consensus.nih.gov/2005/2005MenopausalSymptomsProgram.pdf.

25. "You Have to Be Soy Careful," *Washington Post*, Jan. 30, 2001.

26. "What We Still Don't Know About Soy," *Harvard Women's Health Watch*, August 2001.

27. Richard Chua, Kitty Anderson, Jun Chen, and Ming Hu, "Quality, Labeling, Accuracy, and Cost Comparison of Purified Soy Isoflavonoid Products," *Journal of Alternative and Complementary Medicine* 10 (6) (2004); 1053–1060.

28. *Harvard Women's Health Watch*, December 2001.

29. R. Chenoy, S. Hussain, Y. Tayob, P. M. O'Brien et al., "Effect of Oral Gamolenic Acid from Evening Primrose Oil on Menopausal Flushing," *British Medical Journal* 308 (6927) (Feb. 19, 1994): 50–53.

30. J. D. Hirata, L. M. Swiersz, B. Zell, R. Small, and B. Ettinger, "Does Dong Quai Have Estrogenic Effects in Postmenopausal Women?: A Double-Blind, Placebo-Controlled Trial," *Fertility and Sterility* 68 (1997): 981–986.

31. National Women's Health Network, *The Truth about Hormone Replacement Therapy*, (Roseville, CA: Prima Publishing, 2002), 105–106.

32. I. K. Wiklund, L. A. Mattsson, R. Lindgren, and C. Limoni, "Effects of a Standardized Ginseng Extract on Quality of Life and Physiological Parameters in Symptomatic Postmenopausal Women: A Double-Blind, Placebo-Controlled Trial," *International Journal of Clinical Pharmacological Research* 19 (1999): 89–99.

33. "Selecting a CAM Practitioner," National Center for Complementary and Alternative Medicine, http://nccam.nih.gov/health/practitioner/.

34. "An Introduction to Acupuncture," National Center for Complementary and Alternative Medicine, http://nccam.nih.gov/health/acupuncture/.

35. Janet S. Carpenter, "Other Complementary and Alternative Medicine Modalities: Acupuncture, Magnets, Reflexology and Homeopathy," NIH State-of-the-Science Conference on Management of Menopause-Related Symptoms, conference abstracts, 103. (See note 24, p.440, for link.)

36. J. Williamson, A. White, A. Hart, and E. Ernst, "Randomized Controlled Trial of Reflexology for Menopausal Symptoms," *British Journal of Obstetrics and Gynaecology* 109 (2002): 1050–1055.

37. Hurley, *Natural Causes,* 54–71.

38. Garrard, Harms, Eberly, and Matiak, "Variations in Product Choices," 2290–2295.

39. M. Hardy and A. McQuade-Crawford, "Women's Health: The Role of Alternative Medicines," paper presented at the American Pharmaceutical Association, Annual Meeting, Mar. 10–14, 2000, Washington, D.C.

40. Garrard, Harms, Eberly, and Matiak, "Variations in Product Choices," 2290–2295.

41. Wayne B. Jonas, "Alternative Medicine—Learning From the Past, Examining the Present, Advancing to the Future," *Journal of the American Medical Association* 280 (1998): 1616–1618.

12. The Skinny on Menopausal Weight: Is Gain Really Just Part of the Change?

1. Susun S. Weed, *New Menopausal Years the Wise Woman Way* (Woodstock, NY: Ash Tree Publishing, 2001).

2. Mayo Clinic, "Menopause and Weight Gain: Reverse the Middle Age Spread," Sept. 3, 2004, www.mayoclinic.com.

3. K. M. Flegal, M. D. Carroll, R. J. Kuczmarski et al., "Overweight and Obesity in the United States: Prevalence and Trends, 1960–1994, *International Journal of Obesity Related Metabolic Disorders* 22 (1) (1998): 39–47.

4. Laurey R. Simkin-Silverman and Rena R. Wing, "Weight Gain During Menopause," *Postgraduate Medicine* 108 (3) (Sept. 1, 2000).

5. Artemis Simopoulos, in conversation with the authors, January 10, 2006.

6. S. S. Hedge and S. R. Ahuja, "Assessment of Percent of Body Fat Content in Young and Middle Aged Men: Skinfold Method vs. Girth Method, *Journal of Postgraduate Medicine* 42 (4) (1996): 97–100. This study was performed on Indian men, who may have significantly different lifestyles than American men.

7. "Weight Management: It's Official—Men are Fatter Than Women!" *Obesity, Fitness and Wellness Week,* Jul. 16, 2005: 1691.

8. Mayo Clinic, "Metabolism and Weight Loss: How You Burn Calories," Oct. 5, 2005, www.mayoclinic.com.

9. Ian Maclean Smith, "Aging Begins at 30: Muscle Loss," University of Iowa Virtual Hospital, September 2001, http://www.uihealthcare.com/vh/.

10. National Library of Medicine, "Obesity," Medline Plus, http://www.nlm.nih.gov/medlineplus/obesity.html.

11. Simkin-Silverman and Wing, "Weight Gain."

12. Julia Tolliver Maranan, "Mind Your Metabolism; Weight Gain and Loss of Lean Muscle Mass Often Start in Your 30's—But You Can Fight Both with These Measures," *Boston Globe Magazine*, Dec. 4, 2005, 37.

13. "Thyroid and Weight," The American Thyroid Association, 2005, http://www.thyroid.org/patients>brochures/Thyroid_and_Weight.pdf.

14. Ethne Barnes, *Diseases and Human Evolution* (Albuquerque: University of New Mexico Press, 2005), 333.

15. N. R. Kleinfield, "Diabetes and Its Awful Toll Quietly Emerge as a Crisis," *New York Times*, Jan. 9, 2006.

16. *Your Guide to Diabetes: Type 1 and 2*, National Diabetes Information Clearinghouse, National Institutes of Health, NIH pub. no. 05-4016, November 2004.

17. "By the Number: One Scourge in Two Forms," *New York Times*, Jan. 9, 2006.

18. Kleinfield, "Diabetes and Its Awful Toll."

19. *Your Guide to Diabetes: Type 1 and 2*.

20. David S. Ludwig, "Glycemic Index," *Journal of the American Medical Association* 287 (18) (May 8, 2002), http://www.glycemicindex.com.

21. Ibid.

22. A. Michael Wallace, Alex D. McMahon, Chris J. Packard, Anne Kelly et al., "Plasma Leptin and the Risk of Cardiovascular Disease in the West of Scotland Coronary Prevention Study," *Circulation* 104 (2001): 3052–3056.

23. "Dr. Jeffrey Friedman Discusses New Research on the Hormone Leptin, Which Helps Regulate Body Weight," *Talk of the Nation*, National Public Radio, April 2, 2004.

24. Ibid.

25. Karine Spiegel, Esra Tasali, Plamen Plamen Penev, and Eve van Couter, "Brief Communication: Sleep Curtailment in Healthy Young Men Is Associated with Decreased Leptin Levels, Elevated Ghrelin Levels, and Increased Hunger and Appetite," *Annals of Internal Medicine* 141 (11) (2001): 846–850.

26. Mads Tang-Christensen et al., "Central Administration of Ghrelin and Agouti-Related Protein (83–132) Increases Food Intake and Decreases Spontaneous Locomotor Activity in Rats," *Endocrinology* 145 (10) (2004): 4645–4652.

27. Shahrad Taheriental, "Short Sleep Duration Is Associated with Reduced Leptin, Elevated Ghrelin, and Increased Body Mass Index," *PLoS Medicine* 1 (3) (2004): c62, http://medicine.plosjournals.org/.

28. Delores Corella, Lu Qi, Jose V. Sorli, Diego Godoy et al., "Obese Subjects Carrying the 11482G>A Polymorphism at the Perilipin Locus Are

Resistant to Weight Loss after Dietary Energy Restriction," *Journal of Clinical Endocrinology* 90 (9) (June 28, 2005): 5121–5126.

29. Amanda Onion, "Can Geneticists Cure Obesity?" *ABC News*, Jan. 11, 2006: http://abcnews.go.com/Technology/Health/story?id=1477757.

30. Gene Borio, "Tobacco Timeline: The Twentieth Century 1900–1948—The Rise of the Cigarette," 1993–2003, www.tobacco.org.

31. Eric Coleman, "Anorectics on Trial: Half a Century of Federal Regulation of Prescription Appetite Suppressants," *Annals of Internal Medicine* 143 (5) (Sept. 6, 2005): 380–385.

32. W. Van Winkle, letter to Endo Products, January 5, 1946, New Drug Application, no. 5632, vol. 1.1 (Rockville, MD: U.S. Food and Drug Administration, 1943).

33. Bridget M. Kuehn, "The Gut Yields Clues to Obesity, Therapies," *Journal of the American Medical Association* 293 (18) (May 11, 2005): 2200–2201.

34. David E. Arteburn, Paul K. Crane, and David L. Veenstra, "The Efficacy and Safety of Sibutramine for Weight Loss: A Systematic Review," *Archives of Internal Medicine* 164 (May 10, 2004): 994–1003.

35. Brian Vastag, "Experimental Drugs Take Aim at Obesity," *Journal of the American Medical Association* 289 (14) (Apr. 9, 2003): 1763–1764.

36. Eric Coleman, "Anorectics on Trial," 380–385.

37. Kuehn, "Gut Yields Clues," 2200–2201.

38. Arya M. Sharma, "Effect of Orlistat-Induced Weight Loss on Blood Pressure and Heart Rate in Obese Patients with Hypertension," *Journal of Hypertension* 20 (9) (2002): 1873–1878.

39. Jean-Pierre Chanoine, Sarah Hampl, Craig Jensen, Mark Boldrin, and Jonathan Hauptman, "Effect of Orlistat on Weight and Body Composition in Obese Adolescents," *Journal of the American Medical Association* 293 (2005): 2873–2883.

40. Melissa Dahl, "Diet Pill's Icky Side Effects Keep Users Honest," *Today*, Jul. 6, 2007, http://today.msnbc.msn.com/id/19587389/.

41. Vastag, "Experimental Drugs."

42. F. Xavier Pi-Sunyer et al., "Effect of Rimonabant, a Cannabinoid-1 Receptor Blocker, on Weight and Cardiometabolic Risk Factors in Overweight or Obese Patients," *Journal of the American Medical Association* 295 (2006): 761–775; and Denise G. Simons-Morton, "Obesity Research—Limitations of Methods, Measurements and Medications," *Journal of the American Medical Association* 295 (2006): 826–828.

43. Jeanne Whalen, " 'Miracle' Obesity Pill Looks Less Miraculous," *Wall Street Journal*, Mar. 29, 2007.

44. Michael L. Dansinger, Joi Augustin Gleason, John L. Griffith, Harry P. Selker, and Ernest J. Schaefer, "Comparison of the Atkins, Ornish, Weight Watchers and Zone Diets for Weight Loss and Heart Disease Reduction," *Journal of the American Medical Association* 293 (1) (Jan. 5, 2005): 43–53.

45. Amanda Spake, "Stop Dieting!" *U.S. News and World Report*, Jan. 16, 2006.

46. Ibid.

47. Dansinger, Gleason, Griffith et al., "Comparison."

48. Ibid.

13. Minding Your Peas and Caveats: Menopause Nutrition and Eating Healthfully in the Second Half of Life

1. Michael Pollan, "Unhappy Meals," *New York Times*, Jan. 28, 2007.

2. U.S. Department of Agriculture and Government of Health and Human Services, *Dietary Guidelines for Americans 2005*, "Chapter 2: Adequate Nutrients Within Calorie Needs," http://www.health.gov/dietaryguidelines/dga2005/document/html/chapter2.htm.

3. Ethne Barnes, *Diseases and Human Evolution* (Albuquerque: University of New Mexico Press, 2005), 331–333.

4. Matt McGowan, "What's Not on the Menu?" *University of Arkansas Research Frontiers*, Fall 2005.

5. Ibid.

6. National Heart, Lung, and Blood Institute and the National High Blood Pressure Education Program, "Stay Young at Heart, Portion Distortion," http://hp2010.nhlbihin.net/oei_ss/PD1/pdiwebtxt.htm.

7. McGowan, "What's Not on the Menu?"

8. Dan Hurley, *Natural Causes* (New York: Broadway Books), 38.

9. U.S. Food and Drug Administration, "Overview of Dietary Supplements," Center for Food and Applied Nutrition, Jan. 3, 2001, http://www.cfsan.fda.gov/~dms/ds-oview.html.

10. Hurley, *Natural Causes*, 164.

11. Ibid.

12. Artemis Simopoulos and Jo Robinson, *The Omega Diet* (New York: HarperCollins, 1999), 16.

13. Mayo Clinic, "Dietary Fats: Know Which Types to Choose," Jan. 31, 2007, http://www.mayoclinic.com/health/fat/NU00262.

14. Judith Groch, "New York City Bans Artificial Trans Fats in Restaurants," *Medpage Today*, Dec. 6, 2006, http://www.medpagetoday.com/Cardiology/AcuteCoronarySyndrome/tb/4641.

15. Simopoulos and Robinson, *Omega Diet*, 25.

14. Change of Pace: Menopause and Exercise

1. National Institute on Aging, *Exercise: A Guide From the National Institute on Aging*, NIH pub. no. 01-4258, reprinted April 2004.

2. Mayo Clinic, "Fitness Center," www.mayoclinic.com/health/fitness/SM99999.

3. National Institute on Aging, *Exercise*.

4. Bruce Weber, "Losing Patience, Not Weight: Guidelines for Exercise May Discourage Activity," *New York Times*, Apr. 21, 2005.

5. Ibid.

6. Martha Gulati et al., "The Prognostic Value of a Nomogram for Exercise Capacity in Women," *New England Journal of Medicine* 353 (Aug. 4, 2005): 468–475.

7. "Groundbreaking Study of 5,700 Women Finds Not Enough Exercise Means Serious Risk for Heart Problems, Death; All Current Exercise Guidelines Based on Study of Only 224 Men, No Women," *Ascribe*, Aug. 2, 2005.

8. National Institute on Aging, *Exercise*.

9. Ibid.

10. Mayo Clinic, "Adjust Your Workout: Why Warming Up and Cooling Down Help Keep You on the Go," Mar. 4, 2005: http://www.cnn.com/HEALTH/library/SM/00067.html.

11. Ibid.

12. National Institute on Aging, *Exercise*.

13. Ibid.

14. Jack Williams, "Balance Often a Missing Ingredient in Fitness," Copley News Service, July 31, 2005, http://www.copleynews.com.

15. B. C. Stillman, "Making Sense of Proprioception," *Physiotherapy*, 88(11) (Nov. 1, 2002): 667–676.

16. "Balance Training to Maintain Mobility and Prevent Disability," *American Journal of Preventive Medicine* 25 (3) (2003): 150–156.

17. L. Wolfson, R. Whipple, C. Derby, J. Judge et al., "Balance and Strength Training in Older Adults: Intervention Gains and Tai Chi Maintenance," *Journal of the American Geriatrics Society* 44 (5) (May 1996): 498–506.

18. Maria Howard, "Get Better Posture, Prevent Pain with Balance Training: A Leg Up" (Richmond, VA) *Times Dispatch*, Jun. 29, 2005.

19. Lewis Bowling, "Try a Three-Pronged Approach to Exercise" (Durham, NC) *Herald-Sun*, Jul. 14, 2005.

20. Mayo Clinic, "Fitness on a Budget: Low Cost Ideas for Getting in Shape," Aug. 19, 2004: http://www.mayoclinic.com/health/fitness/HQ00694_D.

15. Mindful Menopause: Memory, Cognition, and Alzheimer's Disease

1. A. Paganini-Hill and V. W. Henderson, "Estrogen Deficiency and Risk of Alzheimer's Disease in Women," *American Journal of Epidemiology* 140 (1994): 256–261.

2. N. F. Woods, E. S. Mitchell, and C. Adams, "Memory Functioning

among Midlife Women: Observations from the Seattle Midlife Women's Health Study," *Menopause* 7 (4) (July/August 2000): 257–265.

3. Ibid.

4. Robert Sapolsky, "Taming Stress," *Scientific American* 289 (3) (Sept. 2003): 88–95.

5. Ibid.

6. R. S. Wilson, D. A. Evans, J. L. Bienias, C.F. Mendes de Leon et al., "Proneness to Psychological Distress Is Associated with Risk of Alzheimer's Disease," *Neurology* 61 (2003): 1479–1485.

7. Christine Gorman, Dan Cray, Simon Crittle et al., "Why We Sleep," *Time,* Dec. 20, 2004.

8. Ibid.

9. V. W. Henderson, J. R. Guthrie, E. C. Dudley, H. G. Burger, and L. Dennerstein, "Estrogen Exposures and Memory at Midlife," *Neurology* 60 (2003): 1369–1371.

10. Susana M. Phillips and Barbara B. Sherwin, "Effects of Estrogen on Memory Function in Surgically Menopausal Women," *Psychoneuroendocrinology* 17 (5) (1992): 485–495.

11. Cathryn Jakobson Ramin, *Carved in Sand: When Attention Fails and Memory Fades at Midlife* (New York: HarperCollins, 2007).

12. Rebecca Rupp, *Committed to Memory: How We Remember and Why We Forget* (New York: Crown Publishers, 1998), 24–25.

13. Ibid.

14. Daniel Schacter, *The Seven Sins of Memory: How the Mind Forgets and Remembers* (Boston and New York: Houghton Mifflin, 2001), 33–34.

15. Ibid., 51.

16. Ibid., 55.

17. D. A. Bennett, J. A. Schneider, J. L. Bienias, D. A. Evans, and R. S. Wilson, "Mild Cognitive Impairment Is Related to Alzheimer Disease Pathology and Cerebral Infarctions," *Neurology* 64 (2005): 834–841.

18. Catherine Arnst, "I Can't Remember," *Business Week,* Sept. 1, 2003.

19. Oscar L. Lopez, William J. Jagust, Steven T. Dekosky et al., "Prevalence and Classification of Mild Cognitive Impairment in the Cardiovascular Health Study Cognition Study," *Archives of Neurology* 60 (10) (October 2003): 1385–1389.

20. Gary W. Small, Vladimir Kepe, Linda M. Ercoli et al., "PET of Brain Amyloid and Tau in Mild Cognitive Impairment," *New England Journal of Medicine* 355 (25) (Dec. 21, 2006): 2652–2663.

21. Ramin, *Carved in Sand,* 46.

22. "Researchers Find Definitive Proof that Repetitive Head Injury Accelerates the Pace of Alzheimer's Disease," *Science Daily*, Jan. 17, 2002, www.sciencedaily.com.

23. "New Study at UNC Shows Concussions Promote Dementias in Retired Professional Football Players," University of North Carolina press release, Oct. 10, 2005, http://www.unc.edu/news/archives/oct05/guskie101005.htm.

24. "Crucial Step Towards Better Diagnosis of Alzheimer's," *Medical News Today*, Mar. 11, 2007, www.medicalnewstoday.com.

25. L. J. Launer, K. Andersen, M. E. Dewey et al., "Rates and Risk Factors for Dementia and Alzheimer's Disease: Results from EURODEM Pooled Analyses," *Neurology* 52 (1999): 78–84.

26. Ramin, *Carved in Sand*, 92–97.

27. Mellanie V. Springer, Anthony R. McIntosh, Gordon Winocur, and Cheryl L. Grady, "The Relation Between Brain Activity During Memory Tasks and Years of Education in Young and Older Adults," *Neuropsychology*, 19 (2) (March 2005): 181–192.

28. Lisa Melton, "Use It Don't Lose It," *New Scientist*, Dec. 17, 2005.

29. Ramin, *Carved in Sand*, 31–32.

30. Alison Motluk, "Got a Minute?," *New Scientist*, Jun. 24, 2006.

31. Edward M. Hallowell, "Why Smart People Underperform," *Harvard Business Review*, January 2005.

32. U.S. Congress. Office of Technology Assessment, *Losing a Million Minds: Confronting the Tragedy of Alzheimer's Disease and Other Dementias: Congressional Summary* (Washington D.C.: US Government Printing Office, 1987).

33. Richard J. Hodes, "Public Funding for Alzheimer Disease Research in the United States," *Nature Medicine* 12 (July 2006): 770–773.

34. Claire Mount and Christian Downton, "Alzheimer Disease: Progress or Profit?," *Nature Medicine* 12 (July 2006): 780–784.

35. Stephen R. Rapp, Mark A. Espeland, Sally A. Shumaker et al., "Effect of Estrogen plus Progestin on Global Cognitive Function in Postmenopausal Women: The Women's Health Initiative Memory Study: A Randomized Controlled Trial," *Journal of the American Medical Association* 289 (May 2003): 2663–2672; and Michael C. Craig, Pauline M. Maki, and Declan G. M. Murphy, "The Women's Health Initiative Memory Study: Findings and Implications for Treatment," *Lancet Neurology* 4 (2005): 190–194.

36. Mount and Downton, "Alzheimer Disease."

37. Hodes, "Public Funding."

38. Stephen S. Hall, "The Quest for a Smart Pill," *Scientific American* 289 (3) (September 2003).

39. Ibid.

40. James L. McGaugh, "Remembering and Forgetting: Physiological and Pharmacological Aspects," Transcript of address, Session 3, The President's Council on Bioethics, Oct. 17, 2002.

41. "Stroke: A Cause of Dementia You Can Do Something About," Mt. Sinai School of Medicine: Focus on Healthy Aging, February 2002.

42. Barbara Seaman, *The Greatest Experiment Ever Performed on Women: Exploding the Estrogen Myth* (New York: Hyperion, 2003).

43. G. Logroscigno et al., "Diabetes May Influence Cognitive Decline," *British Medical Journal* 328 (7439) (Mar. 6, 2004): 548.

44. Rupp, *Committed to Memory*.

16. Loving the Skin You're In: Skin, Hair, and Midlife Beauty

1. Robert Wilson, *Feminine Forever*, (New York: M. Evans and Company, 1966).

2. Orly Etingin, "Ask Dr. Etingin," *Cornell Women's Health Advisor*, January 2000.

3. Mayo Clinic, "Know Your Skin, Hair and Nails," Dec. 19, 2003, www.mayoclinic.com.

4. Ibid.

5. Etingin, "Ask Dr. Etingin."

6. Miriam Stoppard, *Menopause* (New York: DK Publishing, 2002).

7. Etingin, "Ask Dr. Etingin."

8. Ibid.

9. Joan Liebmann-Smith and Jacqueline Nardi Egan, *Body Signs* (New York: Random House, 2007), 275.

10. Ibid.

11. M. Krug, A. Wunsche, and A. Blum, "Addiction to Tobacco and the Consequences for the Skin," *Hautarzt* 55 (3) (March 2004): 301–315.

12. Mayo Clinic, "Over-the-Counter Wrinkle Creams: Miracle or Marketing Myth?," Jan. 19, 2005, www.mayoclinic.com.

13. Ibid.

14. Ibid.

15. Ibid.

16. Etingin, "Ask Dr. Etingin."

17. Mayo Clinic, "Over-the-Counter Wrinkle Creams."

18. M. G. Shah and H. I. Maibach, "Estrogen and Skin. An Overview," *American Journal of Clinical Dermatology* 2 (2001): 143–150.

19. M. J. Thornton, "The Biological Actions of Estrogens on Skin," *Experimental Dermatology* 11 (6): 487–502.

20. Chhon Shik Youn, Oh Sang Kwon, Chong Hyun Won et al., "Effect of Pregnancy and Menopause on Facial Wrinkling in Women," *Acta Dermato-Venereologica* 83 (2003): 419–424.

21. K. Tsukahara, H. Nakagawa, S. Moriwaki et al., "Ovariectomy Is Sufficient to Accelerate Spontaneous Skin Ageing and to Stimulate Ultraviolet Irradiation-induced Photoaging or Murine Skin," *British Journal of Dermatology* 151 (5) (November 2004): 948.

22. Youn, Kwon, Won et al., "Effect of Pregnancy and Menopause," 419–424.

23. Etingin, "Ask Dr. Etingin."

24. L. B. Dunn, M. Damesyn, A. A. Moore et al., "Does Estrogen Prevent Aging Skin? Results from the First National Health and Nutrition Examination Survey," *Dermatology* 133(3) (1997): 1459–1460.

25. Mayo Clinic, "Smooth Moves: Medical Treatments for Facial Wrinkles," Aug. 10, 2004: www.mayoclinic.com.

26. Ibid.

27. Ibid.

28. Ibid.

29. "Chloasma," The New England Dermatological Society, www.derm netz.org.

30. "What Is Rosacea?," The National Rosacea Society, www.Rosacea .org.

31. "Questions and Answers about Rosacea," The National Institute of Arthritis and Musculoskeletal and Skin Diseases, National Institutes of Health, NIH pub. no. 02-5038, June 2002.

32. Ibid.

33. "Questions and Answers about Rosacea," The National Institute of Arthritis and Musculoskeletal and Skin Diseases.

34. "What Is Rosacea?"

35. Ibid.

36. "Getting to the Roots of Female Hair Loss," Mt. Sinai School of Medicine: Focus on Healthy Aging, April 2000.

37. "Hair Loss," Dermatology, *Harvard Women's Health Watch,* May 1995.

38. Ibid.

39. Richard K. Scher (speech at the American Academy of Dermatology's summer scientific session, July 2005).

40. Mayo Clinic, "What Your Fingernails Can Tell You about Your Health," Dec. 11, 2003.

41. Scher, speech.

17. The Great Pretender: Thyroid Disease and Menopause

1. "Thyroid Fact Sheet," The American Association of Clinical Endocrinologists," 2005.

2. Kenneth Ain and M. Sara Rosenthal, *The Complete Thyroid Book* (New York: McGraw Hill, 2005), 37.

3. Nancy Ross-Flanigan, "All in the Family," *Arthritis Today,* The National Arthritis Foundation, November 2005.

4. Martin I. Surks, Eduardo Ortiz, Gilbert H. Daniels et al., "Sub-clinical Thyroid Disease: Scientific Review and Guidelines for Diagnosis and Management," *Journal of the American Medical Association* 291 (2) (Jan. 14, 2004): 228–238.

5. Ibid.

6. Anne R. Cappola, Linda P. Fried, Alice M. Arnold et al., "Thyroid Status, Cardiovascular Risk, and Mortality in Older Adults," *Journal of the American Medical Association* 295 (9) (Mar. 1, 2006): 1033–1041.

7. American Thyroid Association, "Thyroid and Weight," 2005, www .thyroid.org.

8. Marion Nestle, *Food Politics* (Berkeley, CA: University of California Press, 2003).

9. Ain and Rosenthal, *The Complete Thyroid Book,* 43.

10. Ibid.

11. Ralph Faggotter, "Theories on Thyroid Condition," e-mail message to BRS, April 2, 2007.

12. David Cooper, "Hashimoto's Thyroiditis," *National Women's Health Information Center,* January 2006: www.WomensHealth.gov.

13. Ross-Flanigan, "All in the Family."

14. Ibid.

15. Mayo Clinic, "Graves' Disease," Jul. 7, 2005, www.mayoclinic.com.

16. Ibid.

17. The Thyroid Foundation of America, "Thyroid Problems Over 50," 2004, www.allthyroid.org.

18. Louise Davies and H. Gilbert Welch, "Increasing Incidence of Thyroid Cancer in the United States," *Journal of the American Medical Association* 295 (18) (May 10, 2006): 2164–2167.

19. Jacobijn Gussekloo, Eric Van Exel, Anton J. M. de Crean, Arend E. Meinders, Marijke Frolich and Rudi G. J. Westendorp, "Thyroid Status, Disability and Cognitive Function, and Survival in Old Age," *Journal of the American Medical Association* 292 (21) (Dec. 1, 2004): 2591–2599.

20. Ross-Flanigan, "All in the Family."

21. Ain and Rosenthal, *The Complete Thyroid Book.*

18. Taking Heart: Menopause and Heart Disease

1. "Heart and Cardiovascular Disease," National Women's Health Information Center, Office on Women's Health, U.S. Department of Health and Human Services, November 2002.

2. "Heart Disease and Heart Attacks: What Women Need to Know," The American Academy of Family Physicians, www.familydoctor.org.

3. "Women and Heart Disease Fact Sheet," Centers for Disease Control and Prevention, U.S. Department of Health and Human Services, http://www.cdc.gov.

4. Patrick Y. Yee, Karen P. Alexander, Bradley G. Hammill, Sara K. Pasquali, and Eric D. Peterson, "Representation of Elderly Persons and Women in Published Randomized Trials of Acute Coronary Syndromes," *Journal of the American Medical Association* 286 (6) (Aug. 8, 2001): 708–713.

5. Sharonne Hayes, "Protecting Women's Hearts: An Interview with a Mayo Clinic Specialist," Jan. 18, 2005, www.mayoclinic.com.

6. Jane Brody, "Women Struggle for Parity of the Heart," *New York Times,* Apr. 12, 2005.

7. Ibid.

8. "Insights from the NHLBI-Sponsored Women's Ischemia Syndrome

Evaluation (WISE) Study," Parts I and II, *Journal of the American College of Cardiology* 47 (3) (Feb. 7, 2006): supplement 1.

9. "Heart and Cardiovascular Disease," National Women's Health Information Center, Office on Women's Health, U.S. Department of Health and Human Services, November 2002.

10. Harriet Rosenberg and Danielle Allard, "Evidence for Caution: Women and Statin Use," submitted to Women and Health Protection, Health Canada, Mar. 14, 2007.

11. W. P. Castelli, "Making Sense of Clinical Trial Data in Decreasing Cardiovascular Risk," *American Journal of Cardiology* 88 (4A) (2001): 16F–20F.

12. Boston Women's Health Book Collective, *Our Bodies, Ourselves: Menopause* (New York: Touchstone Books, 2006), 246–247.

13. John Abramson, *Overdosed America: The Broken Promise of American Medicine* (New York: HarperCollins, 2004), 129.

14. Akira Endo, "The Discovery and Development of HMG-CoA Reductase Inhibitors," *Journal of Lipid Research* 33 (1992): 1569–1582.

15. Ibid.

16. H. Ulmer, C. Kelleher, G. Diem et al., "Why Eve Is Not Adam: Prospective Follow Up in 14,650 Women and Men of Cholesterol and Other Risk Factors Related to Cardiovascular and All-Cause Mortality," *Journal of Women's Health* 13(1) (2004): 41–53.

17. Rosenberg and Allard, "Evidence for Caution."

18. Judith M. E. Walsh and Michael Pignone, "Drug Treatment of Hyperlipidemia in Women," *Journal of the American Medical Association* 291 (2004): 2243–2252.

19. Ibid.

20. "Statin Information," Statin Effects Study, University of California, San Diego, http://medicine.ucsd.edu/ses/adverse_effects.htm.

21. Maryann Napoli, "(Almost) Everything You Need to Know About Statin Drugs," *Health Facts*, November 2003.

22. Greg Crister, *Generation RX* (New York: HoughtonMifflin, 2005), 192.

23. "Well-Known Side Effects," Statin Effects Study, University of California, San Diego, http://medicine.ucsd.edu/ses/adverse_effects.htm.

24. P. S. Phillips, R. H. Hass, S. Bannykh, S. Hathaway, N. L. Gray, B. J. Kimura, G. D. Vladutiu, and J. D. F. England, Scripps Mercy Clinical Research Center, "Muscle Abnormalities in Four Patients Taking Statins to Treat Unfavorable Cholesterol Levels," *Annals of Internal Medicine* 137 (7) (October 1, 2002): 1–45.

25. D. Gaist, U. Jeppesen, M. Andersen, L. A. Garcia-Rodriguez, J. Hallas, and S. H. Sindrup, "Statins and Risk of Polyneuropathy," *Neurology* 58 (2002): 1333–1337.

26. H. Sinzinger and H. O'Grady, "Professional Athletes Suffering from Familial Hypercholesterolaemia Rarely Tolerate Statin Treatment Because of

Muscular Problems," *British Journal of Clinical Pharmacology* 57 (4) (April 2004): 525.

27. Susan S. Tomlinson and Kathleen K. Mangione, "Potential Adverse Effects of Statins on Muscle," *Physical Therapy* 85 (5) (May 2005): 459–465.

28. Eleanor Laise, "The Lipitor Dilemma," *Smart Money*, November 2003.

29. M. F. Muldoon, S. D. Barger, C. M. Ryan, J. D. Flory, J. P. Lahoczky, K. A. Mathews, and S. B. Manuck, "Effects of Lovastatin on Cognitive Function and Psychological Well-Being," *American Journal of Medicine* 108 (7) (May 2000): 538–46.

30. Laise, "The Lipitor Dilemma."

31. "Statin Adverse Effects," Statin Effects Study, University of California, San Diego, http://medicine.ucsd.edu/ses/adverse_effects.htm.

32. B. A. Golomb, T. Kane, and J. E. Dimsdale, "Severe Irritability Associated with Statin Cholesterol-Lowering Drugs," *Quarterly Journal of Medicine* 97 (Jan. 2004): 229–235.

33. Mayo Clinic, "Co-Enzyme Q-10," May 1, 2006, www.mayoclinic.com/health/coenzyme-q10/NS_patient-coenzymeq10.

34. James J. Nawarskas, "HMG-CoA Reductase Inhibitors and Coenzyme Q-10," *Cardiology in Review* 13 (2) (March-April 2005): 76–79.

35. S. Lewis et al., "Effect of Pravastatin on Cardiovascular Events in Women after Myocardial Infarction: The Cholesterol and Recurrent Events (CARE) Trial," *Journal of American Cardiology* 32 (1998): 140–146.

36. James Shepherd, Gerard J. Blauw, Michael B. Murphy et al., "Prevastatin in Elderly Individuals at Risk of Vascular Disease (PROSPER): A Randomized Controlled Trial," *Lancet* 360 (2002): 1623–1630.

37. Uffe Ravnskov, Paul J. Rosch, Morley C. Sutter, and Mark C. Houston, "Should We Lower Cholesterol as Much as Possible?," *British Medical Journal* 332 (2006): 1330–1332.

38. Laise, "The Lipitor Dilemma."

39. Duff Wilson, "New Blood Pressure Guidelines Pay Off—For Drug Companies," *Seattle Times*, Jun. 26, 2005.

40. Ibid.

41. Ray Moynihan and Alan Cassels, *Selling Sickness* (New York: Nation Books, 2005).

42. "Metabolic Syndrome—A Low Profile, High Risk Combination of Disorders," *Mayo Clinic Women's HealthSource*, July 2005.

43. Laura Tarkan, "Low cholesterol? Don't Brag Quite Yet," *New York Times*, May 10, 2005.

44. "Metabolic Syndrome."

45. P. A. Tataranni, "Metabolic Syndrome: Is There a Pathophysiological Common Denominator in Nutrition and Fitness: Obesity, the Metabolic Syndrome, Cardiovascular Disease and Cancer," *World Review of Nutrition and Dietetics*, ed. A. P. Sinopoulos (Basel: Karger, 2005) 94:75–83.

46. Kristen Bibbens-Domingo, Feng Lin, Eric Vittinghoff et al., "Predic-

tors of Heart Failure among Women with Coronary Disease," *Circulation* 100 (2004): 1424–1430.

47. "Diabetes and Heart Health," *Johns Hopkins Medical Letter: Health After 50* 13 (1) (March 2001).

48. "Diabetes Complications: Diabetes a Bigger Heart Disease Risk for Women than for Men," *Heart Disease Weekly*, Mar. 20, 2005.

49. Feng Lin, Eric Vittinghoff, Elizabeth Barrett-Connor et al., "Predictors of Heart Failure Among Women with Coronary Artery Disease," *Circulation* 110 (2004): 1424–1430.

50. "Heart and Cardiovascular Disease," National Women's Health Information Center, Office on Women's Health, U.S. Department of Health and Human Services, November 2002.

51. T. R. Wessel, C. R. Arant, M. B. Olsen et al., "Relationship of Physical Fitness vs. Body Mass Index with Coronary Artery Disease and Cardiovascular Events in Women, *Journal of the American Medical Association* 292 (10) (2004): 1179–1187.

52. Evelyn O. Talbott, Davia S. Guzick, Kim Sutton-Tyrrell et al., "Evidence for Association between Polycystic Ovary Syndrome and Premature Carotid Atherosclerosis in Middle-Aged Women," *Atherosclerosis, Thrombosis, and Vascular Biology* 20 (2000): 2414.

53. "New Coronary Culprit: The Surprising Role of Inflammation," *Mt. Sinai School of Medicine: Focus on Healthy Aging* 3 (3) (March 2000).

54. Jennifer K. Pai, Tobias Pischon, Jing Ma et al., "Inflammatory Markers and the Risk of Coronary Heart Disease in Men and Women," *New England Journal of Medicine* 351 (Dec. 16, 2004): 25.

55. "Your Heart Attack Risk: Inflammation Counts," *Harvard Women's Health Watch* 10 (6) (February 2003).

56. "Emerging Risk Factors for Heart Disease," *Mayo Clinic Women's Health Watch* 6 (1) (January 2002).

57. K. S. McCully, "Vascular Pathology of Homocysteinemia: Implications for the Pathogenesis of Arteriosclerosis," *American Journal of Pathology* 56 (1969): 111–128.

58. Ottar Nygard, Jan Erik Nordrehaug, Helga Refsum et al., "Plasma Homocysteine Levels and Mortality in Patients with Coronary Artery Disease," *New England Journal of Medicine* 337 (1997): 230–237.

59. Paul M. Ridker, Charles H. Hennekens, Julie E. Buring and Nader Rifai, "C-Reactive Protein and Other Markers of Inflammation in the Prediction of Cardiovascular Disease in Women," *New England Journal of Medicine* 342 (Mar. 23, 2000): 836–843.

60. "Homocysteine, Folic Acid, and Cardiovascular Disease," The American Heart Association, 2008, http://americanheart.org./presenter.jhtml?identifier=4677.

61. Elizabeth Agnvall, "Taking the Message to Heart," *Washington Post*, May 3, 2005.

62. "In a Heartbeat: Act in Time—You Could Avoid Dying From A Heart Attack," *Cornell Women's Health Advisor*, November 2001.

63. Agnvall, "Taking the Message to Heart."

64. Ibid.

65. "Surviving a Heart Attack," *Cornell Women's Health Advisor*, December 1999, 7.

66. Mayo Clinic, "Stroke," July 5, 2006, http://www.mayoclinic.com/health/stroke/DS00150.

67. John Abramson, *Overdosed America: The Broken Promise of American Medicine* (New York: HarperCollins, 2005), 221.

68. Jacques E. Rossouw, Ross L. Prentice, JoAnn E. Manson et al., "Post-menopausal Hormone Therapy and Risk of Cardiovascular Disease by Age and Years Since Menopause," *Journal of the American Medical Association* 297 (13) (Apr. 4, 2007): 1465–1477.

19. Close to the Bone: Osteoporosis, Bone Density, and Menopause

1. Gillian Sanson, *The Myth of Osteoporosis* (Ann Arbor, MI: MCD Publications, 2003), 12.

2. "BMD Testing: What the Numbers Mean," The National Osteoporosis Foundation, http://www.nof.org/osteoporosis/bmd test.htm.

3. Robert P. Heaney, "Bone Mass, Bone Fragility and the Decision to Treat," *Journal of the American Medical Association* 280 (1998): 2119–2120.

4. Gillian Sanson, "Osteoporosis: Blowing the Whistle on an Epidemic," www.gilliansanson.com.

5. National Women's Health Network, *The Truth about Hormone Replacement Therapy* (Roseville, CA: Prima Publishing, 2002), 146.

6. Gina Kolata, "Bone Diagnosis Gives New Data But No Answers," *New York Times*, Sept. 28, 2003.

7. Joan M. Neuner, Neil Binkley, Rodney A. Sparapani et al., "Bone Density Testing in Older Women and Its Association with Patient Age," *Journal of the American Geriatrics Society* 54(3) (March 2006): 485–489.

8. C. I. Green, K. Bassett, V. Foerster, and A. Kazanjian, "Bone Mineral Testing: Does the Evidence Support Its Selective Use in Well Women?" B.C. Office of Health Technology Assessment, December 1997: www.chspr.ubc.ca.

9. Sanson, *The Myth of Osteoporosis*, 37.

10. S. Pors-Nielsen, "The Fallacy of BMD: A Critical Review of the Diagnostic Use of Dual X-ray Absorptiometry," *Clinical Rheumatology* 19 (2000): 174–183.

11. C. D. Marci, M. B. Viechnicki, and S. L. Greenspan, "Bone Mineral Densitometry Substantially Influences Health Related Behaviours of Post-menopausal Women," *Calcified Tissue International* 66 (2) (Feb. 19, 2004): 113–118.

12. Renee M. Brennan, Jean Wactawski-Wende, Carlos J. Crespo, and Jacek Dmochowski, "Factors Associated with Treatment Initiation after Os-

teoporosis Screening," *American Journal of Epidemiology* 160 (5) (2004): 475–483.

13. Margaret-Mary G. Wilson, Douglas K. Miller, Elana M. Anderson et al., "Fear of Falling and Related Activity Restriction Among Middle-Aged African Americans," *Journal of Gerontology* 60: 355–360.

14. T. D. Faber, D. C. Yoon, S. K. Service, S. C. White, "Fourier and Wavelet Analyses of Dental Radiographs Detect Trabecular Changes in Osteoporosis," *Bone* 35 (2) (2004): 403–411.

15. Gina Kolata, "Bone Diagnosis Gives New Data But No Answers," *New York Times*, Sept. 28, 2003.

16. Ibid.

17. Laufey Steingrimsdottir, Orvar Gunnarsson, Olafur S. Indridason et al., "Relationship Between Serum Parathyroid Hormone Levels, Vitamin D Sufficiency and Calcium Intake," *Journal of the American Medical Association* 294(18) (November 2005): 2336–2341.

18. Ibid.

19. D. M. Hegsted, "Calcium and Osteoporosis," *Journal of Nutrition* 116 (1986): 2316–2319.

20. Sanson, *The Myth of Osteoporosis*, 135.

21. Loren Cordain, "Are Higher Protein Intakes Responsible for Excessive Calcium Excretion?," 1999, http://www.beyondveg.com/cordain-1/prot-calc/prot-calcium-loss-1a.shtml.

22. Roland L. Weinsier and Carlos L. Krumdieck, "Dairy Foods and Bone Health: Examination of the Evidence," *American Journal of Clinical Nutrition* 72 (2000): 681-689.

23. Sanson, *The Myth of Osteoporosis*, 129.

24. Ibid., 131.

25. Robert P. Heaney, "Excess Dietary Protein May Not Adversely Affect Bone," *Journal of Nutrition* 128 (1998): 1054–1057.

26. Uriel S. Barzel and Linda K. Massey, "Excess Dietary Protein Can Adversely Affect Bone," *Journal of Nutrition* 128 (1998): 1051–1053.

27. D. J. A. Jenkins, C. W. C. Kendall, E. Vidgen, L. A. S. Austen et al., "Effect of High Vegetable Protein Diets on Urinary Calcium Loss in Middle-Aged Men and Women," *European Journal of Clinical Nutrition* 57 (2003): 376–382.

28. R. L. Wolf, J. A. Cauley, M. Pettinger et al., "Lack of a Relation Between Vitamin and Mineral Antidepressants and Bone Mineral Density: Results from the Women's Health Initiative," *American Journal of Clinical Nutrition* 82 (2005): 581–588.

29. Diane Feskanich, Walter Willett, Meir J. Stampfer, and Graham Colditz, "Milk, Dietary Calcium and Bone Fractures in Women: A 12-Year Prospective Study," *American Journal of Public Health* 87 (1997): 992–997.

30. Elizabeth R. Bertone-Johnson, Susan E. Hankinson, Adrianne Bendich et al., "Calcium and Vitamin D Intake and Risk of Incident Premenstrual Syndrome," *Archives of Internal Medicine* 165 (11) (Jun. 13, 2005): 1246–1252.

31. Joel S. Finkelstein, "Calcium plus Vitamin D for Postmenopausal Women—Bone Appetit?" *New England Journal of Medicine* 354 (Feb. 16, 2006): 750–752.

32. R. J. Ingelzi, "Time to Bone Up On Skeletal Health," Copley News Service, Nov. 6, 2005.

33. Oliver Ganry, Claude Baudoin, and Patrice Fardellone, "Effect of Alcohol Intake on Bone Mineral Density in Elderly Women," *American Journal of Epidemiology* 151 (2000): 773–780.

34. "Balance of Essential Fats May Prevent Bone Loss After Menopause," Purdue News Service, Jul. 11, 2005, press release, http://www.foodsci.purdue.edu/news/showarticle.cfm?id=61.

35. Joyce B. J. Van Meurs et al., "Homocysteine Levels and the Risk of Osteoporotic Fracture," *New England Journal of Medicine* 350 (May 13, 2004): 2033–2041.

36. Harry K. Genant et al., "Quantitative Computed Tomography of Vertebral Spongiosa: a Sensitive Method for Detecting Early Bone Loss After Oophorectomy," *Annals of Internal Medicine* 97 (1982): 699–705.

37. Jane Cauly, John Robbins, Zhao Chen et al., "Effects of Estrogen Plus Progestin on Risk of Fracture and Bone Mineral Density," *Journal of the American Medical Association* 290 (13) (October 1, 2003): 1729–1738.

38. Bruce Ettinger et al., "Reduction of Vertebral Fracture Risk in Postmenopausal Women With Osteoporosis Treated With Raloxifene," *Journal of the American Medical Association* 282 (7) (Aug. 18, 1999): 637–645.

39. Ray Moynihan and Alan Cassels, *Selling Sickness* (Vancouver and Toronto: Greystone Books, 2005), 139–155.

40. John Abramson, *Overdosed America: The Broken Promise of American Medicine* (New York: Harper Perennial, 2005), 213–215.

41. Henry G. Bone, David Hosking, Jean-Pierre Devogelaer et al., "Ten Years' Experience with Alendronate for Osteoporosis in Postmenopausal Women," *New England Journal of Medicine* 350 (12) (Mar. 18, 2004): 1189–1199.

42. Abby Lippman, letter to *New York Times*, March 20, 2004.

43. S. Komatsubara, S. Mori, T. Mashiba et al., "Suppressed Bone Turnover by Long-Term Bisphosphonate Treatment Accumulates Microdamage But Maintains Intrinsic Material Properties in Cortical Bone of Dog Rib," *Journal of Bone Mineral Research* 19 (6) (January 19, 2004): 999–1005.

44. A. Sarathy, S. Bourgeois Jr., and S. Goodell, "Bisphosphonate-associated Osteonecrosis of the Jaws and Endodontic Treatment: Two Case Reports," *Journal of Endodontics* 31 (10) (October 2005): 759–763.

45. Sanson, *The Myth of Osteoporosis*, 112–113.

46. Alan Cassels, personal correspondence with authors, Apr. 18, 2005.

47. Gillian Sanson, "Bisphosphonate Fact Sheet," www.gilliansanson.com.

48. Yu-Xiao Yang, James D. Lewis, Solomon Epstein, and David C. Metz, "Long-Term Proton Pump Inhibitor Therapy and Risk of Hip Fracture," *Journal of the American Medical Association* 296 (24): 2947–2953.

49. M. R. McClung, P. Geusens, P. D. Miller et al., "Effect of Risedronate

on the Risk of Hip Fracture in Elderly Women," *New England Journal of Medicine* 344(5) (2001): 333–340.

50. John Abramson, *Overdosed America: The Broken Promise of American Medicine* (New York: HarperCollins, 2004), 210–220.

51. Jo Revill, "How the Drugs Giant and a Lone Academic Went to War," *The Observer,* Dec. 4, 2005.

52. Eric Orwoll, Mark Ettinger, Stuart Weiss et al., "Alendronate for the Treatment of Osteoporosis in Men," *New England Journal of Medicine* 343 (2000): 604–610.

53. Neil Gonter, "Forteo: Do the Benefits Outweigh the Risks?," Nov. 13, 2006, www.osteoporosisconnection.com.

54. R. Bowen, "Calcitonin," October 11, 2003: www.vivo.colostate.edu/.

55. Andrea Z. LaCroix, Jane A. Cauley, Mary Pattinger et al., "Statin Use, Clinical Fracture and Bone Density in Postmenopausal Women: Results from the Women's Health Initiative Observational Study," *Annals of Internal Medicine* 139 (2) (July 15, 2003): 97–104.

56. Daniel H. Solomon, Jerry Avorn, Jeffrey N. Katz et al., "Compliance with Osteoporosis Medications," *Archives of Internal Medicine* 165 (Nov. 14, 2005): 2414–2419.

57. E. Israel, T. R. Banerjee, G. M. Fitzmaurice et al., "Effects of Inhaled Glucocorticoids on Bone Density in Premenopausal Women," *New England Journal of Medicine* 345 (13) (Sept. 2001): 941–947.

58. J. Brent Richards, Alexandra Papiaioannou, Jonathan D. Adachi et al., "Effect of Selective Seretonin Reuptake Inhibitors on the Risk of Fracture," *Archives of Internal Medicine* 167 (2) (Jan. 22, 2007): 188–194.

59. "Antidepressants may raise risk of broken bones," Associated Press, Jan. 25, 2007, www.msnbc.com.

60. Sandra Coney, *The Menopause Industry* (North Melbourne: Spinifex Press, 1993).

61. D. C. Bauer, B. Ettinger, M. C. Nevitt, "Risk for Fracture in Women in the Low Serum Levels of Thyroid Stimulating Hormone," *Annals of Internal Medicine* 134 (7) (April 2001): 561–568.

62. Patrizia D'Amelio, Gian Piero Pescarmona, Angela Garibolodi, and Gian Carlo Isaia, "High Density Lipoproteins (HDL) in Women with Postmenopausal Osteoporosis: A Preliminary Study," *Menopause* 8 (6) (2001): 429–432.

63. L. B. Tanko et al., "Relationship between Osteoporosis and Cardiovascular Disease in Postmenopausal Women," *Journal of Bone Mineral Research* 20 (11) (2005): 1912–1920.

64. Zhao Chen, Michael Maricic, Mary Pettinger et al., "Osteoporosis and Rate of Bone Loss Among Postmenopausal Survivors of Breast Cancer," *Cancer* 104 (2005): 1520–1530.

65. Denise E. Bonds, Joseph C. Larson, Ann V. Schwartz et al., "Risk of Fracture in Women with Type 2 Diabetes: the Women's Health Initiative Observational Study," *The Journal of Clinical Endocrinology and Metabolism* 91(9) (2006): 3404–3410.

66. W. G. Beamer, L. R. Donahue, C. J. Rosen, and D. J. Baylink, "Genetic Variability in Adult Bone Density Among Inbred Strains of Mice," *Bone* 18 (5) (May 1996): 397–403.

67. Jane A. Cauley, Li-Yung Lui, Katie L. Stone et al., "Longitudinal Study of Changes in Hip Bone Mineral Density in Caucasian Women and African American Women," *Journal of the American Geriatrics Society* 53 (2) (Feb. 2005): 183.

68. R. G. Miller et al., "Disparities in Osteoporosis Screening Between At-Risk African-American Women and White Women," *Journal of General Internal Medicine* 20 (9) (2005): 847–851.

69. P. M. Mayhew, C. D. Thomas, J. G. Clement et al., "Relation Between Age, Femoral Neck Cortical Stability and Hip Fracture," *Lancet* 366 (9480) (July 2005).

70. S. Mehrsheed, P. C. Wollan, R. W. Scott et al., "Can Strong Back Extensions Prevent Vertebral Fractures in Woman with Osteoporosis?" *Mayo Clinic Proceedings* 71 (1996): 951–956.

71. Barbara Seaman, *The Greatest Experiment Ever Performed on Women* (New York: Hyperion, 2003), 188.

20. The Golden Bowl: Incontinence and Menopause

1. "Urinary Incontinence," University of Maryland Medical Center, 2007, http://www.umm.edu/patiented/articles/who_has_urinary_incontinence_000050_6.htm.

2. "Staying Dry," *Harvard Women's Health Letter*, December 1995.

3. Ibid.

4. Craig C. Freudenrich, "How Your Kidneys Work," HowStuffWorks, Inc., 1998–2005, http://www.howstuffworks.com/kidney.htm.

5. "Bladder Control for Women," National Institutes of Health, National Kidney and Urologic Diseases Information Clearinghouse. NIH pub. no. 03-4195, May 2003.

6. "Urinary Incontinence in Women," National Institutes of Health, National Kidney and Urologic Diseases Information Clearinghouse. NIH pub. no. 04-4132, September 2004.

7. Ibid.

8. Ibid.

9. Public Citizen Health Research Group, *Health Letter* 8 (2) (February 1992).

10. "Urinary Incontinence in Women."

11. "Staying Dry."

12. "Urinary Incontinence in Women."

13. "Staying Dry."

14. Public Citizen Health Research Group.

15. Ibid.

16. Ibid.

17. William H. Parker, MD, with Rachel L. Parker, *A Gynecologist's Second Opinion* (New York: Plume Books, 1996), 189.

18. Ibid., 189–190.

19. Ibid., 192.

20. "Urinary Incontinence in Women."

21. "Urinary Incontinence: Bladder Training," American Academy of Family Physicians, 2004–2005, http//www.familydoctor.org.famdocen/home/seniors/common=older/798.html.

22. Ibid.

23. P. E. Keegan, K. Atiemo, J. Cody et al., "Periurethral Therapy for Urinary Incontinence in Women," *Cochrane Database of Systematic Reviews* 2 (2003).

24. Sandra Emmons and Lesley Otto, *Obstetrics and Gynecology* 106 (July 2005): 138–143.

25. Maryann Napoli, "Some Drugs Cause Urinary Incontinence," *Health Facts* (July 1999).

26. Susan L. Hendrix, Barbara B. Cochrane, Ingrid E. Nygaard et al., "Effects of Estrogen With and Without Progestin on Urinary Incontinence," *Journal of the American Medical Association* 293 (8) (2005): 935–948.

21. Male Menopause: How the Other Half Changes

1. Nancy Gibbs, "Midlife Crisis? Bring It On!" *Time*, May 16, 2005.

2. "The 5th World Congress on the Aging Male," Salzburg, Austria, February 9–12, 2006.

3. "Male Menopause: Myth or Reality?," *University of Chicago Better Health Newsletter* (January 1996): 4.

4. Ibid.

5. Josh Fischman, "Do Men Experience Menopause?," *US News and World Report*, Jul. 30, 2001.

6. A. Morales, J. Heaton, and C. Carson III, "Andropause: A Misnomer for a True Clinical Entity," *The Journal of Urology* 163 (3) (2000): 705–712.

7. Rob Hicks, "Male Menopause," BBC, October 1997.

22. Half the Sky: Menopause Around the World

1. Margaret Morganroth Gullette, *Declining to Decline: Cultural Combat and the Politics of the Midlife* (Charlottesville: University of Virginia, 1997).

2. Margaret Morganroth Gullette, "Mid-Life Discourses in the Twentieth-Century United States: An Essay on the Sexuality, Ideology and Politics of 'Middle-Ageism,'" in *Welcome to Middle Age: And Other Cultural Fictions*, Richard A. Shweder, ed. (Chicago: The University of Chicago Press, 1998).

3. Lynette Leidy Sievert, *Menopause: A Biocultural Approach* (New Brunswick, New Jersey, Rutgers University Press, 2006), 61.

4. Yewoubdar Beyene, *From Menarche to Menopause: Reproductive Histories of Peasant Women in Two Cultures* (Albany: State University of New York Press, 1989).

5. Sievert, *Menopause*, 61–62.

6. Margaret Lock, "Menopause: Lessons from Anthropology," *Psychosomatic Medicine* 60 (4) (July-August 1998): 410–419.

7. Sievert, *Menopause*, 112–117.

Afterword. Becoming a No-Nonsense Patient: A Crash Course in the Basics of Health Literacy

1. "How Good Is Your Doctor?," *Consumer Reports on Health*, April 1996.

2. Ibid.

3. Ibid.

4. National Practitioner Data Bank: http://www.npdb-hipdb.com/.

5. "How Good is Your Doctor?"

6. If you want to be really careful, you can check that your hospital is properly accredited as well by looking it up in a national directory, such as the Joint Commission on Accreditation in Healthcare Organizations, in the local library.

7. *University of Texas Lifetime Health Letter*, April 1998.

8. The National Library of Medicine PubMed Data Base: http://www.ncbi.nim.nih.gov/sites/entrez.

9. M. K. Marvel, R. M. Epstein, K. Flowers, H. B. Beckman, "Soliciting the Patient's Agenda: Have We Improved?" *Journal of the American Medical Association* 281 (3) (1999): 283–287.

10. Barbara Seaman, "Charting the Doctor/Patient Relationship," March 2005.

11. M. K. Marvel et al., "Soliciting the Patient's Agenda: Have We Improved?"

12. Seaman, "Charting the Doctor/Patient Relationship."

13. Alan N. Schwartz, "Are You Getting Less Than the Best From Your Doctor?," *Bottom Line/Health*, October 1998.

14. *Johns Hopkins Medical Letter: Health After Fifty*, November 1994.

15. Ibid.

16. *Cornell Women's Health Advisor*, May 2000.

17. Harry L. Greene, "Questions and Answers," *HealthNews*, September 2000.

18. Michael Mason, "One for the Ages: A Prescription That May Extend Life," *New York Times*, Oct. 31, 2006.

19. Nicholas Wade, "Yes, Red Wine Holds the Answer. Check Dosage," *New York Times*, Nov. 2, 2006.

20. Klaus Hinklemann, in John L. Fennick, *Studies Show: A Popular Guide to Understanding Scientific Studies* (Amherst, NY: Prometheus Books, 1997), 7.

21. We have made up this example.

22. S. Hulley, D. Grady, T. Bush et al., "Randomized Trial of Estrogen Plus Progestin for Secondary Prevention of Coronary Heart Disease in Post Menopausal Women," *Journal of the American Medical Association* 280(7) (1998): 605–613.

23. Romano Deghenghi, interview with the authors, June 2, 2005.

24. John C. Bailar, "The Promise and Problems of Meta-analysis," *New England Journal of Medicine* 337 (8) (Aug. 21, 1997): 559–561.

25. "WSU Study Shows Benefits of Birth Control Pills," Wayne State University Prognosis E-news, http://prognosis.med.wayne.edu/article/wsu-study-shows-benefits-of- birth-control-pill.

index

Menogen, 178
menopause
aging associated with, 280
biology of, 19–20
and culture, 391–95
differences in experiences of, 34
disease model of, 33, 34
early and premature, 29
emergence of term, 17–18
as estrogen deficiency disease, 33, 150
history of, 13–23
as inappropriate topic of discussion, 13
language of, 24–26, 393–94
as "living decay," 154
male, 387–90
meaning of, 26–27
medicalization of, 363
natural distinguished from induced, 20
as psychological, 34
as public topic of discussion, 391
questions about, 21–23
signs/symptoms of, 16, 26–27, 29, 30, 33, 36
similarities between puberty and, 49–50
Taylor and Sumrall stories about, 20–21
as vehicle for transformation of women, 16
menorrhagia. *See* bleeding: excessive
menstruation, as means for cleansing body, 16
Merck, 151, 318, 362, 363, 364
Merck Manual, 151
Meridia (sibutramine), 228
metabolic syndrome, 331–32
metabolism, 218–20, 221, 244, 246, 268, 309, 331–32
methimazole, 308
methyl-testosterone, 178, 179
metronidazole, 292
Mevacor (lovastatin), 317, 318
Mevastatin, 317–18
Micardis (telmisartan), 329
microdermabrasion, 289, 290
Micronor, 186
Microzide, 328
migraines. *See* headaches
mild cognitive impairment (MCI), 267–70
Million Woman Study, 170, 182
mindfulness, 266
Minipress (prazosin), 330
minocycline, 292
Mirena, 187
Miscalcin, 368
Mitchell, Ellen, 21, 47
mnemonics, 266

moles, 283
monkey, and history of menopause, 14–16
monosaturated fat, 240
moods. *See* depression/mood
Moore, Demi, 84
Morales, Alvaro, 389
Mori, Satoshi, 365
Motens (lacidipine), 331
mother hypothesis, 15
motion-sickness pills, 269
Motluk, Alison, 272
Motrin, 366
Moynihan, Ray, 107, 326, 327
MPA. *See* medroxyprogesterone acetate
Muldoon, Matthew, 322–23
"multiple sleep latency test," 82
muscles/joints, 218–20, 303, 321–22, 325, 329, 380
Mykrox, 328
myolysis, 138
myomectomy, 136–37
myxedema, 307

nails, 297–98
Namenda (memantine), 274–75
Napheys, George H., 47–48
Napoli, Maryann, 122, 129, 320, 382
naproxen sodium, 366
narcolepsy, 75, 82
National Association for Continence, 374
National Cancer Institute, 152
National Center for Complementary and Alternative Medicine (NCCAM), 211, 212
National Cholesterol Education Program (NCEP), 316–17, 325
National Diabetes Information Clearinghouse, 222
National Heart, Lung, and Blood Institute (NHLBI), 235–36
National Institute on Aging, 244, 250, 409
National Institute of Arthritis and Musculoskeletal and Skin Diseases, 292
National Institute of Diabetes and Digestive and Kidney Diseases, 222
National Institutes of Health (NIH), 33, 45, 47, 61–62, 94, 111, 116–17, 149, 199, 243, 248, 292, 326, 358, 412, 414
National Kidney and Urological Diseases Information Clearinghouse, 376
National Library of Medicine, 211, 212, 219, 403–4
National Osteoporosis Foundation, 346